Thoracoscopic Spine Surgery

Thoracoscopic Spine Surgery

Edited by

Curtis A. Dickman, M.D.

Director of Spinal Research
Associate Chief, Spine Section
Division of Neurological Surgery
Barrow Neurological Institute
St. Joseph's Hospital and Medical Center
Phoenix, Arizona

Daniel J. Rosenthal, M.D.

Bad Homburg Clinic
Division of Neurosurgery
Chief of Spinal Surgery
Hochtaunus Regional Clinics
Bad Homburg, Germany

Noel I. Perin, M.D., F.R.C.S.

Assistant Professor and Director
Division of Spinal Surgery
Department of Neurosurgery
Mount Sinai Medical Center
New York, New York

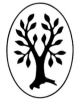

1999

Thieme
New York • Stuttgart

Thieme New York
333 Seventh Avenue
New York, NY 10001

Thoracoscopic Spine Surgery
Curtis A. Dickman, M.D.
Daniel J. Rosenthal, M.D.
Noel I. Perin, M.D.

Editorial Director: Avé McCracken
Editorial Assistant: Mindy Scalzetti
Director, Production & Manufacturing: Maxine Langweil
Senior Production Editor: Eric L. Gladstone
Marketing Director: Phyllis Gold
Sales Manager: David Bertelsen
Chief Financial Officer: Seth S. Fishman
President: Brian D. Scanlan
Compositor: Preparé, Inc.
Printer: G. Canale & C.

Library of Congress Cataloging-in-Publication Data

Thoracoscopic spine surgery / edited by Curtis A. Dickman, Daniel J.
　Rosenthal, Noel I. Perin.
　　　p.　　cm.
　　Includes bibliographical references and index.
　　ISBN 0-86577-785-3 (TNY).--ISBN 3-13-107931-2 (GTV)
　　1. Spine--Surgery.　2. Thoracoscopic.　3. Spine--Endoscopic
surgery.　I. Dickman, Curtis A.　II. Rosenthal, Daniel J.
III. Perin, Noel I.
　　[DNLM: 1. Spine--surgery.　2. Thoracoscopy.　3. Surgical
Procedures, Endoscopic.　WE 725 T4877 1999]
RD768.T487　1999
617.5'6059--dc21
DNLM/DLC
for Library of Congress　　　　　　　　　　99-19799
　　　　　　　　　　　　　　　　　　　　　　CIP

Important note: Medical knowledge is ever-changing. As new research and clinical experience broaden our knowledge, changes in treatment and drug therapy may be required. The authors and editors of the material herein have consulted sources believed to be reliable in their efforts to provide information that is complete and in accord with the standards accepted at the time of publication. However, in view of the possibility of human error by the authors, editors, or publisher of the work herein, or changes in medical knowledge, neither the authors, editors, publisher, nor any other party who has been involved in the preparation of this work, warrants that the information contained herein is in every respect accurate or complete, and they are not responsible for any errors or omissions or for the results obtained from use of such information. Readers are encouraged to confirm the information contained herein with other sources. For example, readers are advised to check the product information sheet included in the package of each drug they plan to administer to be certain that the information contained in this publication is accurate and that changes have not been made in the recommended dose or in the contraindications for administration. This recommendation is of particular importance in connection with new or infrequently used drugs.

Some of the product names, patents, and registered designs referred to in this book are in fact registered trademarks or proprietary names even though specific reference to this fact is not always made in the text. Therefore, the appearance of a name without designation as proprietary is not to be construed as a representation by the publisher that it is in the public domain.

Printed in Italy

5　4　3　2　1

TNY ISBN 0-86577-785-3

GTV ISBN 3-13-107931-2

To our families for their endless love and support.

To our patients for their faith and courage and for the privilege of caring for them and learning from them.

To our mentors for providing us with the foundations, skills, and curiosity to envision improved treatments for our patients.

Curtis A. Dickman, M.D.
Daniel J. Rosenthal, M.D.
Noel I. Perin, M.D.

Contents

Foreword by Richard G. Fessler ix

Foreword by Regis W. Haid xi

Preface xiii

Contributors xv

1. **The History of Thoracoscopic Spine Surgery** 1
   Daniel J. Rosenthal and Curtis A. Dickman

2. **General Principles of Thoracoscopy** 7
   Curtis A. Dickman

3. **Education and Credentialing for Thoracoscopic Spine Surgery** 19
   Curtis A. Dickman and Richard G. Fessler

4. **Instrumentation and Equipment for Thoracoscopic Spine Surgery** 27
   Curtis A. Dickman and Noel I. Perin

5. **Thoracoscopic Perspectives of Thoracic and Mediastinal Anatomy** 49
   Randall K. Wolf, Toshiya Ohtsuka, and Alvin H. Crawford

6. **Surgical Anatomy of the Thoracic Spine** 57
   T. Glenn Pait, Ugur Türe, Kenan I. Arnautović, and Ron M. Tribell

7. **Microanatomy of Thoracic Spine Foramina and Ligaments** 69
   Gökhan Akdemir, Mukesh Misra, Manuel Dujovny, and M. Serdar Alp

8. **Anesthetic Considerations for Thoracoscopic Spine Surgery** 79
   Volker Lischke, Paul Kessler, Klaus Westphal, and Gerhard Matheis

9. **Anesthetic Management and Intraoperative Monitoring** 83
   Paul W. Detwiler, Randall W. Porter, Michael Lemole, and Steven Shedd

10. **Perioperative Management for Thoracoscopic Spine Surgery** 87
    Noel I. Perin, Curtis A. Dickman, Stephen M. Papadopoulos, and Daniel J. Rosenthal

11. **Operating Room Setup and Patient Positioning** 95
    Daniel J. Rosenthal and Curtis A. Dickman

12. **Thoracoscopic Access Strategies: Portal Placement Techniques and Portal Selection** 107
    Curtis A. Dickman and Daniel J. Rosenthal

13. **Spinal Exposure and Pleural Dissection Techniques** 125
    Curtis A. Dickman and Daniel J. Rosenthal

14. **Thoracoscopic Sympathectomy** 143
    Stephen M. Papadopoulos and Curtis A. Dickman

15. **Anterior Release of Spinal Deformities** 161
    Alvin H. Crawford

16. **Endoscopic Anterior Correction of Idiopathic Scoliosis** 183
    Ronald G. Blackman and Eduardo Luque

17. **Biopsy of Vertebral Lesions** 213
    Noel I. Perin

18. **Thoracoscopic Microsurgical Discectomy** 221
    Curtis A. Dickman, Daniel J. Rosenthal, and Noel I. Perin

19. **Thoracoscopic Resection of Intrathoracic Neurogenic Tumors** 245
    Curtis A. Dickman and Ronald I. Apfelbaum

20. **Thoracoscopic Corpectomy** 271
    Curtis A. Dickman and Daniel J. Rosenthal

21. **Thoracoscopic Spinal Reconstruction Techniques** 293
    Curtis A. Dickman and Daniel J. Rosenthal

22. **Thoracoscopic Internal Fixation Techniques** 323
    Daniel J. Rosenthal and Curtis A. Dickman

23. **Future Directions for Spinal Thoracoscopy** 355
    Curtis A. Dickman, Daniel J. Rosenthal, and Noel I. Perin

Index 361

Foreword

by Richard G. Fessler

Over the last decade we have experienced a remarkable renewed interest in minimally invasive spine surgery. Ultimately, our interest stems from what we believe to be significant benefits for our patients. These benefits include less pain, less disruption of normal anatomy, less time in intensive care, less hospitalization, less medication, less disability, and less expense. Currently, minimally invasive spine surgery is being evaluated at every level of the spine for many types of procedures. However, unlike previous attempts at minimally invasive spine surgery, many current techniques may become permanent parts of our surgical armamentarium. The key difference between current attempts and previous attempts of this type of surgery is improved technology. In many cases we are now able to perform the same types of procedures that have been traditionally performed as open minimally invasive techniques.

Among the types of minimally invasive spine surgeries, thoracoscopy has played an early and prominent role. There are several reasons for this. First, functional endoscopes and many soft tissue instruments had previously been developed for thoracoscopic surgery. Therefore, only "bone and disc" instruments required development. Second, thoracic endoscopy can be performed in a large cavity that is ideal for visualization and working space. Third, this large working space gives us relatively direct access to relevant anatomy. Finally, we had the advantage of collaborating with experienced thoracoscopic "chest" surgeons.

Early procedures performed on the spine included sympathectomy, vertebral biopsy, and anterior release scoliosis. Thoracoscopic discectomy evolved shortly thereafter. Additional procedures that have evolved using endoscopic techniques are vertebrectomy, tumor resection, vertebral reconstruction, and internal fixation.

However, along with new techniques come new challenges and responsibilities: Endoscopic surgery requires the acquisition of a new set of surgical skills, which require a relatively long learning curve. Initially, therefore, surgical procedures take longer to complete and may affect compensation, which lead to increased frustration during the early stages of this learning curve. In addition, it is likely that there is an increased risk of complications during the early learning phase. For these reasons these techniques have remained in the hands of a relatively limited number of surgeons. However, if minimally invasive spine surgery follows the same utilization curve as endoscopic cholecystectomy, patients will demand the less invasive procedures, and utilization is likely to become more frequent and widespread.

Thus, we must determine how to train and credential individuals to do this surgery. For residents the training is relatively easy. Training programs can slowly increase the didactic and technical knowledge of residents as they progress through the years of their training. Practicing surgeons, however, are more difficult to train. Training for all individuals must include didactic lectures of indications, contraindications, techniques, complications and their avoidance, equipment, risks, benefits, intraoperative and postoperative care, and collaborative surgery. This training also must include inanimate trainers, practice on human cadavers, and live animal surgery. Methods for preceptorship proctoring also would be advisable. These steps are not intended to discourage surgeons from learning these techniques but to ensure patient safety: Complications usually occur in the early phases of learning a new technique, but with adequate training, we can avoid unnecessary complications.

This text is timely in its publication. Many minimally invasive spine procedures, not just thoracoscopic ones, are becoming more widely accepted and increasingly utilized. By steadfastly focusing on what we as responsible physicians must do to acquire a firm foundation in these new techniques, as well as to keenly study all aspects of each specific technique, we can safely usher in this new era of surgical care of our patients.

Foreword

by Regis W. Haid

How ironic that Bozzini, the inventor of the first "endoscope," was censured by his local surgical academy for "undue curiosity." Although not officially censured, Curtis Dickman faced significant skepticism upon embarking in the field of thoracoscopic spine surgery. I was his most vociferous critic–as only a true friend could be. However, Dr. Dickman has silenced the nonbelievers among us.

This excellent monograph has reacquainted us with Dr. Dickman's personal quest to establish thoracoscopic approaches to the spine as a "standard of care." The contents are arranged in the same thoughtful, logistic fashion as Dr. Dickman's scientific approach to maximize the advantages of spinal endoscopy, while minimizing the numerous obstacles. To wit, Dr. Dickman and his co-authors were the initial developers of the indications, strategies, and instrumentation to attack thoracic spinal pathologies via an endoscopic approach.

The discipline and honesty of their endeavor has borne fruit in the likeness of thoracoscopic sympathectomy, discectomy, scoliotic release, and reconstruction techniques. *Thoracoscopic Spine Surgery* is the culmination of these efforts. Much is to be gleaned from this text, ranging from general principles to astute clinical pearls. I congratulate Curtis Dickman and his collaborators for their dedication; while many may envision the future, few have the tenacity to shape reality. The credit belongs to the devoted.

Preface

This textbook is intended to provide a comprehensive foundation of the principles and surgical techniques that are required to apply microsurgical endoscopy to pathology affecting the thoracic spine. Thoracoscopy only became popular in surgery in the early 1990s. Since then, however, the field has burgeoned, reflecting related advances in technology, imaging equipment, surgical tools, and endoscopic surgical techniques.

Thoracoscopy has widespread applications for use in the treatment of the spine by neurosurgeons and orthopaedic spine surgeons. Anterior transthoracic endoscopy can be used to perform sympathectomies and the anterior release of spinal deformities, to biopsy vertebral lesions, to decompress the nerve roots and spinal cord, to resect neoplasms and infections, to remove nerve sheath tumors, to resect herniated thoracic discs, to decompress and stabilize spinal fractures, to perform corpectomies, to reconstruct the vertebrae, and to apply internal fixation devices to the spine.

Anterior transthoracic endoscopy (thoracoscopy) provides a direct view of the ventral surface of the thoracic spine and spinal cord, requiring only small incisions in the intercostal spaces. The cosmetic effects, although of most concern to the patient, are only one obvious advantage. Compared to thoracotomy and to posterior and posterolateral approaches to the spine, endoscopy benefits patients in several other ways. The smaller incisions used in thoracoscopy reduce the amount of tissue dissection, muscular transection, and rib retraction. Normal tissues are preserved even while extensive access to the thoracic spine is provided. Consequently, patients experience less postoperative pain and recover and return to their normal activities more quickly than after conventional surgery.

Thoracoscopy represents a new and revolutionary alternative for treating thoracic spinal pathology. It is critical, however, to recognize the educational, ethical, and technical challenges that accompany this new technology. The basic principles, psychomotor skills, and surgical techniques of spinal endoscopy are unfamiliar to most spinal surgeons, and the associated learning curve is steep and requires significant adaptations on the part of the surgeon. Thoracoscopy is performed with very long tools, which are placed through restricted "windows" of access using endoscopes that provide a focal perspective of the anatomy. These techniques must be practiced in the laboratory before they are attempted in a clinical setting. Nonetheless, thoracoscopy definitely can be mastered with dedicated training. We recommend intensive hands-on laboratory experience with live animal models and human cadavers where navigational and triangulation skills, tissue dissection, and hemostatic techniques can be practiced in an environment that simulates a clinical surgical setting.

Thoracoscopy is technically more difficult for the surgeon to perform than open surgery. Why, then, should we make our jobs as surgeons tougher? The answer is that we believe that these techniques benefit our patients substantially. Consequently, spinal surgeons cannot shirk the challenge of acquiring these new skills.

Completing this project would have been impossible without the efforts of the members of Neuroscience Publications Office of the Barrow Neurological Institute. We thank them all for their outstanding work on this project. Shelley A. Kick, Ph.D., Senior Editor; Dawn Mutchler, Assistant Editor; and Judy Wilson and Eve DeShazer, Editorial Assistants, meticulously prepared and edited the text. Medical Illustrators Mark Schornak, M.S., and Aileen Conley, M.S., helped to produce the extensive and outstanding illustrations of the intraoperative anatomy for the book. Pamela A. Smith, Medical Photographer/Videographer, provided many of the photographs and compiled the accompanying surgical video atlas.

Outside the Neuroscience Publications Office, Medical Illustrator, Deborah Ravin, M.F.A., contributed the majority of the fine illustrations in this book.

We also would like to express our gratitude to Avé McCracken, Editorial Director, and the editorial staff at Thieme New York for their comprehensive and generous support in the development of this project.

This textbook and the accompanying surgical video atlas are complementary educational tools. The text describes the fundamental anatomy, principles, pathology, and surgical approaches involved with thoracoscopy. The video atlas offers further insights into the surgical anatomy, surgical strategies, and dissection techniques. We are strongly committed to clinical education and hope to encourage and to facilitate the practice of these valuable surgical techniques among qualified spine surgeons. Our goal is to enhance the learning process for surgeons so that they, in turn, might enhance the outcome, recovery, and lives of their patients.

Curtis A. Dickman, M.D.
Daniel J. Rosenthal, M.D.
Noel I. Perin, M.D.

Contributors

Gökhan Akdemir, M.D.
Research Assistant
Department of Neurosurgery
The University of Illinois at Chicago
Chicago, Illinois

M. Serdar Alp, M.D.
Resident
Department of Neurosurgery
The University of Illinois at Chicago
Chicago, Illinois

Ronald I. Apfelbaum, M.D.
Professor
Department of Neurological Surgery
University of Utah
Salt Lake City, Utah

Kenan I. Arnautović, M.D.
Resident
Department of Neurosurgery
University of Arkansas Medical Sciences
College of Medicine
Little Rock, Arkansas

Ronald G. Blackman, M.D.
Director of Scoliosis Surgery
Children's Hospital
Oakland, California

Alvin H. Crawford, M.D.
Professor, Pediatrics and Orthopedic Surgery
Director, Department of Pediatric Orthopedic Surgery
Children's Hospital Medical Center
University of Cincinnati
Cincinnati, Ohio

Paul W. Detwiler, M.S., M.D.
Resident
Division of Neurological Surgery
Barrow Neurological Institute
St. Joseph's Hospital and Medical Center
Phoenix, Arizona

Curtis A. Dickman, M.D.
Director of Spinal Research
Associate Chief, Spine Section
Division of Neurological Surgery
Barrow Neurological Institute
St. Joseph's Hospital and Medical Center
Phoenix, Arizona

Manuel Dujovny, M.D.
Professor and Associate Head
Department of Neurosurgery
The University of Illinois at Chicago
Chicago, Illinois

Richard G. Fessler, M.D., Ph.D.
Dunspaugh Dalton Chair in Brain and Spinal Surgery
Department of Neurological Surgery
College of Medicine, University of Florida
Gainesville, Florida

Regis W. Haid, M.D.
Associate Professor
Department of Neurosurgery
The Emory Clinic
Atlanta, Georgia

Paul Kessler, M.D.
Zentrum der Anesthesiologie und Wiederbelebung
Klinikum der Johann Wolfgang Goethe Universität
Frankfurt am Main, Germany

Michael Lemole, M.D.
Resident
Division of Neurological Surgery
Barrow Neurological Institute
St. Joseph's Hospital and Medical Center
Phoenix, Arizona

Volker Lischke, M.D.
Zentrum der Anesthesiologie und Wiederbelebung
Klinikum der Johann Wolfgang Goethe Universität
Frankfurt am Main, Germany

Eduardo Luque, M.D.
Director
Medico Hospital
Mexico City, Mexico

Gerhard Matheis, M.D.
Abteilung für Thorax-, Herz- und Gefäßchirurgie
Klinikum der Johann Wolfgang Goethe Universität
Frankfurt am Main, Germany

Mukesh Misra, M.D.
Resident
Department of Neurosurgery
The University of Illinois at Chicago
Chicago, Illinois

Toshiya Ohtsuka, M.D.
Assistant Professor
Department of Cardiothoracic Sugery
University of Tokyo
Tokyo, Japan

T. Glenn Pait, M.D.
Associate Professor
Department of Neurosurgery
University of Arkansas Medical Sciences
College of Medicine
Little Rock, Arkansas

Stephen M. Papadopoulos, M.D.
Associate Professor, Surgery
Section of Neurosurgery
University of Michigan
Ann Arbor, Michigan

Noel I. Perin, M.D., F.R.C.S.
Assistant Professor and Director
Division of Spinal Surgery
Department of Neurosurgery
Mount Sinai Medical Center
New York, New York

Randall W. Porter, M.D.
Resident
Division of Neurological Surgery
Barrow Neurological Institute
St. Joseph's Hospital and Medical Center
Phoenix, Arizona

Daniel J. Rosenthal, M.D.
Bad Homburg Clinic
Division of Neurosurgery
Chief of Spinal Surgery
Hochtaunus Regional Clinics
Bad Homburg, Germany

Steven Shedd, M.D.
Division of Neuroanesthesia
Barrow Neurological Institute
St. Joseph's Hospital and Medical Center
Phoenix, Arizona

Ron M. Tribell
Chief Medical Illustrator
Department of Neurosurgery
University of Arkansas Medical Sciences
College of Medicine
Little Rock, Arkansas

Ugur Türe, M.D.
Research Staff
Department of Neurosurgery
University of Arkansas Medical Sciences
College of Medicine
Little Rock, Arkansas

Klaus Westphal, M.D.
Zentrum der Anesthesiologie und Wiederbelebung
Klinikum der Johann Wolfgang Goethe Universität
Frankfurt am Main, Germany

Randall K. Wolf, M.D.
Professor
Department of Cardiothoracic Surgery
University of Cincinnati
Cincinnati, Ohio

CHAPTER **1**

The History of Thoracoscopic Spine Surgery

Daniel J. Rosenthal, M.D. and Curtis A. Dickman, M.D.

The word *endoscopy* is derived from the ancient Greek word that means visualization (*scopien*) from inside (*endo*). A primitive form of endoscopy was performed by the ancient Romans who used special instruments called *specula* (mirror), predecessors of contemporary specula, to look inside the human body.[1] Abulkasim from Córdoba in the 10th century A.D. wrote about illuminating dark cavities of the body, reflecting light into the body from one of these instruments.[1]

ORIGINS OF ENDOSCOPY

The origin of medical endoscopy can be traced to 1806 when Philipp Bozzini from Frankfurt am Main, Germany, developed a novel invention called the *Lichtleiter* (light conductor).[2,3] This invention is considered the first endoscopic instrument (Table 1–1). It consisted of a candle attached to a thin cannula that enabled the light to be projected into body orifices or viscera (i.e., the rectum, urethra, vagina, or bladder) to provide visualization of the internal anatomy. The device was limited by its lack of an optical or magnifying system. The *Lichtleiter* was not accepted by physicians because visibility was poor, and it was painful for the patient to have the cannula inserted into the body. Bozzini's work was censured by the Viennese Surgical Academy because of his "undue curiosity."[3] He died soon thereafter in 1809 at the age of 35 years.

During the first decade of the development (i.e., the 1800s) of the endoscope, the visualization devices predominantly were used to view anatomic cavities through physiological orifices (i.e., the rectum, urethra, bladder, oral cavity, esophagus, and vagina). The cystoscope was the principal technological device used medically.

Desormeaux has been considered the "father of Endoscopy." In 1853, he first introduced an endoscope that used a lens to focus, direct a light source, and provide a clearer

image. In 1868, Bevan first employed an esophagoscope to remove foreign bodies and visualize esophageal strictures.[1] Two years later, Kussmaul performed the first esophagogastroscopy; his patient was a professional sword swallower.[1]

In 1879, the first cystoscope was developed by Nitze, a urologist from Berlin, Beneche, an optician from Berlin, and Leiter, who produced instruments in Vienna.[4] This development represented a major advance for endoscopy. The instrument had a hollow center with an outer diameter of 7 mm. It incorporated a working channel, an illumination source, and an optical lens system at one end through which light was deflected through the cystoscope. The light source was a heated platinum wire. In 1887, the cystoscope was improved by adding a miniaturized light bulb at the distal end. The first flexible endoscope was developed by Kelling in 1929. It had a 45° angle, a 360° rotating lens, and the working channel could be bent 135°. The optics, however, were poor and distorted.

TWENTIETH-CENTURY DEVELOPMENTS

The 1900s heralded the introduction of the endoscope for diagnostic and therapeutic intracavitary use, examination of the viscera through incisions, and for the treatment of pathology. At the turn of the century, three techniques were developed: ventroscopy (intrapelvic endoscopy), laparoscopy (intraabdominal endoscopy), and thoracoscopy (intrathoracic endoscopy). In 1901, Ott from Petrograd, Russia, reported the technique of ventroscopy.[5] Ott introduced the cystoscope into the pelvic cavity to view the viscera through a culdotomy. This technique was not widely adopted by the medical community.

In 1902, Kelling performed the first experimental laparoscopic surgery in dogs.[6] Subsequently, he published his clinical results, obtained after 14 years of clinical

1

TABLE 1–1 Time Line for the Development of Endoscopic Technology

Year	Author (Ref)	Event
10th century A.D.	Romans[1]	Specula and light illumination first used to look into human body
1806	Bozzini[2,3]	Developed the *Lichtleiter*, a hollow cannula that used illumination from a candle to examine body orifices.
1853	Desmoreaux[1]	Introduced the first lens system to focus image and transmit light. Dubbed the "father of Endoscopy"
1877	Bruck[1]	Introduced an electrified platinum wire loop for cavitary illumination
1879	Nitze[4]	Developed first cystoscope for urologic use. Incorporated an optical lens system, a hollow cannula with a working channel, and a heated platinum wire as a light source
1883	Newman[1]	Light bulb incorporated into the cystoscope
1901	Ott[5]	Introduced intracavitary endoscopy called ventroscopy to view the pelvic viscera. Endoscope inserted after performing a culdotomy incision
1902	Kelling[6]	Developed laparoscopy in dogs using a cystoscope. Introduced pneumoperitoneum using needle insufflation. Called *Koeliscopie* (celioscopy)
1910	Jacobeus[7,8]	Performed first thoracoscopic and laparoscopic procedures on humans. Published reports of laparoscopic treatment of ascites. His thoracoscopic bedside procedure became mainstay of diagnosis and treatment of pulmonary tuberculosis (intrapleural pneumolysis) in 1920s, 1930s, and 1940s until it was replaced with drug therapy
1950s	Hopkins et al.[1]	Introduced Hopkins Lens System: quartz and air lenses developed and vastly improved optical images
mid1980s	Semm[43]	Performed first laparoscopic appendectomy
	Mouret[12]	Performed first laparoscopic cholecystectomy
1988	Reddick and Olsen[10]	Popularized techniques for laparoscopic cholecystectomy
1990	–	Video-assisted thoracoscopy introduced. Modern era of thoracoscopy began. Rapid development of sophisticated endoscopic surgical tools to perform dissection
1992	Rosenthal et al.[35]	Performed first thoracoscopic spine procedure in Europe
	Mack et al.[36]	Performed first thoracoscopic spine procedure in the United States

laparoscopy in humans. Kelling was the first to use insufflation to provide a pneumoperitoneum and to introduce his endoscope through a trocar into the abdominal cavity. He named this method *Koelioskopie*, which is the origin of the word *celioscopy.*

The first laparoscopic procedure and the first thoracoscopic procedure in humans were both performed by Jacobeus, a professor of internal medicine in Stockholm, Sweden. Jacobeus learned the experimental intracavitary endoscopic technique from Kelling. In 1910, Jacobeus published his experience treating patients with ascites using laparoscopy.[7] Of the 115 laparoscopic cases that he reported, only one patient sustained a complication (bleeding) serious enough to require conversion to an open laparotomy.

In 1900, Jacobeus introduced thoracoscopy to medical practice for the diagnosis and treatment of pulmonary tuberculosis.[7,8] He popularized thoracoscopy as a bedside procedure under local anesthesia. The endoscope was inserted into the thorax through a small incision in an intercostal space. Illumination and cauterization were provided by a heated platinum loop inserted through a second incision. The endoscopic procedure was performed to lyse tuberculous pleural adhesions (intrapleural pneumolysis), which became the principal therapeutic tool employed in the treatment of tuberculosis from the 1920s through the 1940s.

After pharmacological agents for the treatment of tuberculosis became available, intrapleural pneumolysis was no longer used (Fig. 1–1).

Interest in thoracoscopy waned. During the 1950s, it was rarely used, except for the diagnosis of pleural diseases and trauma and occasionally to drain hemothoraces, pleural effusions, and empyemas. In the 1960s, 1970s, and 1980s, thoracoscopy was almost replaced entirely by open surgical techniques for thoracotomy.

The resurgence in the clinical use of thoracoscopy in the 1990s was preceded by the explosive growth of endoscopic techniques in other medical and surgical specialties in the 1960s, 1970s, and 1980s. Marked technical improvements in the optical lens systems, fiber optic illumination systems, and improvements in the manipulability and steerability of endoscopes (i.e., flexible steerable endoscopes) fostered the growth of endoscopy in medicine. Its predominant medical uses included gastrointestinal medicine (esophagogastroscopy, proctoscopy, colonoscopy), ear–nose–throat surgery, pulmonary medicine, and thoracic surgery (larygnoscopy, sinus endoscopy, bronchoscopy, mediastinoscopy), and urology (cystoscopy).

Before the 1970s, the use of endoscopy was hindered by the need for the endoscopist to look directly into an eyepiece (objective) on the end of the telescope to view an endoscopic procedure. The proximity of the surgeon's face

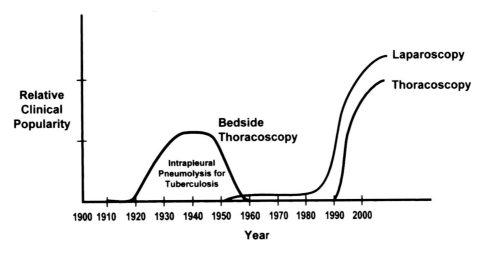

Figure 1–1. The relative popularity of endoscopic procedures as a function of time. Intrapleural pneumolysis for the treatment of tuberculosis was popular between 1920 and the late 1940s. Subsequently, it was supplanted by pharmaceutical treatment. Laparoscopic procedures became widely used in the late 1980s and led the way for the resurgence of thoracoscopy in the early 1990s.

to the end of the endoscope interfered with maintaining a sterile surgical field and prevented endoscopy from becoming popular in surgical specialties. This disadvantage, however, was not a major deterrent for bronchoscopy, cystoscopy, laryngoscopy, colonoscopy, or upper gastrointestinal endoscopy where a completely sterile field was unnecessary.

CONTEMPORARY ENDOSCOPY

The modern era of surgical endoscopy was initiated by the introduction of video-assisted endoscopic techniques in the late 1970s and early 1980s. A video camera was mounted on the endoscope to relay the endoscopic images to a video screen. The video screen allowed endoscopists to view the procedure without looking into an objective lens on the endoscope. Video-assisted endoscopy facilitated the development of sterile endoscopic surgical procedures and fostered teaching and intraoperative documentation of the procedure (via photography and videography).

Orthopedic surgery was one of the first surgical specialties to advance endoscopic surgery in the 1970s and 1980s. Arthroscopy grew and essentially replaced open techniques for the reconstruction of ligaments of the knee and shoulder.

In the late 1980s, the explosive growth of laparoscopy in general surgery was a major factor that facilitated the growth of thoracoscopy in cardiothoracic surgery. Gynecology deserves credit for being the first specialty to routinely use laparoscopy. Gynecologists embraced this technique before general surgery, using it to explore the pelvic organs.[9]

The revolutionary growth of laparoscopy in general surgery began in the late 1980s with the introduction of the laparoscopic cholecystectomy procedure in 1987. The laparoscopic technique for cholecystectomy was shown to have substantial clinical advantages compared with open cholecystectomy, including less postoperative pain, briefer hospitalizations and recovery times, and significantly lower medical costs.[10–12] This technique was wholeheartedly embraced by the surgical community and the public and has become the preferred method for cholecystectomy. Today, most cholecystectomies are performed endoscopically rather than via open procedures.

Concurrent with the massive growth of the laparoscopic cholecystectomy procedure was the development of new endoscopic soft-tissue dissection tools, including stapling devices, suturing tools, anastomosis tools, ligatures, and other devices. These tools permitted a wider application of endoscopic surgery for many other types of surgical procedures (e.g., hernia repair, bowel resection, fundoplasty, tubal ligation).

VIDEO-ASSISTED THORACOSCOPY

The development of sophisticated endoscopic dissection tools and video-assisted imaging by general surgeons spawned the development of video-assisted thoracoscopic surgery (VATS) by cardiothoracic surgeons around 1990. Initially, thoracoscopy was used to biopsy peripheral lung lesions, to ligate apical blebs with surgical loops, and to treat pleural pathology (e.g., drain empyemas, hemothoraces, effusions, perform sclerotherapy). Compared with open thoracotomy, VATS had marked clinical benefits: less postoperative pain, faster recoveries, briefer hospitalizations, and less postoperative pulmonary and shoulder girdle dysfunction.[13–16]

Subsequently, the role of VATS and the variety of procedures performed have expanded considerably.[17–19] Applications for thoracoscopy in cardiothoracic surgery now include resecting lung nodules, tumors, blebs, and bullae; sealing lung lacerations that cause pneumothoraces; performing talc sclerotherapy (pleurodesis); performing lobectomies for the treatment of pleural diseases; treating mediastinal pathology; biopsying lymph nodes; removing neoplasms; and performing thymectomies. Other procedures include creating pericardial windows, performing sympathectomies, ligating the thoracic duct, and performing esophageal procedures, among others.[20] VATS now has a prominent role in cardiothoracic surgery.

The history of spinal endoscopy began in the 1930s with the introduction of spinoscopy and myeloscopy [21–25] as diagnostic tools that never gained widespread clinical utility. Not until the 1970s and 1980s were percutaneous access techniques attempted to perform endoscopic, minimally invasive dissections in the lumbar spine.[25–31] Although these techniques have evolved for lumbar discectomy, they have not yet become used widely. During the early 1990s, laparoscopic and endoscopic retroperitoneal approaches also were developed to access the lumbar spine to perform discectomy and interbody fusion and spinal fixation.[32–34] These techniques have tremendous potential and have evolved rapidly.

In the early 1990s, thoracoscopy for the treatment of spinal pathology was developed independently by Daniel Rosenthal and colleagues [35] in Germany and by Michael Mack, John Regan, and coworkers [36] in the United States. Initially, it was used to biopsy vertebrae, to perform anterior releases of scoliotic or kyphotic deformities, and to perform transthoracic microsurgical discectomies.[35–37] The role of spinal thoracoscopy has now been expanded to include corpectomy, vertebral reconstruction, internal fixation, hardware application, and resection of neurogenic, spinal, and paraspinal tumors.[38–41] Although first described in 1954, thoracoscopic sympathectomy has been simplified and popularized by the recent advances in thoracoscopy.[42] For a variety of pathologies, thoracoscopic techniques for spinal surgery have gained considerable clinical momentum as an alternative to thoracotomy. Both surgical techniques and instrumentation have become quite sophisticated, and the field of thoracoscopy has evolved rapidly in the last several years.

CONCLUSION

Endoscopy has a rich history and has undergone a slow, gradual evolution. Spinal endoscopy is possible because of advances in technology related to imaging, optics, illumination, and video systems. Physicians and surgeons have long attempted to maximize the therapeutic benefit of interventional procedures for their patients while minimizing the disruption of normal healthy tissue. Currently, endoscopy permits extensive microsurgical dissection to be performed with wide exposures through minimal incisions in the surfaces of the body. Undoubtedly, endoscopic surgical techniques will continue to evolve.

REFERENCES

1. Smythe WR, Kaiser LR: History of thoracoscopic surgery. In Kaiser LR, Daniel TM, eds: *Thoracoscopic Surgery.* Boston: Little, Brown; 1993: 1–16.
2. Bozzini PD: Lichtleiter, eine Erfindung zur Anschauung innerer Teile und Krankheiten nebst Abbildung. *J Prakt Arztkunde* 1806; 24:107.
3. Bush RB, Leonhardt H, Bush IV, et al: Dr. Bozzini's Leichtleiter. A translation of his original article (1806). *Urology* 1974; 3(1):119–123.
4. Nitze M: Eine neue Boebachtungs- und Untersuchungsmethode für Harnröhre, Harnblase und Rectum. *Wien Med Wochenschr* 1879; 24:649–652.
5. Ott DV: Illumination of the abdomen (ventroscopia). *J Akusk Ahensk Boliez* 1901; 15:1045–1049.
6. Kelling G: Über Oesophagoskopie, Gastroskopie, und Koelioskopie. *Münich Med Wochenschr* 1902; 52:21.
7. Jacobeus HC: Possibility of the use of the cystoscope for investigation of serious cavities. *Münich Med Wochenschr* 1910; 57:2090–2092.
8. Jacobeus HC: The practical importance of thoracoscopy in surgery of the chest. *Surg Gynecol Obstet* 1921; 32:493–500.
9. Steptoe PC, Edwards RG: Laparoscopic recovery of preovulatory human oocytes after priming of ovaries with gonadotrophins. *Lancet* 1970; 1(649):683–689.
10. Reddick EJ, Olsen DO: Laparoscopic laser cholecystectomy. A comparison with mini-lap cholecystectomy. *Surg Endosc* 1989; 3(3): 131–133.
11. The Southern Surgeon's Club: A prospective analysis of 1518 laparoscopic cholecystectomies. *N Engl J Med* 1991; 324(16): 1073–1078.
12. DuBois F, Icard P, Berthelot G, et al: Coelioscopic cholecystectomy. Preliminary report of 36 cases. *Ann Surg* 1990; 211(1):60–62.
13. Regan JJ, Mack MJ, Picetti GD, III, et al: A comparison of video-assisted thoracoscopic surgery (VATS) with open thoracotomy in thoracic spinal surgery. *Today's Therapeutic Trends* 1994; 11:203–218.
14. Landreneau RJ, Hazelrigg SR, Mack MJ, et al: Postoperative pain-related morbidity: Video-assisted thoracic surgery versus thoracotomy. *Ann Thorac Surg* 1993; 56(6):1285–1289.
15. Hazelrigg SR, Landreneau RJ, Boley TM, et al: The effect of muscle-sparing versus standard posterolateral thoracotomy on pulmonary function, muscle strength, and postoperative pain. *J Thorac Cardiovasc Surg* 1991; 101(3):394–401.
16. Ferson PF, Landreneau RJ, Dowling RD, et al: Comparison of open *versus* thoracoscopic lung biopsy for diffuse infiltrative pulmonary disease. *J Thorac Cardiovasc Surg* 1993; 106(2): 194–199.
17. Kaiser LR: Video-assisted thoracic surgery. Current state of the art. *Ann Surg* 1994; 220(6):720–734.

18. Coltharp WH, Arnold JH, Alford WC, Jr., et al: Videothoracoscopy: Improved technique and expanded indications. *Ann Thorac Surg* 1992; 53(5):776–779.

19. Mack MJ, Aronoff RJ, Acuff TE, et al: Present role of thoracoscopy in the diagnosis and treatment of diseases of the chest. *Ann Thorac Surg* 1992; 54(3):403–409.

20. Krasna MJ, Mack MJ: *Atlas of Thoracoscopic Surgery*. St. Louis: Quality Medical; 1994.

21. Burman MS: Myeloscopy or the direct visualization of spinal cord. *J Bone Joint Surg* 1931; 13:695–696.

22. Stern E: Spinascope, new instrument for visualizing the spinal canal and its contents. *Med Rec (NY)* 1936; 143:31–32.

23. Pool JL: Myeloscopy: Diagnostic inspection of the cauda equina by means of the endoscope. *Bull Neurol Inst New York* 1938; 7:178–189.

24. Ooi Y, Satoh Y, Sugawara S, et al: Myeloscopy. *Internat Orthop (SICOT)* 1977; 1:107–111.

25. Blomberg R: A method of epiduroscopy and spinaloscopy. Presentation of preliminary results. *Acta Anaesthesiol Scand* 1985; 29(1):113–116.

26. Kambin P, Gellman H: Percutaneous lateral discectomy of the lumbar spine. A preliminary report. *Clin Orthop* 1983; 174:127–132.

27. Hijikata S, Toyama Y: A clinical experience of percutaneous nucleotomy for scoliosis with special reference to its indication and technical problems (abstract). *25 Jahrestagung der Japanischen Skoliosegesellschaft, Kyoto, Japan* 1991;

28. Schreiber A, Suezawa Y: Transdiscoscopic percutaneous nucleotomy in disc herniation. *Orthop Rev* 1986; 15(1):35–38.

29. Maroon JC, Onik GM: Percutaneous automated discectomy: A new method for lumbar disc removal. Technical note. *J Neurosurg* 1987; 66(1):143–146.

30. Leu HJ, Schreiber A: Biportal approach to the lumbar intervertebral discs: Nucleotomy, arthrodesis and percutaneous pedicle fixation. *Sem Orthop* 1991; 6:118–120.

31. Matthews HH, Kyles MK, Long BH: Arthroscopic assisted percutaneous interbody fusion with percutaneous internal fixation (PIF) (abstract). Sixth International Symposium Arthroscopic Microdis-section, the Graduate Hospital, University of Philadelphia, November 1991.

32. Obenchain TG: Laparoscopic lumbar disectomy: Case report. *J Laparoendosc Surg* 1991; 1(3):145–149.

33. Obenchain TG, Cloyd D: Outpatient lumbar discectomy: Description of the technique and review of the first twenty-one cases. *Surg Techn Int* 1994; 2:415–418.

34. Rosenthal D: Retroperitoneal approach to the lower lumbar spine using microsurgical endoscopy. Presented at the AO/ASIF Course on Minimal Invasive Spine Surgery, Davos, Switzerland, December 1995.

35. Rosenthal D, Rosenthal R, De Simone A: Removal of a protruded thoracic disc using microsurgical endoscopy. A new technique. *Spine* 1994; 19(9):1087–1091.

36. Mack MJ, Regan JJ, Bobechko WP, et al: Application of thoracoscopy for diseases of the spine. *Ann Thorac Surg* 1993; 56(3):736–738.

37. Horowitz MB, Moossy JJ, Julian T, et al: Thoracic discectomy using video assisted thoracoscopy. *Spine* 1994; 19(9):1082–1086.

38. Rosenthal D: Microsurgical endoscopic tumor resection and stabilization for neoplastic disease of the dorsal spine. Second Annual Symposium SSAF, New York, December 1993.

39. Dickman CA, Rosenthal D, Karahalios DG, et al: Thoracic vertebrectomy and reconstruction using a microsurgical thoracoscopic approach. *Neurosurgery* 1996; 38(2):279–293.

40. McAfee PC, Regan JR, Zdeblick T, et al: The incidence of complications in endoscopic anterior thoracolumbar spinal reconstructive surgery. A prospective multicenter study comprising the first 100 consecutive cases. *Spine* 1995; 20(14): 1624–1632.

41. Rosenthal D, Marquardt G, Lorenz R, et al: Anterior decompression and stabilization using a microsurgical endoscopic technique for metastatic tumors of the thoracic spine. *J Neurosurg* 1996; 84(4):565–572.

42. Kux E: *Thorakoskopische Eingriffe am Nervensystem*, Stuttgart: Georg Thieme Verlag; 1954.

43. Semm K: Endoscopic appendectomy. *Endoscopy* 1983; 15(2): 59–64.

CHAPTER **2**

General Principles of Thoracoscopy

Curtis A. Dickman, M.D.

Endoscopic techniques have substantially affected almost every sphere of medicine and surgery. The impetus for this movement is multifaceted. Patients find minimally incisional techniques attractive from cosmetic and aesthetic perspectives. The clinical benefits include minimal dissection of superficial tissues, which can result in less postoperative pain, less blood loss, shorter hospital stays, and faster recovery times than are associated with open procedures. In turn, these techniques have the potential for lowering the costs of health care and hastening a patient's recovery and return to normal activities.

DEVELOPMENT OF ENDOSCOPY

Technological advances in endoscopic imaging devices have played a critical role in the development of minimally invasive surgery. The resolution of endoscopic images now far surpasses those obtained earlier because technology such as computer interfacing, optical chips, fiber-optic cables, video endoscopy, and three-dimensional (3-D) imaging has improved. Endoscopes provide illumination, visualization, magnification, as well as a conduit for accessing almost every region of the human body through very small skin incisions. Because "conventional" operations with extensive anatomical dissections can be performed through very small incisions, we prefer the term minimally *incisional* surgery rather than minimally *invasive* surgery.

In almost every surgical specialty, endoscopes are used as diagnostic and therapeutic tools. An increasing number of surgical procedures, once performed solely with open techniques, are now performed almost exclusively with endoscopic techniques. Endoscopes have been used extensively as arthroscopes in orthopedics, as laparoscopes in general surgery and gynecology, as cystoscopes and ureteroscopes in urology, and as thoracoscopes in cardiothoracic surgery. Endoscopic approaches have radically altered the way many surgical procedures are performed, including cholecystectomy, hernia repair, tubal ligation, knee and shoulder reconstruction, and prostatectomy, among other procedures. Only recently has endoscopy found its respective niche for spinal surgery, but successful treatment of spinal pathology has expanded rapidly.

During the past decade, cardiothoracic surgeons used thoracoscopy widely, and the techniques for thoracoscopic spinal surgery are adapted from their methodologies.[1-4] Endoscopic approaches to the spine include posterolateral percutaneous approaches to the lumbar disc spaces and neural foramina, anterior laparoscopic and anterolateral retroperitoneal endoscopic approaches to the lumbar spine, and thoracoscopic approaches to the thoracic spine.[5-18] All these techniques primarily use rigid rod-lens endoscopes for visualization of the anatomy and pathology. Flexible fiber-optic endoscopes are also used as adjuncts to open spinal surgical procedures for inspection of the cauda equina, spinal cord, and neural foramina and assessment of the internal anatomy of syringomyelic cavities.[11-14,17,19] The clinical uses of flexible fiber-optic endoscopes are more limited than rigid endoscopes because their resolution and image quality are poorer.

DEVELOPMENT OF THORACOSCOPY

Thoracoscopy was introduced in the early 1900s and was initially used as a diagnostic tool for the evaluation of pleural diseases.[20-23] During the late 1980s, techniques and instrumentation for laparoscopic surgical procedures improved dramatically, facilitating new applications for thoracoscopy. During the early 1990s, thoracoscopic techniques evolved rapidly and were applied to a broad spectrum of pathology involving the thorax.[1-4] Today, many thoracic procedures previously performed via thoracotomy are routinely performed preferentially using thoracoscopy. These procedures include biopsy or resection of pleural or lung lesions, biopsy of lymph nodes, dissection for tumor staging, biopsy and resection of mediastinal masses, lobectomy, pneumonectomy, pleural sclerotherapy, treatment of blebs, esophageal procedures, sympathectomy, and other procedures.[1-4,24]

Clinical studies have found that thoracoscopy has significant advantages compared with thoracotomy for the treatment of thoracic pathology.[24,25] For example, during the resection of pulmonary lesions, small incisions with minimal dissection and retraction of the chest wall decreased blood loss, reduced postoperative pain, improved postoperative pulmonary and shoulder function, shortened intensive care unit and overall hospital stays, decreased complications, and hastened recovery times.[1-4,24-26] Compared to thoracotomy, morbidity rates, the amount of pain, and length of recovery were significantly lower with thoracoscopy. Thoracoscopy confers the same clinical advantages on the surgical management of spinal pathology.[5-7,27-29]

THORACOSCOPY IN SPINAL SURGERY

Thoracoscopic access is achieved by temporarily deflating the lung on the ipsilateral side of the spinal exposure using a double-lumen endotracheal tube. The chest cavity becomes a wide empty corridor or working space through which to access the thoracic spine. Narrow portals are strategically positioned in small incisions in the intercostal spaces. One portal is used for the endoscope, which is usually a 1-cm diameter, rigid, high-resolution endoscope. Two or three other portals are used to insert working tools. Video cameras mounted on the endoscopes relay the images to video monitors from which the entire surgical team can view the operation.

Thoracoscopy can access the entire thoracic spine from T1 to T12 but only provides unilateral exposure. Thoracoscopy can be used to access the discs, vertebral bodies, and ipsilateral pedicle; however, it cannot access the posterior surfaces of the spine or the contralateral pedicle. A wide variety of thoracic spinal pathology is amenable to treatment using thoracoscopy (Table 2–1). Thoracoscopic approaches have been used to treat herniated thoracic discs;[6-10,30] to drain vertebral epidural abscesses; to debride vertebral osteomyelitis and discitis; to decompress fractures; to biopsy and resect neoplasms;[5-7,30] and to perform vertebrectomies and interbody fusions, vertebral body reconstructions and instrumentation,[5-7,30,31] sympathectomies,[32-34] and anterior releases for the treatment of kyphosis and scoliosis.[6,7,10,30,31]

COMPARISONS OF THORACOSCOPY WITH OTHER SPINAL SURGICAL APPROACHES

The relative merits and disadvantages of thoracoscopy, thoracotomy, and costotransversectomy approaches to the thoracic spine are compared in Figures 2–1, 2–2, 2–3, and Table 2–2. Spinal surgeons have often been reluctant to use thoracotomy for access to the ventral thoracic spine, primarily because of the morbidity associated with thoracotomy (i.e, postthoracotomy pain syndromes, intercostal neuralgia, and pulmonary dysfunction) and the need for a cardiothoracic surgeon for exposure and closure.[26,27,32,35-46] However, an

TABLE 2–1 Clinical Indications for Spinal Thoracoscopy

Procedure	Pathology
Sympathectomy	Palmar hyperhidrosis Raynaud's disease Reflex sympathetic dystrophy
Diagnostic vertebral biopsy	Spinal infections Spinal tumors
Drainage of paravertebral and anterior epidural abscesses	Infections
Resection of intrathoracic nerve sheath tumors	Schwannomas Neurofibromas Primitive neuroectodermal tumors
Thoracic microdiscectomy	Herniated thoracic discs
Thoracic corpectomy, vertebral reconstruction, and internal fixation	Spinal fractures Tumors Osteomyelitis Hemivertebrae resection
Rib head resection	Costovertebral joint syndrome

Spinal deformity correction
  Anterior ligamentous release
  Anterior osteotomy
  Anterior interbody fusion
  Anterior epiphysiodesis
	Rigid kyphosis
	Rigid scoliosis greater than 75°
	Neuromuscular spinal deformity
	Congenital spinal anomalies
	Deformity with skeletal immaturity (prevent Crankshaft phenomena)

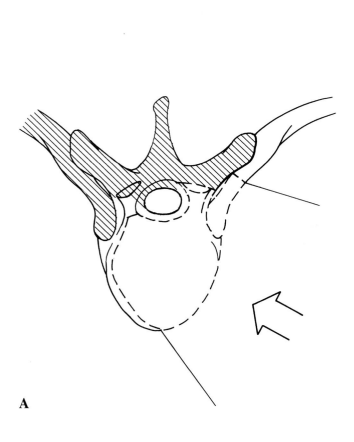

A

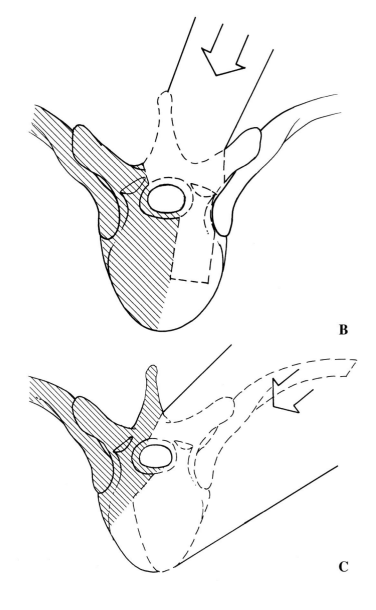

B

C

Figure 2–1. Comparative operative views of **(A)** the anterolateral approaches (thoracotomy and thoracoscopy), **(B)** the transpedicular approach, and **(C)** the costotransversectomy approach. The only approaches that provide a view of the ventral dura are the thoracotomy and thoracoscopic approaches. Each approach has a blind area on the surface of the dura opposite the surgeon's line of view.

TABLE 2–2   Comparison of Operative Approaches to the Thoracic Spine

Feature	Costotransversectomy	Thoracotomy	Thoracoscopy
Direction of approach	Posterolateral	Anterolateral	Anterolateral
View of ventral surface of spinal cord	Oblique, indirect	Full, direct	Full, direct
Size of incisions	4 to 12 inches	6 to 15 inches	$\frac{1}{2}$ inch (x 3–4)
Muscle transection	Moderate or extensive	Extensive	Minimal
Relationship to pleura	Extrapleural	Intrapleural	Intrapleural
Postoperative chest tube	No	Yes	Yes
Access to posterior spinal elements for decompression or fixation	Yes	No	No
Access to vertebral bodies for screw-plate fixation	No	Yes	Yes
Extent of rib resection or rib retraction	3 to 7 inches of rib removed/moderate retraction	6 to 12 inches of rib removed/extensive retraction	1 inch of rib head and proximal rib removed/no retraction
Incidence of postoperative intercostal neuralgia	Uncommon, often transient	Common, often prolonged	Uncommon, usually transient

[From Dickman CA, Karahalios D: Thoracoscopic spinal surgery, *Clin Neurosurg* 1996; 43:392–422. Reprinted with permission of Williams & Wilkins.]

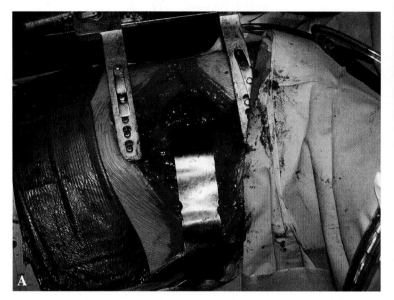
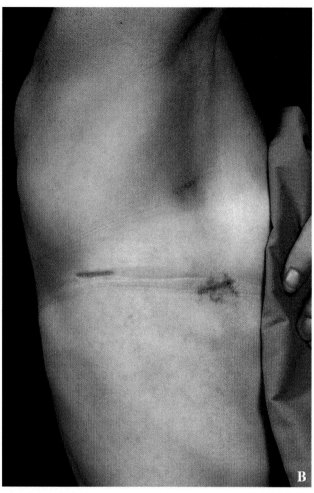

Figure 2–2. **(A)** Intraoperative photograph of a thoracotomy incision used to perform a T7–T8 discectomy. The incision is 12 inches long. The retractor is opened 6 inches wide, which displaces the chest wall and ribs to provide exposure that enables surgeons to insert their hands into the thoracic cavity. **(B)** Postoperative view of the lateral surface of the thorax after a thoracoscopic microdiscectomy has been performed at T7–T8. Three 15-mm incisions were made in the intercostal spaces to insert portals for the endoscope and dissection tools. This approach provided the same ventral view and access for dissection as the thoracotomy incision, but required no rib retraction. Furthermore, the postoperative scars were much smaller.

anterior transthoracic approach provides the only way for directly visualizing the ventral surfaces of the thoracic spine and spinal cord to facilitate decompression, reconstruction, and internal fixation of ventral spinal pathology.

Thoracoscopy has advantages (i.e., minimal muscular incisions, no rib retraction, and minimal rib resection) that both thoracotomy and costotransversectomy lack. Thoracoscopy reduces the morbidity and pain associated with the anterior transthoracic approach while preserving the broad, direct view and unobstructed surgical access to the entire ventral surfaces of the spine and spinal cord. Complex dissections of the spine, such as spinal cord decompression, reconstruction, and instrumentation, can be performed using thoracoscopy. Unlike costotransversectomy, thoracoscopy offers a direct, complete view of the entire ventral surface of the spinal cord (Figs. 2–1 and 2–3).

Thoracoscopy Compared to Laparoscopy

Laparoscopic surgery usually requires CO_2 insufflation to create a working space within the peritoneal cavity. Consequently, rigid sealed trocars must be used, and they restrict the use of suction to maintain the pressurization. The need

for pressurized CO_2 insufflation to maintain the surgical exposure has several disadvantages. It alters cardiovascular hemodynamics and intracranial pressure. It decreases venous return and causes venous stasis. It also restricts the types of surgical strategies that can be used to maintain a clear, bloodless field. The CO_2 pressure (usually 10 to 15 mm Hg) can also obscure sources of venous bleeding because the pressure of the intraabdominal compartment matches or exceeds central venous pressure. Delayed venous hemorrhage can occur after laparoscopy unless meticulous hemostasis is achieved during the dissection. The pressurized CO_2 can cause hypercapnia from diffuse intravascular absorption; it can also cause a CO_2 embolism if a large bolus of gas is absorbed intravascularly. Gasless laparoscopic techniques have been developed to reduce the problems associated with an insufflated, pressurized compartment.

In contrast, thoracoscopy does *not* require an insufflated, pressurized compartment. Blocking ventilation to the lung on the side of surgical access using a double-lumen endotracheal tube deflates the ipsilateral lung. The passive pneumothorax created by the densely atelectatic lung gives rise to a large, empty working space within the thoracic cavity.

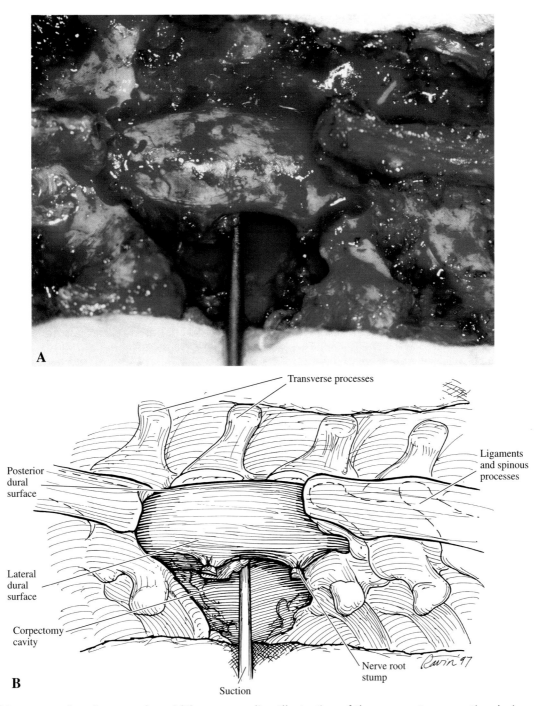

Figure 2–3. **(A)** Intraoperative photograph and **(B)** corresponding illustration of the surgeon's perspective during a costotransversectomy approach for a T6–T7 corpectomy and fusion for metastatic breast cancer. The T6 and T7 nerve roots were ligated to improve the access to the vertebral bodies. The dura has been decompressed. The spinous processes, laminae, facets, and transverse processes are viewed dorsally adjacent to the dura. A large cavity made into the T6 and T7 vertebrae enabled resection of the neoplasm and decompression of the spinal cord. The suction tip is positioned against the ventral surface of the dura. During the costotransversectomy approach, the surgeon can view *only* the posterior and lateral surfaces of the dura and is blind to the ventral surface of the dura.

The surgeon has the freedom to use suction, retractors, drills, tools, and cauterization in an unrestricted way without interfering with the exposure. Eliminating the sealed, pressurized environment provides tremendous freedom for dissection, allowing the same surgical strategies to be used as in open surgery. The portals do not need to be rigid or to have a sealing mechanism (i.e., valve, diaphragm) or a valve for gas insufflation. The portals for thoracoscopy are simple, flexible protective sheaths that provide conduits of access through the intercostal spaces into the thorax.

Occasionally, CO_2 insufflation may temporarily be required for thoracoscopy to accelerate the collapse of the lung or create more operative space if the lung is partially ventilated because the endotracheal tube has been malpositioned or the patient is unable to tolerate ventilation. If CO_2 insufflation is used with thoracoscopy, sealed rigid trocars, which increase the incidence of intercostal neuralgia, must be used.

The pressure achieved with intrathoracic CO_2 insufflation should *not* exceed 15 mm Hg. Insufflation of CO_2 up to 10 to 15 mm Hg is safe. Intrathoracic pressures *above* 15 to

20 mm Hg cause mediastinal shift and hemodynamic compromise—an iatrogenic effect comparable to a tension pneumothorax.[47] If intraoperative hypotension occurs during intrathoracic CO_2 insufflation, the pressurization should be discontinued immediately.

Thoracoscopic Surgical Skills Compared to Open Surgery

The endoscopic sequencing of the surgical steps and the types of dissection for the soft tissues and spine are no different from those used in open surgery. Operative maneuvers that would not be used during open surgery should *never* be performed endoscopically. The normal anatomical structures should always be clearly identified first. The surgeon should then work from the regions where the anatomy is clearly identified toward the pathology so that critical structures (e.g., the spinal cord, aorta) can be preserved. Dissection, too, should *never* be performed blindly. All maneuvers must be clearly visualized, and the tools must be used accurately.

If the visual perspective is inadequate to allow assessment during dissection, then a different perspective should be implemented, either by inserting a new portal or by opening the chest using a thoracotomy. Converting to a thoracotomy is not a failure of the endoscopic procedure. If the dissection cannot be safely performed, visibility is compromised, or the tissue planes are scarred and distorted by the pathology, an open procedure may become necessary. If the surgeon cannot achieve the desired goals of the operation endoscopically, an open thoracotomy should be used.

Hemostasis is obtained using the same techniques and tools (albeit longer versions) as used during open surgery. Monopolar cauterization is used to incise the pleura or cauterize the segmental vessels, but it should be avoided near the nerve roots, the sympathetic chain, and the spinal cord. Fine-tipped insulated bipolar forceps are used for hemostasis near nerves and the spinal cord, especially for hemostasis of the epidural veins. Small pieces of hemostatic agents (i.e., gelfoam, Nu-Knit™ [Johnson & Johnson, Arlington, TX], Avitene,® and so on) are applied precisely and carefully with $\frac{1}{2} \times \frac{1}{2}$ - inch or $\frac{1}{2} \times 1$ - inch cottonoid patties to control epidural bleeding (Fig. 2–4). Large patties are avoided so that the application of hemostatic agents is clearly visualized and precisely applied to avoid inadvertent compression of the dura. Bone bleeding is controlled with bone wax applied on an endoscopic cotton-tipped dissector (Fig. 2–5). The segmental vessels are secured with hemoclips for permanent ligation.

The endoscopic sequencing of spinal dissection is identical to the sequence used in open thoracotomy. If the spinal cord is to be decompressed, the first maneuver is to resect the rib head and pedicle at the level of compression to identify the dura and spinal cord clearly. All subsequent dissection steps can be performed with *direct* visual reference of the maneuvers relative to the position of the spinal cord to protect the spinal cord. Also, if the spinal cord is compressed, a cavity must be created to make a *working space* in the bone adjacent to the pathology. This working space allows the compressive material to be delivered away from the spinal cord, minimizing the dissection within the compromised spinal canal. This space allows pathology to be decompressed, using only the tips of fine microsurgical dissectors so that the spinal cord will not be further compressed by the dissection tools. The bone dissection tools are used as in open surgery. Curettes and other microsurgical dissection tools are used to decompress the pathology *away* from the spinal cord (not toward the spinal canal).

Although the sequences and dissection techniques for thoracoscopy closely resemble those used during open surgery, thoracoscopy requires several new skills, psychomotor strategies, and perceptions of the anatomy that differ substantially from open surgery. The portals provide narrow windows of restricted access (and no direct visualization) through the chest wall. Trajectories are restricted and confined, based on the position and trajectory of the portals. A "virtual reality" surgical environment is created because the surgeon cannot directly see through the chest wall. They do not see the tools directly but rather depend on the video endoscopic projection of the surgical view. During the operation, the surgeon looks directly ahead at the monitor rather than down at the anatomy or at his or her hands (Fig. 2–6). To become competent at endoscopic surgery, surgeons need to develop new skills: endoscopic navigation; triangulation (i.e., determining the trajectory, angulation, and depth of tools toward the pathology based on surface landmarks); operating while looking forward to watch a video screen; maintaining a stable, clear, oriented endoscopic image; stabilizing, controlling, and moving long tools precisely; controlling the amplification of movements; readjusting visual–motor and sensorimotor feedback loops; localizing the spinal levels based on internal landmarks; coordinating the different phases of dissection performed by different surgeons working simultaneously with different tools; and relearning all phases of the operative dissection based on these new technique parameters. To develop these skills requires dedicated practice in a surgical skills laboratory. We cannot overemphasize this point. The "learning curve" for acquiring these psychomotor and technical skills for thoracoscopy is *steep*.

Endoscopic surgical tools must be held and manipulated differently from the shorter tools used in open surgery. The long endoscopic dissection tools are often more difficult to learn to control because their increased length amplifies movements. These tools may also be heavier (Fig. 2–7). Two hands are often used to maneuver bone dissection tools (i.e., Kerrison rongeurs, curettes) when precise control is needed near the spinal cord. The surgeon controls the tools with two hands and further stabilizes them against the chest wall within the portal to achieve three-point anchoring of the tools (Fig. 2–8). With practice, the surgeon can control the endoscopic dissection tools with exquisite precision.

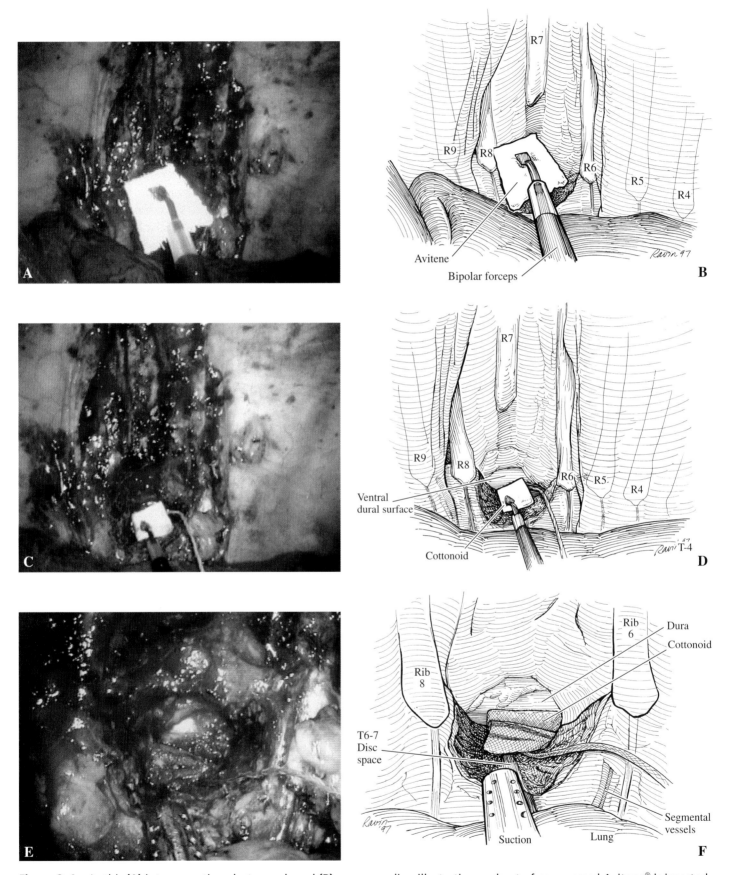

Figure 2–4. In this **(A)** intraoperative photograph and **(B)** corresponding illustration, a sheet of compressed Avitene® is inserted with endoscopic bipolar forceps. **(C)** Intraoperative photograph and **(D)** corresponding illustration showing the small sheet of hemostatic material precisely delivered to the epidural space and covered gently with a small cottonoid patty. In this **(E)** intraoperative photograph and **(F)** corresponding illustration, the epidural space is visible adjacent to the patty after hemostasis was obtained. The dura was exposed to remove a herniated thoracic disc. R = rib.

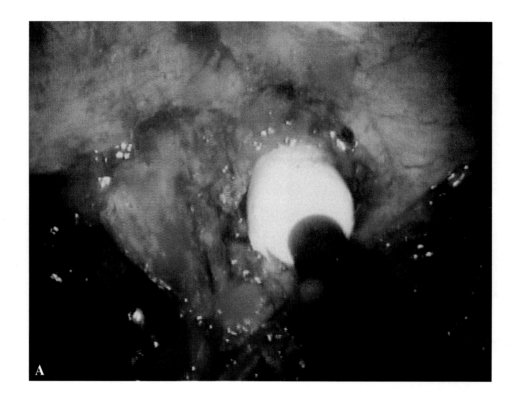

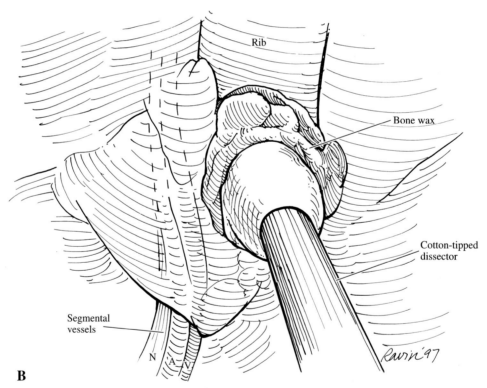

Figure 2–5. **(A)** Intraoperative photograph and **(B)** corresponding illustration showing a piece of bone wax applied to a bleeding rib surface with an endoscopic cotton-tipped dissector.

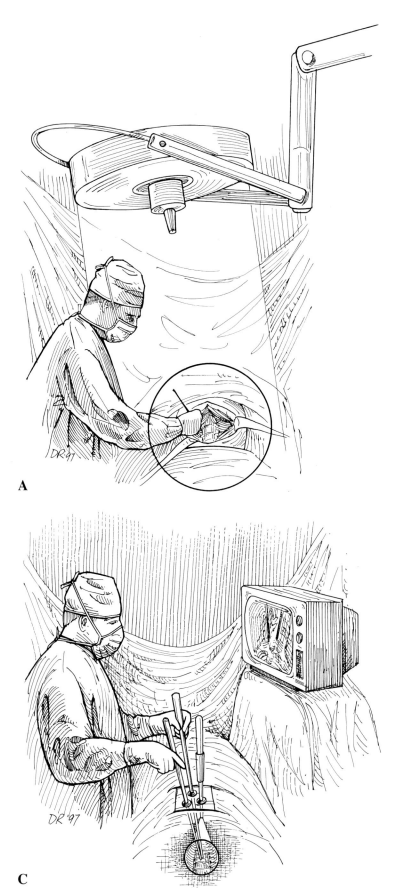

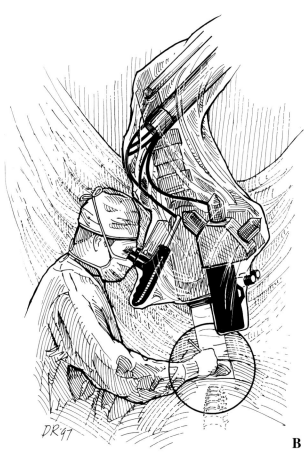

A

B

C

Figure 2–6. Comparison between **(A)** thoracotomy, **(B)** microsurgery with thoracotomy, and **(C)** video-assisted thoracoscopic microsurgery. The microsurgical approaches use smaller incisions and provide a magnified, illuminated operative field. The operating microscope and the thoracoscope both require a surgeon to look straight ahead rather than down at the operating field during the procedure. Thoracoscopy requires no retraction of the ribs or chest wall.

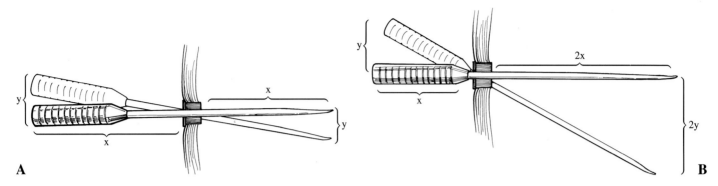

Figure 2–7. The surgeon's movements of the tools are amplified in thoracoscopic procedures because the distance from the chest wall to the pathology is increased. Similarly, in thoracoscopic procedures, pathologies that are **(A)** close to the chest wall will amplify movement less than pathologies that are **(B)** distant to the chest wall. Amplification of the movements of tools requires a two-handed strategy to stabilize and precisely control the dissection tools, especially near the spinal cord and major blood vessels.

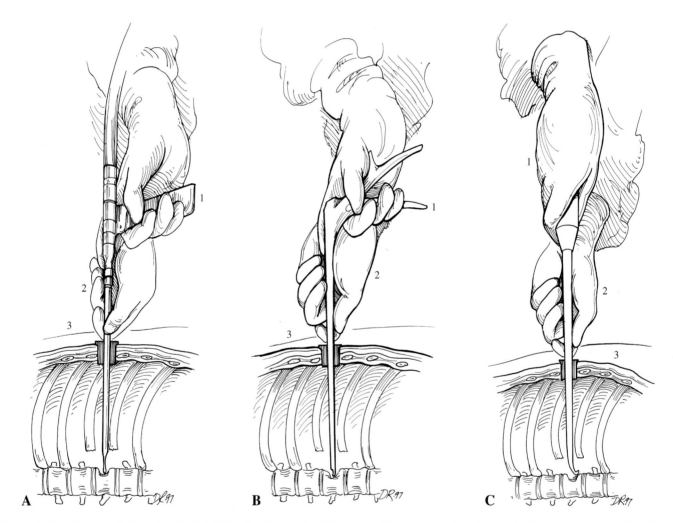

Figure 2–8. Three-point mechanical stabilization is required for several thoracoscopic spine tools. The surgeon uses two hands to control **(A)** the pneumatic drill, **(B)** Kerrison rongeurs, and **(C)** curettes as well as other bone dissection tools. The shaft of the tool is further anchored against the patient's chest wall within the portal.

ADVANTAGES OF THORACOSCOPY

1. Thoracoscopy is based on preserving all normal healthy tissue of the chest while completely treating the pathology surgically. This has been a long-standing goal for surgeons throughout time.
2. Thoracoscopy reduces trauma to the chest, which, in turn, reduces pain, facilitates recovery, reduces pulmonary dysfunction, and provides cosmetic benefits.
3. Thoracoscopy provides a full, direct, unobstructed anterior view of the spinal cord that allows extensive dissection and decompression and reconstruction to be performed under full visualization.
4. Reconstructing the spine ventrally along its weight-bearing axis (where more than 80% of loads are borne) has structural and biomechanical advantages for restoring spinal stability.

DISADVANTAGES OF THORACOSCOPY

1. This technique cannot be performed if the patient has dense, extensive pleural adhesions (i.e., from a prior thoracotomy, emphysema, hemothorax, or pleurodesis) or severe pulmonary disease (e.g., chronic obstructive pulmonary disease, parenchymal disease).
2. Thoracoscopy provides no access to the posterior spinal elements (i.e., laminae, spinous processes) or the contralateral pedicle.
3. The technology and equipment for thoracoscopy are expensive; however, most operating rooms already have most of the tools and equipment for thoracoscopy without needing to make further capital expenditures.
4. Application of thoracoscopy requires patience and dedicated laboratory practice to acquire the needed surgical skills. Initially, the operations take longer than open surgery and are technically more difficult for surgeons to perform. With experience and time, however, the difficulty of the surgical procedures is reduced significantly.

CONCLUSION

Thoracoscopic spinal surgical techniques are based on skills and principles borrowed from several other surgical specialties. To become a competent thoracoscopic spinal surgeon, several unique strategies and dedicated practice are needed to master the techniques.

REFERENCES

1. Kaiser LR: Video-assisted thoracic surgery. Current state of the art. *Ann Surg* 1994; 220(6):720–734.
2. Landreneau RJ, Mack MJ, Hazelrigg SR, et al: Video-assisted thoracic surgery: Basic technical concepts and intercostal approach strategies. *Ann Thorac Surg* 1992; 54:800–807.
3. Coltharp WH, Arnold JH, Alford WC, Jr., et al: Videothoracoscopy: Improved technique and expanded indications. *Ann Thorac Surg* 1992; 53:776–779.
4. Mack MJ, Aronoff RJ, Acuff TE, et al: Present role of thoracoscopy in the diagnosis and treatment of diseases of the chest. *Ann Thorac Surg* 1992; 54:403–409.
5. Dickman CA, Rosenthal D, Karahalios DG, et al: Thoracic vertebrectomy and reconstruction using a microsurgical thoracoscopic approach. *Neurosurgery* 1996; 38(2):279–293.
6. McAfee PC, Regan JR, Zdeblick T, et al: The incidence of complications in endoscopic anterior thoracolumbar spinal reconstructive surgery. A prospective multicenter study comprising the first 100 consecutive cases. *Spine* 1995; 20(14):1624–1632.
7. Regan JJ, Mack MJ, Picetti GD, III, et al: A comparison of video-assisted thoracoscopic surgery (VATS) with open thoracotomy in thoracic spinal surgery. *Today's Therapeutic Trends* 1994; 11:203–218.
8. Horowitz MB, Moossy JJ, Julian T, et al: Thoracic discectomy using video assisted thoracoscopy. *Spine* 1994; 19(9):1082–1086.
9. Rosenthal D, Rosenthal R, de Simone A: Removal of a protruded thoracic disc using microsurgical endoscopy. A new technique. *Spine* 1994; 19(9):1087–1091.
10. Regan JJ, Mack MJ, Picetti GD, III: A technical report on video-assisted thoracoscopy in thoracic spinal surgery. *Spine* 1995; 20(7):831–837.
11. Burman MS: Myeloscopy or the direct visualization of the spinal canal and its contents. *J Bone Joint Surg* 1931; 13:695–696.
12. Pool JL: Direct visualization of dorsal nerve roots of the cauda equina by means of the myeloscope. *Arch Neurol Psychol* 1938; 39:1308–1312.
13. Pool JL: Myeloscopy: Diagnostic inspection of the cauda equina by means of the endoscope. *Bull Neurol Inst NY* 1938; 7:178–189.
14. Pool JL: Myeloscopy: Intrathecal endoscopy. *Surgery* 1942; 11:169–182.
15. Onik G, Helms CA, Ginsburg L, et al: Percutaneous lumbar discectomy using new aspiration probe. *AJR* 1985; 144:1137–1140.
16. Kambin P, Schaffer JL: Percutaneous lumbar discectomy. Review of 100 patients and current practice. *Clin Orthop* 1989; 238:24–34.
17. Ooi Y, Satoh Y, Morisaki N: Myeloscopy: The possibility of observing the lumbar intrathecal space by use of an endoscope. *Endoscopy* 1973; 5:901–906.
18. Mathews H: First International Symposium on Lasers in Orthopaedics. San Francisco, 1991.
19. McKneally MF: Video-assisted thoracic surgery: Standards and guidelines. *Chest Surg Clin North Am* 1993; 3:345–351.
20. Jacobaeus HC: Possibility of the use of the cystoscope for investigation of serious cavities. *Munch Med Wochenscr* 1910; 57:2090–2092.
21. Jacobaeus HC: The practical importance of thoracoscopy in surgery of the chest. *Surg Gynecol Obstet* 1922; 34:289–296.
22. Jacobaeus HC: The cauterization of adhesions in pneumothorax treatment of tuberculosis. *Surg Gynecol Obstet* 1921; 32:493–500.
23. Jacobaeus HC: Endopleural operations by means of a thoracoscope. *Beitr Klin Tuberk* 1915; 35:1.
24. Landreneau RJ, Hazelrigg SR, Mack MJ, et al: Postoperative pain-related morbidity: Video-assisted thoracic surgery versus thoracotomy. *Ann Thorac Surg* 1993; 56:1285–1289.
25. Ferson PF, Landreneau RJ, Dowling RD, et al: Comparison of open

versus thoracoscopic lung biopsy for diffuse infiltrative pulmonary disease. *J Thorac Cardiovasc Surg* 1993; 106:194–199.

26. Hazelrigg SR, Landreneau RJ, Boley TM, et al: The effect of muscle-sparing versus standard posterolateral thoracotomy on pulmonary function, muscle strength, and postoperative pain. *J Thorac Cardiovasc Surg* 1991; 101:394–401.

27. Bohlman HH, Zdeblick TA: Anterior excision of herniated thoracic discs. *J Bone Joint Surg (Am)* 1988; 70(7):1038–1047.

28. Rosenthal D, Dickman CA: Thoracoscopic microsurgical exicision of herniated thoracic discs. *J Neurosurg* 1998; 89: 224–235.

29. Dickman CA, Karahalios DG: Thoracoscopic spinal surgery. *Clin Neurosurg* 1995; 43:392–422.

30. Mack MJ, Regan JJ, Bobechko WP, et al: Application of thoracoscopy for diseases of the spine. *Ann Thorac Surg* 1993; 56:736–738.

31. Dickman CA, Mican CA: Multilevel anterior thoracic discectomies and anterior interbody fusion using a microsurgical thoracoscopic approach. *J Neurosurg* 1996; 84:104–109.

32. Krasna MJ, Mack MJ: Sympathectomy. In Krasna MJ, Mack MJ, eds: *Atlas of Thoracoscopic Surgery.* St. Louis: Quality; 1994: 139–149.

33. Robertson DP, Simpson RK, Rose JE, et al: Video-assisted endoscopic thoracic ganglionectomy. *J Neurosurg* 1993; 79:238–204.

34. Kao M-C, Tsai J-C, Lai D-M, et al: Autonomic activities in hyperhidrosis patients before, during, and after endoscopic laser sympathectomy. *Neurosurgery* 1994; 34(2):262–268.

35. Benjamin V: Diagnosis and management of thoracic disc disease. *Clin Neurosurg* 1983; 30:577–606.

36. Crafoord C, Hiertonn T, Lindblom K, et al: Spinal cord compression caused by a protruded thoracic disc. Report of a case treated with antero-lateral fenestration of the disc. *Acta Orthop Scand* 1958; 28:103–107.

37. Fidler MW, Goedhart ZD: Excision of prolapse of thoracic intervertebral disc. A transthoracic technique. *J Bone Joint Surg (Br)* 1984; 66(4):518–522.

38. Kaneda K, Abumi K, Fujiya M: Burst fractures with neurologic deficits of the thoraco-lumbar spine. Results of anterior decompression and stabilization with anterior instrumentation. *Spine* 1984; 9:788–795.

39. Kostuik JP: Anterior spinal cord decompression for lesions of the thoracic and lumbar spine, techniques, new methods of internal fixation results. *Spine* 1983; 8(5):512–531.

40. Kostuik JP: Anterior fixation for fractures of the thoracic and lumbar spine with or without neurologic involvement. *Clin Orthop* 1984; 189:103–115.

41. Yuan HA, Mann KA, Found EM: Early clinical experience with the Syracuse I-plate: An anterior spinal fixation device. *Spine* 1988; 2764:13056–13248.

42. Perot PL, Jr., Munro DD: Transthoracic removal of midline thoracic disc protrusions causing spinal cord compression. *J Neurosurg* 1969; 31:452–458.

43. Ransahoff J, Spencer F, Siew F, et al: Transthoracic removal of thoracic disc. Report of three cases. *J Neurosurg* 1969; 31:459–461.

44. Otani K, Nakai S, Fujimura Y, et al: Surgical treatment of thoracic disc herniation using the anterior approach. *J Bone Joint Surg (Br)* 1982; 64(3):340–343.

45. Faciszewski T, Winter RB, Lonstein JE, et al: The surgical and medical perioperative complications of anterior spinal fusion surgery in the thoracic and lumbar spine in adults. A review of 1223 procedures. *Spine* 1995; 20(14):1592–1599.

46. Dajczman E, Gordon A, Kreisman H, et al: Long-term postthoracotomy pain. *Chest* 1991; 99(2):270–274.

47. Jones DR, Graeber GM, Tanguilig GG, et al: Effects of insufflation on hemodynamics during thoracoscopy. *Ann Thorac Surg* 1993; 55(6):1379–1382.

CHAPTER **3**

Education and Credentialing for Thoracoscopic Spine Surgery

Curtis A. Dickman, M.D. and Richard G. Fessler, M.D., Ph.D.

Thoracoscopic spinal surgery is highly technical and is associated with a very steep learning curve. Surgeons should only attempt to use thoracoscopic techniques clinically after pursuing an educational program that includes comprehensive lectures and extensive practice of surgical skills in a surgical laboratory. Surgeons must recognize that their previous surgical experience with open techniques is inadequate preparation for competency with these new surgical techniques.

Many ethical and technical challenges face surgeons in specialties where rapidly evolving procedures literally change our clinical practices overnight. The development of endoscopic spine techniques, however, can be guided by examples from endoscopic general surgeons and thoracic surgeons. Their experiences and problems in developing new skills, new surgical techniques, and new procedures provide valuable information to spinal surgeons.

GUIDELINES FOR THORACOSCOPIC SPINAL SURGERY

In the early 1990s, laparoscopy became extremely popular, especially for cholecystectomy.[1,2] A flood of general surgeons rapidly learned techniques in seminars and began to use them clinically. Subsequently, it became apparent that most serious clinical complications occurred relatively early in the experience of novice laparoscopic surgeons. Their high early complication rates reflected the steep learning curve involved in mastering the technique. Consequently, supervisory practices were instituted. Training, educational, and credentialing requirements were created, and continuing medical education requirements were established.[3–10] Novice laparoscopic surgeons were required to demonstrate endoscopic clinical competence through a variety of mechanisms, which included experience in a residency or fel-

lowship training and attendance at basic didactic workshops that taught endoscopic surgical theory, skills, techniques, and strategies to prevent and treat complications. Preceptorships and supervisory practices were instituted to assess clinical competency and to provide peer review. Ongoing assessment of the clinical results achieved with endoscopic techniques was required. Professional societies were developed to promote education, to establish standards for credentialing, and to assess clinical outcomes. The Society of American Gastrointestinal Endoscopic Surgeons (SAGES) is an example of such an organization.

The development of professional endoscopic surgical societies (SAGES is the model organization) has facilitated the growth and advancement of endoscopic techniques. SAGES provides surgeons with responsible leadership and guidance on a variety of issues: continuing education, guidelines for training, granting of privileges, application of new technology, development of standards of practice, active dialogue with manufacturers, resident and fellow training, assessment of instrument and procedural safety issues, and endoscopic scientific research. SAGES also provides comprehensive educational programs, video and text libraries, preceptorship programs, and an extensive publication program. The publication of guidelines is a particularly important contribution of SAGES.[3,4] The organization serves as a *model* for what is needed in endoscopic spinal surgery in terms of teaching skills, facilitating education, promoting competence, developing guidelines, establishing standards, developing improved techniques, and assessing the clinical impact of the procedures collaboratively.

Thoracic surgeons also developed similar educational and credentialing requirements for video-assisted thoracoscopic surgery. Guidelines have been published with recommendations by cardiothoracic surgeons for endoscopic surgery.[11,12]

Because such a high degree of skill is required for most endoscopic spinal surgery, the major issue confronting spinal surgeons is how endoscopic spinal surgical techniques can be implemented appropriately. This important ethical question must be answered to ensure that high-quality patient care is preserved. The same issues apply to thoracoscopic spinal surgery, laparoscopic spinal surgery, and retroperitoneoscopic spinal surgery.

A team approach should be used for thoracoscopic spinal surgery. An *experienced* endoscopic thoracic surgeon should act as co-surgeon during the clinical initiation of these surgical techniques. After the endoscopic spine surgeon has gained sufficient clinical experience and demonstrated clinical competence with thoracoscopic surgery, the thoracic surgeon may assume a less involved role in the operation. The collaborative relationship, however, should be continued.

An endoscopic thoracic surgeon has valuable skills and may be needed to detach pleural adhesions, to ligate segmental vessels, to mobilize the aorta or azygos vein, or to perform an emergency thoracotomy if a complication occurs. If an endoscopic thoracic surgeon is not needed intraoperatively, he or she should be *on standby* in the hospital in the event of an emergency that would require his or her immediate assistance.

The criteria for determining clinical competency in thoracoscopic spinal surgery include a formal fellowship or residency training in neurosurgery or spinal orthopedic surgery, experience with basic endoscopic skills, and experience with procedures that involve advanced endoscopic skills. Thoracoscopic surgical skills should include portal insertion, adhesiolysis, hemostasis, soft tissue dissection, pleural mobilization, segmental vessel dissection, vessel mobilization, sympathectomy, anterior ligamentous release, discectomy, corpectomy, reconstruction of vertebrae, suturing, lung mobilization, and lung retraction. Therefore, training should include formal endoscopic spinal training during a residency or fellowship, formal courses, participation in skills' laboratories and/or preceptorships, and experience performing *similar* procedures in an *open setting*.

Standards must be uniform to ensure that the quality of patient care is high. Granting privileges is the responsibility of each individual hospital. Proctoring should be performed by a qualified, unbiased physician who is an experienced endoscopic spinal surgeon. Surgeons' endoscopic performance should be monitored on an ongoing basis to maintain their privileges. Existing quality assurance guidelines can be used to assess appropriate utilization, outcomes, complications, and so on. Continuing education is also necessary to help surgeons maintain a high level of knowledge and skill.

EDUCATION IN TECHNIQUES AND SKILL DEVELOPMENT

Thoracoscopic surgery requires surgeons to acquire new psychomotor skills. They must adapt and modify the way they typically manipulate tools, create new ways of per-

ceiving the operative anatomy, develop strategies to maintain a patent image, and navigate in an unfamiliar environment through restricted portals of entry. The entire surgical approach necessitates a challenging reorganization of surgical perceptions and strategies.

Consequently, thoracoscopic surgical techniques must be mastered before they are clinically applied (Table 3–1). The initial learning curve for thoracoscopic spine surgery is steep. Many experienced spinal surgeons have commented that they "felt disoriented, inexperienced, and poorly prepared" to pursue these techniques during their first few laboratory training sessions. Still, surgeons can acquire these skills and develop techniques fairly rapidly (Figs. 3–1 and 3–2).[13] However, each surgeon's aptitude will be different.

The initial learning curve can create frustration for the surgeon until the techniques are mastered. Initially, endoscopic spinal procedures take longer than open spinal procedures, and the initial procedures are more difficult to perform than open surgeries. As surgeons develop competence and confidence with experience, the surgical skills become easy and "second nature." Eventually, the spinal endoscopic procedures can be performed more quickly than open procedures because the length of time associated with opening and closing the incisions is reduced significantly.[13–14]

Instructional courses should teach the fundamental principles of thoracoscopy in a comprehensive fashion. Topics covered should include endoscopic imaging equipment, navigational skills, orientation skills, triangulation skills, and the assembly and use of the components of the endoscopic imaging and video equipment. Relevant anatomy and pathoanatomy should be discussed. Surgeons must acquire a comprehensive understanding of all the new tools and portals and how to select, insert, and use them safely. Operating room setup and patient positioning also must be presented. Methods of anesthesia and perioperative man-

TABLE 3–1 Educational Techniques to Develop Endoscopic Skills for Thoracoscopic Spine Surgery

Residency or spine fellowship training in methods of endoscopic spine surgery

Didactic instructional courses

Thoracoscopic (inanimate) trainer

Cadaver surgical skills laboratories

Animal surgical skills laboratories

Observation of experienced thoracoscopic spine surgeons

Preceptorship with experienced thoracoscopic spine surgeons

Proctoring by experienced thoracoscopic spine surgeons

Collaborative surgery with experienced thoracoscopic thoracic surgeons

Endoscopic visualized open surgical procedures

Initiating thoracoscopy with technically simple procedures (i.e., biopsy, sympathectomy)

Transitioning to complex endoscopic spine procedures after further experience

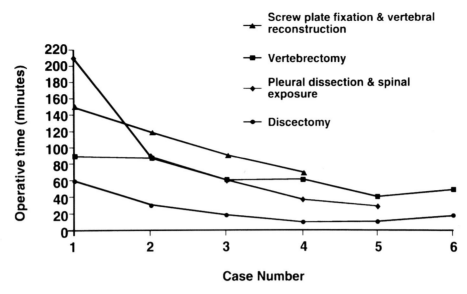

Figure 3–1.   Surgical durations during our initial laboratory training with thoracoscopic spinal surgery in a porcine model. With experience, the operative times were significantly reduced. The acquisition and mastery of the new surgical skills are referred to as the "learning curve."

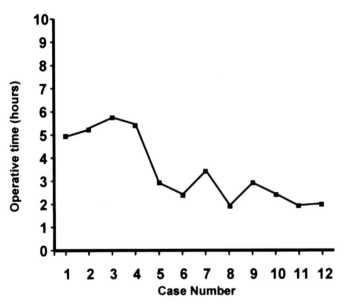

Figure 3–2.   The duration of surgery for clinical cases of thoracoscopic microdiscectomy demonstrates the clinical learning curve associated with the technique. The first few cases lasted 5 to 6 hours. Subsequently, the operative time was reduced to 2 to 3 hours for a one-level thoracic microdiscectomy. [From Dickman CA, Karahalios DG: Thoracoscopic spinal surgery. *Clin Neurosurg* 1996.[14] With permission of Williams & Wilkins.]

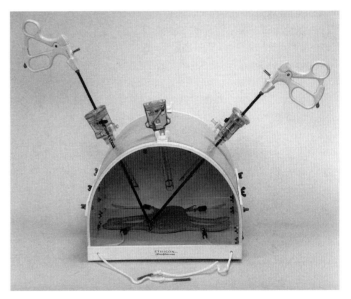

Figure 3–3.   The thoracoscopic trainer is an enclosed simulated thorax that is used to teach endoscopic navigation, triangulation, and dissection skills. The ends of the trainer have a plexiglass window that allows the contents to be viewed externally if desired. The artificial chest wall consists of simulated ribs and intercostal spaces, which are covered by a flexible, soft, and artificial skin-like material. Portals, endoscopes, and tools are inserted into the "thorax" to practice and learn endoscopic surgery. This device is very useful for teaching a novice endoscopist many of the basic surgical strategies.

agement as well as surgical indications and contraindications should be reviewed. Detailed examples of the surgical techniques for spinal exposure and dissection should be taught, along with ways of preventing and treating complications.

After this series of comprehensive lectures, an extensive, practical hands-on skills laboratory should be pursued. Practical laboratories often begin by teaching the basic skills of endoscopic navigation using an endoscopic thoracoscopic trainer to simulate the chest cavity (Fig. 3–3).

After the most basic skills are mastered, it is extremely useful to simulate the clinical scenario with a live animal model. Animal surgery allows the surgeon to practice the important skills needed during actual surgery. The simulation is critical to the development of strategies such as maintaining a patent image, applying a defogging agent, maintaining a bloodless field, retracting the lung, orienting the view to the pathology, ligating the vessels, and dissecting the tissues appropriately with the different surgical tools. Surgeons may also find it helpful to practice with human cadavers. This practice, however, should be a supplement to the animal work because humidity, bleeding, and lung movements cannot be simulated in the cadaver as in the animal model. At a minimum, several days of laboratory experience (i.e., 16 hours or more of practical hands-on experience) are required to develop the initial skills and dexterity necessary to perform thoracoscopic spinal surgery. Attendance at a practical course does not credential surgeons or certify clinical competence; it only documents exposure to the material and the procedures.

A transition from the laboratory to clinical practice is desirable. Preceptorship or supervision from an experienced endoscopic spinal surgeon is important for assessing skills, additional learning, facilitating surgery, and preventing complications.[15] Observing other experienced surgeons perform clinical cases is another useful way to facilitate learning. We also advocate collaborative surgery with a cardiothoracic surgeon so that a thoracotomy can be performed immediately if one is needed.

Initially, surgeons may wish to transition from open thoracotomy to thoracoscopic-assisted open thoracotomy to thoracoscopy. Following this strategy, the surgeon would first insert an endoscope, perform the amount of dissection that felt comfortable, and then complete the surgery via an open thoracotomy under endoscopic visualization. This approach permits the surgeon to inspect the surgical site and progress at a self-established pace. As experience is acquired, the surgeon can increase the amount of endoscopic dissection performed parallel to the development of his or her skills.

The easiest first clinical cases are thoracic sympathectomies or biopsies of a vertebral body. The pathology is located superficially in the vertebrae, and the spinal canal does not have to be exposed. These cases are excellent for refining and improving one's endoscopic surgical skills in a clinical setting. Procedures such as discectomy or corpectomy require more advanced skills and are technically more challenging. Before attempting these procedures, novice

TABLE 3–2 Classification of Thoracoscopic Spine Procedures Based on the Difficulty of the Procedure

Simple Thoracoscopic Spinal Procedures
   Drainage of paravertebral abscess
   Vertebral biopsy
   Sympathectomy
Intermediate Thoracoscopic Spinal Procedures
   Anterior ligamentous release of deformity
   Anterior osteotomy for deformity
   Thoracic microdiscectomy (soft discs)
   Peripheral nerve sheath tumor resection
Complex Thoracoscopic Spinal Procedures
   Thoracic microdiscectomy
      Large discs (>10 mm size)
      Calcified discs
      Intradural discs
      Reoperations (scar)
   Thoracic corpectomy and reconstruction
   Hemivertebrae resection
   Thoracic internal fixation
   Foraminal nerve sheath tumor resection
   Dural suturing and repair techniques

endoscopic surgeons should master the more basic procedures completely (Table 3–2).

LABORATORY MODELS FOR THORACOSCOPY

Goats, sheep, and pigs have provided excellent animal models for thoracoscopic spinal surgery.[16,17] We prefer the porcine model and have developed laboratory protocols for thoracoscopic spine surgery using humane and ethical treatment standards in the surgical laboratory. Swine were chosen because of their ready availability, reasonable cost, large size, and reasonably close resemblance to human thoracic anatomy (Fig. 3–4).

The anatomy of the thorax and thoracic spine in the pig differs from that of humans. Consequently, knowledge of the anatomy and special surgical strategies to facilitate thoracoscopic spine surgery in this model are needed (Table 3–3).

TABLE 3–3 Anatomical Features and Surgical Strategies for Porcine Thoracoscopic Spine Laboratory Procedures

Anatomical Features	Technical Recommendation
Porcine thorax is narrow and oval	Position portals in posterior axillary line for the endoscope, the middle axillary line for tools, and anteriorly for a fan retractor
Porcine intercostal spaces are narrow	Use rigid thoracoports rather than flexible portals. Use rigid 12-mm portals for most access, except for plate and graft insertion. Cut portals to custom length
Cylindrically shaped thoracic vertebral bodies	Drill longitudinally from end plate-to-end plate to perform a corpectomy
Thoracic pedicles are broad, shelf-like, and difficult to remove. Difficult to unroof pedicle because neural foramina are very narrow perforations in the bone	Do not spend excessive time attempting to remove the pedicle. Instead identify the dura by locating the nerve root and foramen with a probe. Then proceed with the vertebral body resection, discectomy, and so on
Thoracic vertebral bodies have a large emissary venous channel	Control bleeding with bone wax on an endoscopic peanut dissector
Moderate epidural bleeding	Control with endoavitene, gelfoam, cottonoids, and bipolar coagulation
Narrow chest. Endoscopes tend to be positioned too close to the spine, giving too close a view, with not enough perspective	Maintain a broader, less magnified perspective by positioning the tip of the endoscope superficially, just inside the thorax. Do not "lose the forest through the trees"

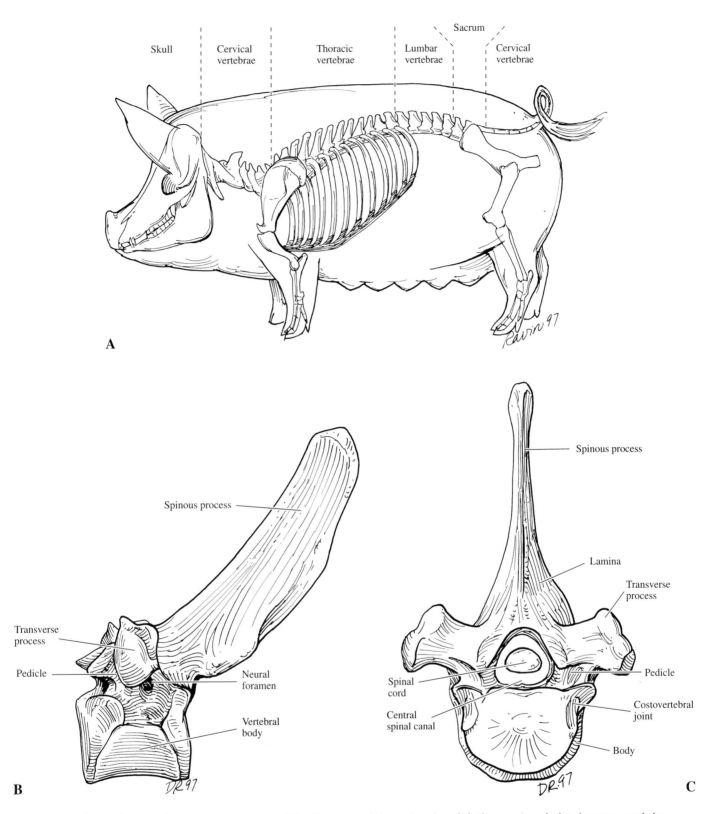

Skull   Cervical   Thoracic   Lumbar   Sacrum   Cervical
         vertebrae   vertebrae   vertebrae   vertebrae

A

Spinous process

Transverse
process

Pedicle

Neural
foramen

Vertebral
body

B

Spinous process

Lamina

Transverse
process

Spinal
cord

Central
spinal canal

Pedicle

Costovertebral
joint

Body

C

Figure 3–4. Illustrations of the porcine anatomy of the thorax and thoracic spine. **(A)** The porcine skeletal system and the shape of the thorax and vertebral column are shown. The intercostal spaces are narrow, the thorax is narrow, and the thoracic spinous processes are elongated. The pig usually has 14 or 15 thoracic vertebrae. **(B)** Lateral view of the porcine thoracic vertebrae. The spinous processes are elongated, the vertebral bodies are cylindrical, and the neural foramina are rudimentary perforations in the bone adjacent to the spinal canal, surrounded by broad thick shelves of bone, and a prominent mammillary process. **(C)** Cross section of the porcine thoracic spinal anatomy at the level of T5.

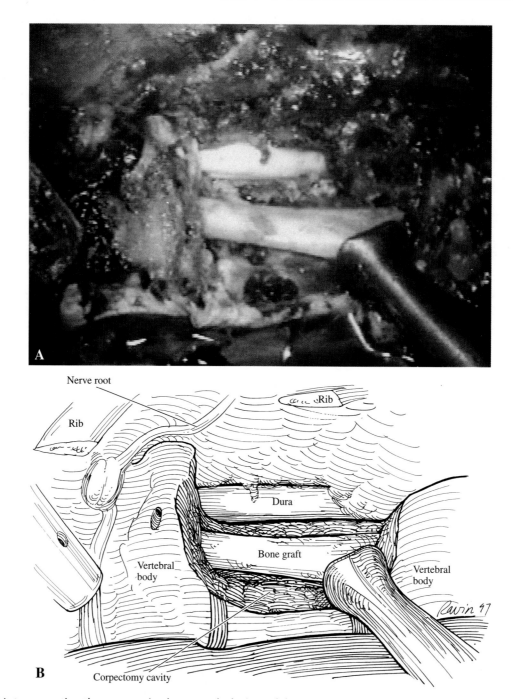

Nerve root

Rib

Rib

Dura

Bone graft

Vertebral
body

Vertebral
body

Corpectomy cavity

B

Figure 3–5. **(A)** Intraoperative thoracoscopic photograph during a laboratory porcine corpectomy and reconstruction and **(B)** corresponding illustration. The corpectomy cavity was created as a rectangular defect, exposing the entire ventral surface of the spinal cord. The corpectomy was reconstructed with a porcine autograft tibial shaft.

Although the pig thoracic vertebrae are cylindrically shaped and more elongated than the human thoracic vertebrae, the resemblance is close enough for them to provide an excellent model for simple and complex spinal procedures (Figs. 3–5, 3–6, and 3–7).

This *in vivo* model allows simulation of surgical techniques and physiological conditions not provided by cadaveric or other models and is an essential experience for developing the skills needed to master the endoscopic spine techniques for clinical application.

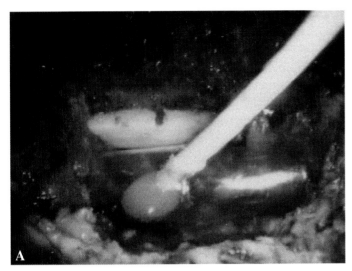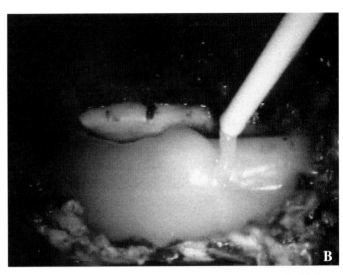

Figure 3–6. **(A)** A porcine corpectomy is reconstructed with methylmethacrylate using a silastic tube for a template to hold the liquefied methacrylate. The slow-setting (cranioplasty type) acrylic is injected into the tube with a long 12- or 14-gauge catheter. **(B)** The acrylic fills the tube and extrudes through the ends of the tube into the cancellous bone of the adjacent vertebrae. Acrylic is also placed anterior and lateral to the tube, preserving the epidural space posteriorly.

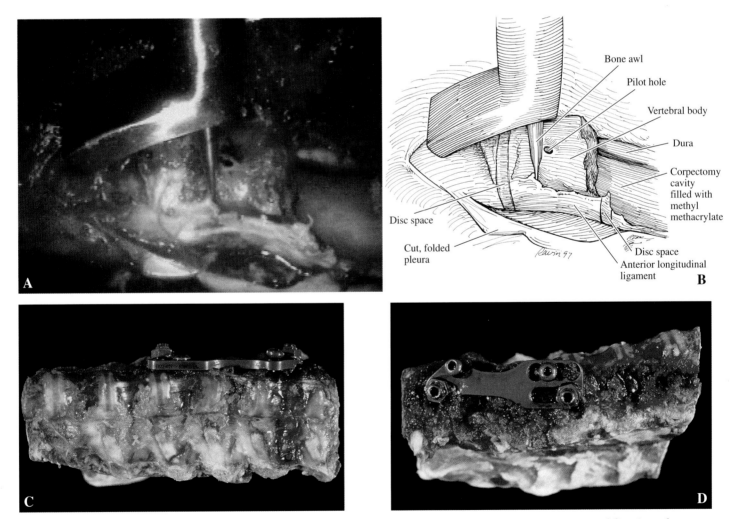

Figure 3–7. **(A)** Intraoperative photograph and **(B)** corresponding illustration showing thoracoscopic internal fixation of a porcine corpectomy with a screw plate. An endoscopic bone awl is used to create a pilot hole in the bone to insert screws. **(C)** Anterior and **(D)** lateral views after the surgery is completed. The spine was harvested so that the position of the screws, bolts, and plate could be inspected. [C and D used with permission of Barrow Neurological Institute.]

CONCLUSION

A high degree of knowledge, skill, expertise, and practice is required to implement thoracoscopic spinal surgery safely. Surgeons should attempt these techniques in a clinical setting only after comprehensive training. Recognition of the intense technical difficulty during the initial acquisition of knowledge and skills will maximize the benefits for patients and minimize associated complications. Spinal surgeons can avoid clinical complications and help patients best by adopting guidelines similar to those followed by our laparoscopic and cardiothoracic endoscopic colleagues.

REFERENCES

1. Reddick EJ, Olsen DO: Laparoscopic laser cholecystectomy. A comparison with a mini-lap cholecystectomy. *Surg Endosc* 1989; 3(3):131–133.
2. The Southern Surgeon's Club: A prospective analysis of 1518 laparoscopic cholecystectomies. *N Engl J Med* 1991; 324(16): 1073–1078.
3. Society of American Gastrointestinal Endoscopic Surgeons: *Granting of Privileges for Gastrointestinal Endoscopy by Surgeons.* Los Angeles, Society of American Gastrointestinal Endoscopic Surgeons; 1992.
4. Society of American Gastrointestinal Endoscopic Surgeons: *Framework for Post-Residency Surgical Education and Training. A SAGES Guideline.* Los Angeles, Society of American Gastrointestinal Endoscopic Surgeons; 1994.
5. American Society of Gastrointestinal Endoscopy: Proctoring and hospital endoscopy privileges. *Gastrointest Endosc* 1991; 37:666–667.
6. Azziz R: Operative endoscopy: The pressing need for a structured training and credentialing process [editorial]. *Fertil Steril* 1992; 58:1100–1102.
7. Dent TL: Training, credentialing, and granting of clinical privileges for laparoscopic general surgery. *Am J Surg* 1991; 161:399–403.
8. Dent TL: Training, credentialing, and evaluation in laparoscopic surgery. *Surg Clin North Am* 1992; 72:1003–1011.
9. Society of American Gastrointestinal Endoscopic Surgeons: Guidelines for submission of continuing medical education seeking SAGES endorsement for courses in laparoscopic surgery. *Surg Endosc* 1993; 7:372–373.
10. Society of American Gastrointestinal Endoscopic Surgeons: Guidelines for granting of privileges for laparoscopic (peritoneoscopic) general surgery. *Surg Endosc* 1993; 7:67–68.
11. McKneally MF: Video-assisted thoracic surgery: Standards and guidelines. *Chest Surg Clin North Am* 1993; 3:345–351.
12. McKneally MF, Lewis RJ, Anderson RP, et al: Statement of the AATS/STS Joint Committee on Thoracoscopy and Video Assisted Thoracic Surgery. *J Thorac Cardiovasc Surg* 1992; 104(1):1.
13. Dickman CA, Rosenthal D, Karahalios DG, et al: Thoracic vertebrectomy and reconstruction using a microsurgical thoracoscopic approach. *Neurosurgery* 1996; 38:279–293.
14. Dickman CA, Karahalios DG: Thoracoscopic spinal surgery. *Clin Neurosurg* 1996; 43:392–422.
15. Moore RG, Adams JB, Partin AW, et al: Telementoring of laparoscopic procedures: Initial clinical experience. *Surg Endosc* 1996; 10(2):107–110.
16. Fedder IL, McAfee PC, Cappuccino A, et al: Thoracoscopic anterior spinal decompression, fusion, instrumentation versus thoracotomy in the thoracic spine. A sheep model. *Proceedings of the 9th Annual North American Spine Society*; 1994.
17. Phillips RE, Jr: *Dissection of the Fetal Pig*, 3rd ed. Burlington, NC: REX Educational Resources; 1985.

CHAPTER *4*

Instrumentation and Equipment for Thoracoscopic Spine Surgery

Curtis A. Dickman, M.D. and Noel I. Perin, M.D.

*T*his chapter reviews the components of endoscopic imaging equipment, the tools used to access the chest, and the tools used to dissect the soft tissue paraspinal structures and thoracic spine. Most of the tools and equipment used for thoracoscopic spinal surgery are also used for thoracoscopy and laparoscopy by other endoscopic surgeons. Consequently, most hospitals already have the basic materials needed to perform endoscopic spinal surgery.

Endoscopic spinal tools differ from those used in open surgery. Because the working distance from the chest wall to the surface of the spine ranges from 14 to 30 cm, spinal dissection tools used for thoracoscopy have been modified in a number of ways. The tools are much longer, and they may have depth markings calibrated on their shafts. Their ends are often slightly angled or curved to facilitate visualization of the tip during dissection (Fig. 4–1).

Because of the long lever arm between the portal and the tip of the tools, the surgeon's hand movements are often amplified. Therefore, surgeons must adopt new strategies for manipulating tools precisely. Often, the surgeon must use both hands to anchor and guide the handle and shaft of the tools. The tool also may need to be steadied by stabilizing the shaft against the endoscopic portal within the chest wall. Usually, lightweight tools (e.g., suctions, bipolar cauterization devices, endoscopic scissors, forceps) can be controlled adequately with one hand. The surgeon can then work simultaneously with tools in both hands for dissection. However, to gain precise control of heavier tools (e.g., Kerrison rongeurs, curettes) or tools used close to the dura, the surgeon often must use both hands.

The tactile feedback from long endoscopic spinal tools differs from that obtained with short tools used in open surgery. Long tools often dampen or reduce the "feel" of tissue planes. This feature also requires the surgeon to develop new psychomotor skills. The surgeon relies heavily on the visual characteristics of the tissue planes and must adapt to the different and more subtle tactile qualities transmitted by endoscopic tools.

Three-dimensional (3-D), visual–spatial orientation, and triangulation are new skills that must be acquired to practice

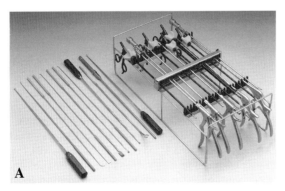
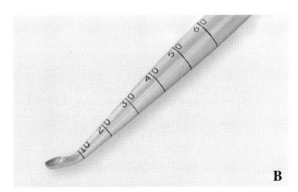

Figure 4–1. **(A)** Spinal tools for endoscopic spinal surgery are much longer than those used for open spinal surgery. Tools stored conveniently on a tool rack are organized and accessed easily during surgery. **(B)** The ends of the tools are calibrated with centimeter markings so that their depth can be judged intraoperatively. The tips of the tools are often curved to allow clear visualization of the tool during dissection.

video-assisted endoscopic spinal surgery. These navigational and psychomotor skills differ substantially from the skills used during open surgery and require dedicated laboratory practice to master. In fact, most experienced spine surgeons comment during their first few laboratory trials with endoscopy that "they feel clumsy, like they never operated before," and that they had to "retrain and reprogram their neural circuitry" to develop comfort with these new dissection skills.

ENDOSCOPIC IMAGING TOOLS

Endoscopes for thoracoscopic spinal surgery are used in the same fashion as an operating microscope is employed for open surgery. They provide a source of illumination and precise visualization, and they magnify the anatomy. These high-resolution endoscopes for spinal thoracoscopy usually do not have working channels within their shaft; therefore, the operative procedures are not performed *through* the endoscope. Rather, the endoscope is inserted through a portal in the chest wall after the ipsilateral lung has been deflated using a double-lumen endotracheal tube. Several other working portals are then placed into the chest wall at different locations for insertion of the tools and retractors.

A high-resolution, rigid endoscope is recommended for thoracoscopic microsurgery. Endoscopes used for thoracoscopy by thoracic surgeons or for laparoscopy by general surgeons can be used for spinal thoracoscopy. The endoscope, however, must provide high-quality, anatomical resolution and tissue definition to facilitate safe, accurate microsurgical dissection, especially near the spinal cord.

A wide-diameter endoscope (1-cm diameter) is preferred to provide a broad field of view and adequate image resolution (Fig. 4–2). Typically, narrow diameter endoscopes (e.g., ventriculoscopes) or flexible endoscopes should be avoided because their image resolution and field of view are inadequate for spinal surgery. High-resolution imaging, a broad field of view of the anatomy, adjustable illumination, zoom capability (adjustable magnification), adjustable focus, image clarity, accurate color reproduction, and 3-D depth perception are desirable features in an endoscope to ensure exquisite definition of the tissues during spinal microsurgery.

The components of the basic surgical endoscopic imaging system include the telescopes (i.e., the rod-lens mechanism), a video camera, a light cable, a light source, a signal processor, video monitors, a videotape recorder, and photographic cameras.

Rod-lens endoscopes were the first endoscopes used in abdominal and thoracic surgery. The Hopkins rod-lens system telescopes are still widely used for endoscopy. Endoscopic optical resolution and image transmission have been improved significantly by the use of fiber-optic cables and

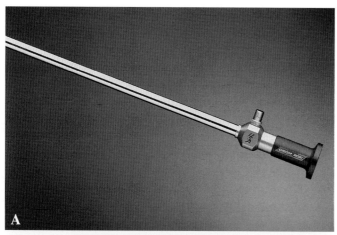

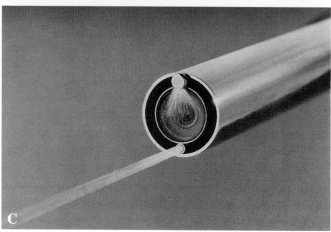

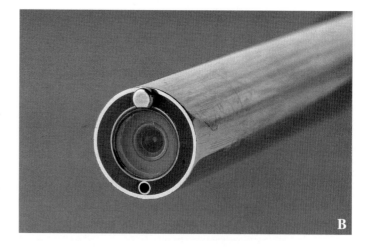

Figure 4–2. **(A)** Typically, video-assisted endoscopes for thoracoscopy are rigid and are 1 cm in diameter. The proximal end of the telescope has adaptors to attach a video camera as well as a fiber-optic light cable. **(B)** The tip of the telescope has a lens that transmits the images and a fiber-optic bundle that transmits the illumination to the operative field. **(C)** The light emanates from the fiber-optic bundle (*bottom*). This endoscope has an integrated irrigation mechanism to clean the lens (*top*). [Photographs courtesy of Circon Corp., Santa Barbara, CA.]

optical chips. Charged coupling devices (CCDs) are silicon optical chips that transmit more reliable, accurate, and high-resolution digital color images.

The early models of endoscopes had an eyepiece or viewing port on one end. This configuration required that the surgeon place his or her face near the sterile endoscope and risk contaminating the operating field. Currently, endoscopes with direct viewing portals are not used for spinal endoscopy. They have been replaced with video endoscopes (Fig. 4–3).

Video-assisted endoscopes integrate a video camera onto the end of the endoscope (Fig. 4–4). The video camera transmits the surgical images to a signal processor, which relays the images to video monitor screens within the operating room. The surgical team then views the operation from the monitors. The images from the camera also can be routed to video recorders and photographic equipment for permanent documentation of the operation (Fig. 4–5). The video monitor, light source, signal processor, and video recorder are usually conveniently stored on a mobile cart (Fig. 4–6).

The telescopes used for endoscopy primarily employ a Hopkins lens system, which integrates air and several quartz rod lenses into a rigid telescope that transmits light and accurate images with minimal optical distortion. The Hopkins lens system uses three separate lenses: a distal objective lens, a relay lens, and a proximal eyepiece lens.

Typically, the *width* of the field of view of the objective lens of the telescope is 80 to 90°. The *angle of view* can vary from 0 to 60° (Fig. 4–7). The 0° endoscope is used to view a field directly ahead of the endoscope. Angled telescopes (off-axis telescope), which are very useful for spinal surgery, allow the surgeon to look around corners or over edges of the operative field. Compared to the zero degree end-viewing scopes, the illumination emanating from angled telescopes is usually less intense. The 30° off-axis telescopes are versatile and very useful for spinal thoracoscopy.

Zero-degree angled endoscopes are simple to use but cannot be utilized to "look around corners." Angled endoscopes, however, are more useful for spinal thoracoscopy because they provide an oblique viewing trajectory to the anatomy and a greater variety of options. They can be inserted through offset working portals or used to look around corners or edges that cannot be viewed with a 0°-angled scope. Angled endoscopes are more difficult to use because they have more variables to control in terms of image orientation, perspective, and navigation. Surgeons should become facile with both 0° and angled endoscopes.

Digital Color Image Generation

The CCD is a recent, revolutionary technological development in optical imaging systems that has greatly improved the quality, resolution, and transmission of endoscopic images. The CCD is often also referred to as an *optical chip* or simply as a *chip*. The CCD digitizes the optical image

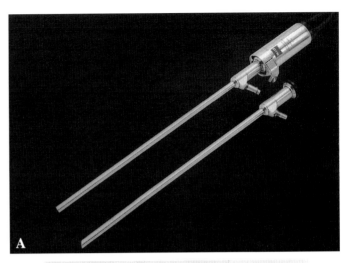

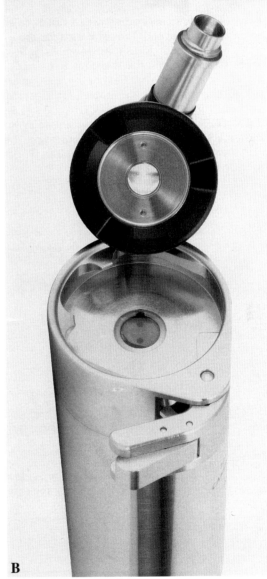

Figure 4–3. **(A)** Video endoscopes use a video camera mounted on the proximal end of the telescope (*top*). The shaft of the telescope has an adaptor for the fiber-optic light cable (Endolive 3-D Endoscopy System, Carl Zeiss, Inc., Thornwood, NY). **(B)** The video camera is coupled to the telescope by a circular attachment with a locking mechanism. The camera may be rotated 360° on the telescope to orient the intraoperative image. [Photographs courtesy of Carl Zeiss, Inc.]

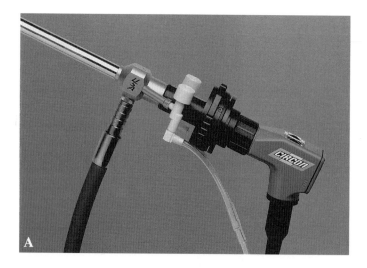

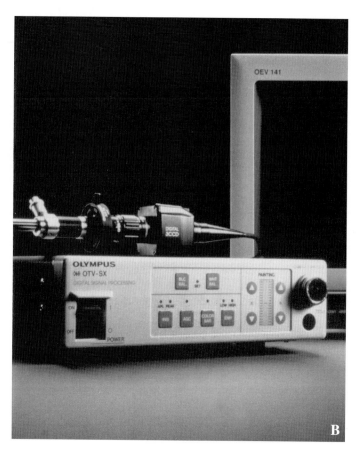

Figure 4–4. **(A)** A video endoscope with a video camera mounted on its proximal end. The video camera also incorporates an adjustable focus mechanism. Irrigation channels are integrated into this telescope to deliver irrigation fluid to the operative field or to clean the end of the telescope. The fiber-optic light cable (*left*) is attached to the telescope. [Photograph courtesy of Circon Corp., Santa Barbara, CA.] **(B)** The video endoscope systems relay the image from the video camera to a signal processor. The images are then transmitted to a video monitor. [Photograph courtesy of Olympus America.]

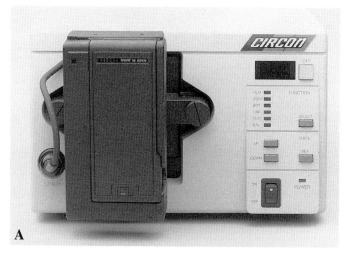

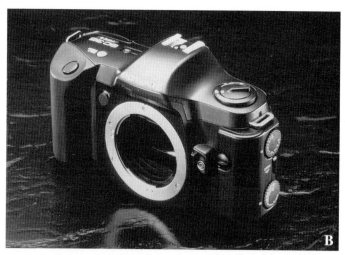

Figure 4–5. **(A)** A video slide-maker (Surgislide® Video Slide Marker, Circon Corp., Santa Barbara, CA) can be used to obtain intraoperative slides or photographs. [Photograph courtesy of Circon Corp.] **(B)** A photographic camera can be mounted on the viewing port on the telescope to obtain intraoperative photographs. Intraoperative photographs may also be obtained from images from the video signal processor. [Photograph courtesy of Olympus America.]

contained in the distal end of the endoscope. The CCD is a photosensitive silicon chip whose surface is divided into thousands of light-sensitive pixels. When photons strike the CCD, a digital electronic signal is generated and sent via wire to a digital image processor. The images are stored in digitized memory and are recombined using analogue reformatting to form a color picture. The processor then reassembles the image and projects it as a television pic-

ture. The digitized system increases the resolution and creates a sharper image compared with optical lens or fiber-optic systems. The CCD chip can be integrated into the tip of the endoscope (called a chip on a stick) or it can be integrated more proximally into the endoscopic camera.

The CCD chip is frequently used in modern endoscopic systems. It has revolutionized endoscopy because it provides superior image quality. It permits high-resolution

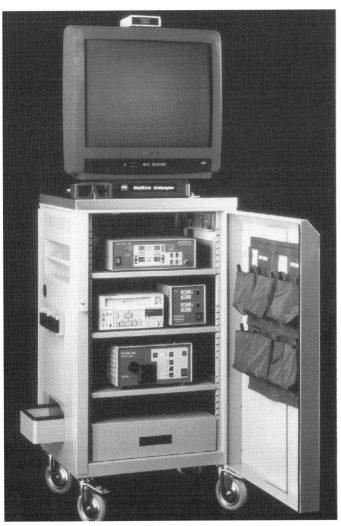

Figure 4–6. A complete video endoscopy system (Endolive 3-D Endoscopy System, Carl Zeiss, Inc., Thornwood, NY) is secured to a mobile video endoscope cart. This three-dimensional (3-D) endoscopy system includes a 3-D monitor, infrared emitter, and eyewear (*top*). The second shelf contains an insufflator. The third shelf contains a videotape recorder (*left*) and the video signal processor. The fourth shelf contains the fiber-optic light source. The bottom shelf contains a drawer for storage. [Photograph courtesy of Carl Zeiss, Inc.]

flexible endoscopes to be manufactured. It also has advanced the development of 3-D stereoscopic endoscopic visualization.

The color images generated by the CCD are produced by three different mechanisms. Two methods use a single CCD (single-chip camera) and one method uses three separate CCDs (three-chip camera). The three-chip endoscope provides the best optical resolution but costs more than the other CCD systems. The three chips each detect, encode, and transmit a separate color—red, green, or blue—to generate the color images.

The simplest single-chip endoscope uses a color grid in front of each CCD chip. Each pixel of the grid differentially senses red, green, or blue light to transmit and create the color image. The cost and the optical resolution of this system are significantly less that those of the three-chip endoscope.

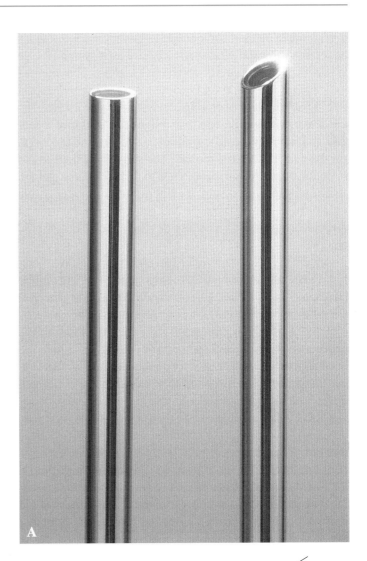

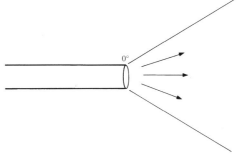

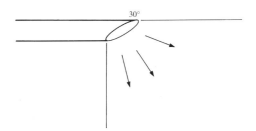

Figure 4–7. (A) The tips of the endoscopes may have a 0° (*left*) or 30° (*right*) angle. **(B)** The field of view associated with the two lenses is different. Angled endoscopes permit the surgeon to bring the endoscope into the field of view from an oblique trajectory that provides more room for the surgeon to work on the surface of the patient's body using his or her hands. [Photograph courtesy of Carl Zeiss, Inc.]

The other method for a single-chip endoscope provides better image resolution than the first one-chip system. It also is less expensive than the three-chip system. This method uses a digitized single CCD with an alternating red, green, or blue strobe light operating at a frequency of 30 Hz. The CCD alternatingly detects green light for 1/30th of a second, red light for the next 1/30th of a second, and blue light for the next 1/30th of a second. The images are then stored in digital memory and recombined to form the color picture.

The digital processors are important components that transform the digital images and provide signal output to the video monitors, recording devices, and photographic equipment.

Recently, video cameras for endoscopes have been improved by integrating CCD components. This integration has dramatically reduced the size and weight of the cameras, which then become easier to use in surgery. The cameras, which are relatively simple to use, are connected to the endoscope with a locking attachment. After the camera has been connected to the endoscope intraoperatively, the optical images must be oriented to verify right, left, up, and down. The surgeon holds the endoscope outside the patient's chest and views an object (e.g., the surgeon's hand or a sterile package with print) to orient the image correctly on the monitor. The camera or the telescope can be rotated separately so that the image appears in its correct orientation. If the orientation of the camera is not verified before proceeding with surgery and the image is inverted, the surgeon could become confused during a procedure. Immediately before the endoscope is used, the color images are white-balanced.

Illumination

Xenon or halogen light sources are integrated into the endoscopes using fiber-optic bundles or liquid-filled cables (Fig. 4–8). The light cables connect the light source to the endoscope and are attached with locking mechanisms. There are two types of light cables: liquid-filled cables and fiber-optic bundles. Liquid-filled light cables are less susceptible to breaking. However, they conduct heat more readily and must be connected to the endoscope immediately after the

light is turned on. Fiber-optic light cables are more fragile and hence susceptible to breaking. The bundles must be inspected for breakage, which would diminish the intensity of the illumination. Typically, these light sources use a 250- to 400-watt bulb, which generates considerable heat. The intensity of the illumination can be varied with an automated or manual control mechanism. The light emanates directly from the end of the endoscope to illuminate the operative field. Xenon provides brighter illumination than halogen and is more useful clinically. With xenon, however, the surgeon must be cautious with the tip of the endoscope, which can become *extremely* hot. If the tip of the endoscope or the tip of the disconnected fiber-optic light cable is placed on the sterile field, xenon fiber-optic light sources can ignite paper drapes and cause an intraoperative *fire*. The tip of the endoscope is not associated with a high risk of thermal damage to the tissue unless contact is prolonged. For a few minutes after removing the endoscope from the chest and turning off the light source, the surgeon should avoid touching its tip. If the end of the endoscope must be touched immediately (i.e., to clean the lens), a saline-moistened gauze or saline irrigation should be used.

Defogging and Cleaning the Lens

Fogging or debris on the telescope lens can degrade the clarity of the image as can pooled blood within the visual field. The latter absorbs light and darkens the image. Fogging is caused by differences in the temperature and humidity between the thoracic cavity and the ambient environment (i.e., the surgical suite). Fogging can be minimized (Table 4–1) by prewarming the end of the endoscope in warm saline and using warm irrigation solution during the procedure. A sterile defogging solution (Fog Reduction and Elimination Device, FRED; Dexide) can be applied to the tip of the endoscope to maintain a clear image. This surfactant can be applied to the lens with a sponge placed on the external operative field (Fig. 4–9A). A small sponge with FRED can also be placed on a tool and inserted through a portal (FRED on a stick) to clean the tip of the endoscope within the chest (Fig. 4–9B and C). This maneu-

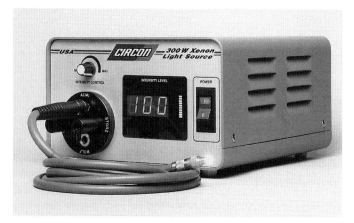

Figure 4–8. An example of a xenon light source and an endoscopic fiber-optic light cable. [Photograph courtesy of Circon Corp.]

TABLE 4–1 Strategies for Defogging and Cleaning Endoscope Lens

Method
External
Endoscope warmers (thermos or electrical)
Prewarming telescope in heated irrigation fluid
Sterile surfactant (FRED) applied with a sponge
Washing lens with irrigation fluid and gauze sponge
Intrathoracic
Using heated irrigation fluid in operative field
Lens cleaning tool (FRED on a stick)
Spraying lens with an irrigation tool
Touching lens to a moist tissue surface (lung or pleura)
Integrated lens washing mechanisms
Disposable plastic sheath with lens-washing jet spray

FRED = fog reduction/elimination device.

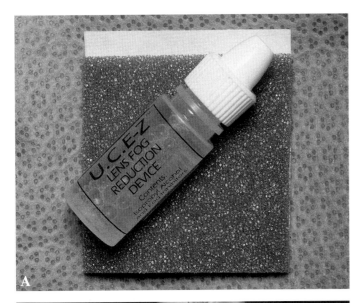

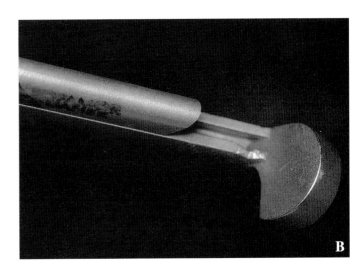

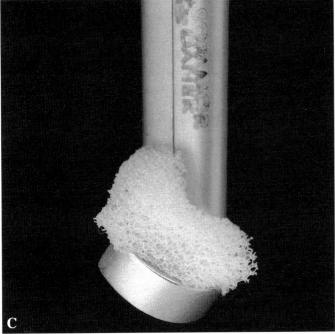

Figure 4–9.   **(A)** Sterile fog reduction solution is applied to the endoscope lens with a sterile sponge that is usually placed on the exterior of the patient's chest. **(B)** This endoscope cleaner has a platform to mount a sponge with the Fog Reduction/Elimination Device (FRED) on the end. **(C)** The sponge is used to clean the lens of the endoscope within the chest. This capability eliminates the need to detach the endoscope from the endoscopic holder for removal and cleaning, which would then require that the endoscope be reinserted and reoriented to the operative anatomy. [Photographs courtesy of Sofamor Danek.]

ver eliminates the need to remove the endoscope and reorient the image after the endoscope has been cleaned. Some endoscopes are equipped with a lens-cleaning mechanism that sprays the tip of the endoscope with irrigation solution (Fig. 4–10). Disposable plastic sheaths, which shoot a jet of irrigation across the lens, also are available to clean the lens of the endoscope.

Endoscope Holders

A stable but adjustable view of the surgical field is critical for facilitating endoscopic spinal surgery. During the initial phases of the operation, when the orientation of the images is changed frequently, a surgical assistant can be devoted to holding the endoscope to maintain a relatively stable perspective. However, an assistant usually fatigues easily and poorly stabilizes images for long procedures. A moving image is difficult to follow and unnecessarily dis-

tracts the surgeon. Therefore, mechanical endoscope holders are extremely useful for reliable fixation of the position of the endoscope in relationship to the patient's chest and spine. These devices use mechanical or pneumatic arms that are mounted onto the operating table (Fig. 4–11). Robotic, voice-activated computerized endoscope holders are also available (Fig. 4–12). Endoscope holders simplify the operation, provide stable images, and free the assistant's hands for other tasks.

3-D Endoscopy

Currently, most surgical endoscopes use two-dimensional imaging to project the view of the surgical field. This approach is adequate for general thoracoscopy and laparoscopy. Recently, 3-D endoscopic systems have been

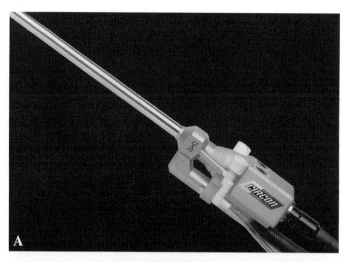
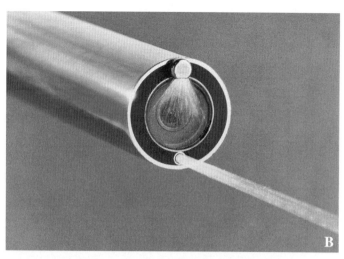

Figure 4–10. The Circon endoscope (Circon Corp., Santa Barbara, CA) provides irrigation channels. **(A)** The sterile irrigation is released by pressing a button on the end of the endoscope. **(B)** The irrigation can be used to spray and clean the lens of the endoscope. A separate irrigation channel is used to irrigate the operative field. [Photographs courtesy of Circon Corp.]

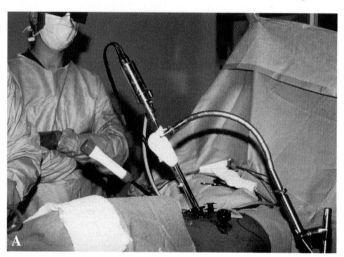
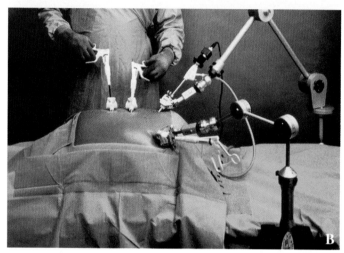

Figure 4–11. Mechanical endoscope holders. **(A)** The Bookwalter endoscope holder has a multiarticulated arm. [Photograph courtesy of Barrow Neurological Institute.] **(B)** This pneumatic endoscope holder is stabilized using a vacuum pump. The locking mechanisms are adjustable. [Photograph courtesy of Leonard Medical, Inc.]

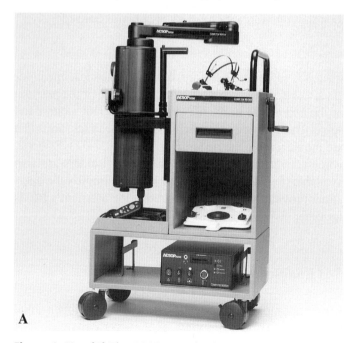
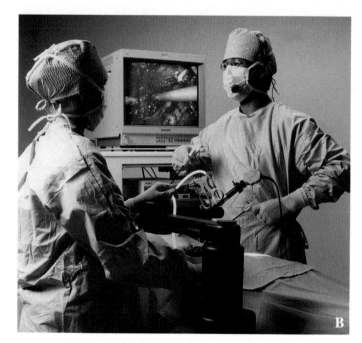

Figure 4–12. **(A)** The AESOP™ robotic arm is used to hold and control the intraoperative movements of the endoscope. **(B)** The robotic arm is activated and deactivated using voice control via a microphone headset worn by the surgeon. [Photographs courtesy of Computer Motion.]

developed to provide stereoscopic visualization of the surgical procedure. This improvement is particularly valuable for facilitating safe, precise, microsurgical dissection around the spinal cord. Precise depth perception is useful for spinal thoracoscopy, analogous to the benefits provided by binocular microscopy for intracranial and spinal microsurgery. To use 3-D endoscopic imaging systems, the surgeon must wear special shutter glasses intraoperatively. The glasses separate and polarize the images to provide depth perception.

Three methods are used to provide 3-D endoscopic imaging (Fig. 4–13). The first method incorporates two separate optical systems into one telescope. The two optical systems view the object from different angles. The handpiece contains two cameras, one for each optical system. Each camera transmits its respective images to the image processor and video monitor (Fig. 4–13A). The second 3-D imaging method incorporates two full-color CCD imagers at the distal end of the telescope. This configuration permits discrete left- and right-eye images to be captured,

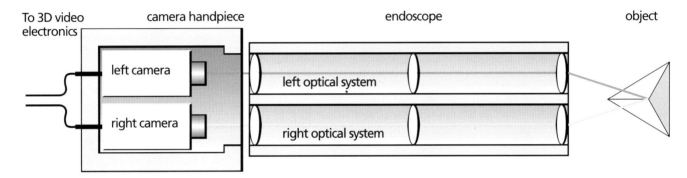

A   **Stereoscopic vision with dual optical channel 3D Video Endoscope**

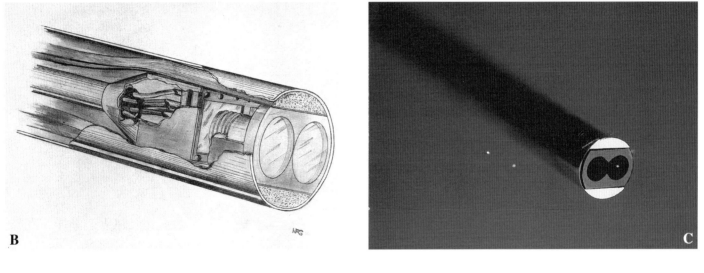

B

C

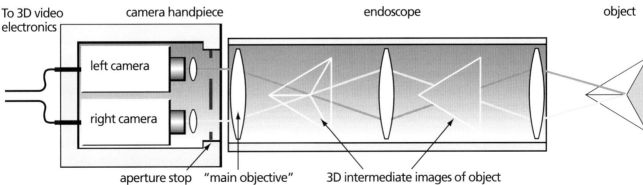

D   **Stereoscopic vision with the single optical channel 3D Video Endoscope**

Figure 4–13. Three-dimensional endoscopic imaging is produced using several methods. **(A)** Two separate video cameras and optical systems are integrated into the endoscope. **(B** and **C)** Two separate charged coupling devices are integrated onto the tip of the endoscope [Photograph courtesy of Midas Rex Pneumatic Tools, Inc.] **(D)** A binocular imaging system is integrated into a single objective lens. [A and D courtesy of Carl Zeiss, Inc.]

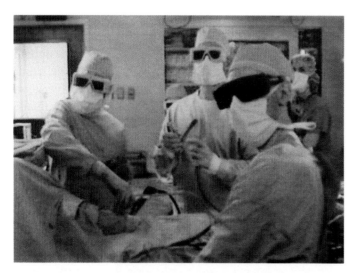

Figure 4–14. Three-dimensional (3-D) endoscopy requires surgeons to wear special glasses to synchronize the 3-D images with the infrared emitter and video monitor. The stereoscopic 3-D image is viewed on a large monitor screen. Depth perception permits precise appreciation of the extent of dissection to facilitate working safely around the spinal cord.

processed, and displayed on the video monitor (Fig. 4–13B and C). The third 3-D imaging method uses a binocular tube to view the images (one on the right and one on the left) through *one* main objective lens. The images are projected from slightly different angles, producing a stereoscopic image (Fig. 4–13D).

All three methods employ an infrared emitter that is placed onto the top of the video monitor screen. The infrared emitter transmits a signal that controls liquid crystal display shutter glasses worn by the user (Fig. 4–14). The shutter glasses synchronize the presentation of the different images to the left and right eyes to create the stereoscopic effect.

ACCESS AND DISSECTION TOOLS

Portals

Portals are protective sheaths with hollow centers that are inserted into the chest wall or abdomen to provide a corridor for the endoscope and tools during a procedure (Fig. 4–15A, B, and C). Portals can be disposable, permanent, rigid, or flexible. A trocar (rigid guide) is inserted into the hollow portal and used to tunnel the portal into its position in the chest wall.

Flexible portals are best for thoracoscopy. Rigid portals, which can compress the intercostal nerves, have been associated with intercostal neuralgia. Flexible, soft, collapsible portals minimize the incidence of intercostal neuralgia. Flexible portals are available in 7-mm, 15-mm, and 20-mm diameters (Fig. 4–15A). If needed, the portals' sleeve can be customized simply by cutting the excess length from the end of the portal with a pair of scissors.

Rigid portals are used more often for laparoscopy than for thoracoscopy and are available in 10-mm, 12-mm, 15-mm and wider diameters. Rigid portals usually have a valve mechanism to seal the portal and maintain pressurization when used with CO_2 insufflation. Pressurized CO_2 insufflation is often used with laparoscopy, but tends to be avoided with thoracoscopy. For thoracoscopy, adequate access to the spine is achieved by deflating the ipsilateral lung and providing a nonpressurized passive pneumothorax. It is easier to work in a noninsufflated, nonpressurized compartment. When CO_2 insufflation is employed, the use of suction to clear blood from the field is restricted; otherwise, the pressurization will be reduced and the working space will collapse.

Like chest tubes, portals are inserted into the chest through the intercostal spaces over the superior surfaces of the ribs to avoid injury to the intercostal neurovascular bundles. We will discuss the insertion of portals more thoroughly in later chapters. Typically, portals have a widened cuff at their base, which maintains their position outside the chest wall. The cuff may be sutured or stapled to the skin to anchor the portal. The sheath of a portal may be smooth or threaded (Fig. 4–15A, B, and C) to stabilize its position in the soft tissues of the chest or abdomen.

Different types of trocars are also available. Optical trocars permit endoscopes to be inserted into the tip of a translucent trocar. These trocars permit the soft-tissue planes to be imaged endoscopically as the portal is tunneled (Fig. 4–16). Trocars with balloon-dilating mechanisms are available for dissecting spaces (i.e., the retroperitoneal or preperitoneal spaces, Fig. 4–17). These trocars are rarely needed for thoracoscopy, but are very useful for approaching the lumbar spine endoscopically.

Soft-Tissue Dissection Tools

A wide array of laparoscopic and thoracoscopic disposable and nondisposable endoscopic soft-tissue dissection tools can be adapted for spinal access. Nondisposable tools tend to minimize procedure-related costs. Sometimes, however, disposable items are needed. The endoscopic soft-tissue dissection tools are used in a manner similar to tools used for open surgery.

Thoracoscopic soft-tissue tools usually have long shafts (20 to 30 cm) with mechanisms that allow the shaft to be rotated (Fig. 4–18). The hand grips may have a ring-forceps grip, a pistol grip, a pencil grip, or a locking mechanism. Combined endoscopic tools that integrate suction, irrigation, and/or cautery mechanisms into the shaft are available so that tissue can be cauterized without inserting a new tool (i.e., cautery-scissors and suction-irrigation-cautery devices, Fig. 4–19).

Lung forceps can be used to grasp lung tissue atraumatically for manipulation, mobilization, or temporary gentle retraction of the lung (Fig. 4–18B). Allis clamps or Babcock clamps may be used to grasp soft tissue, bone grafts, or instrumentation within the thorax.

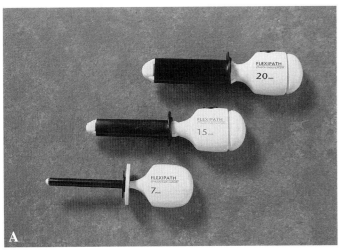

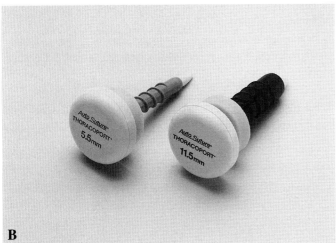

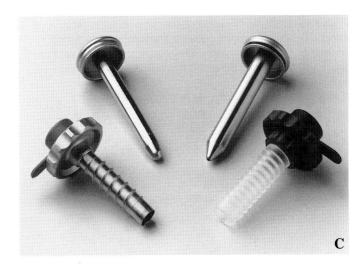

Figure 4–15.   Thoracoscopic portals are made from soft flexible materials to avoid compression of the intercostal nerves and intercostal neuralgia. **(A)** These disposable flexible portals can be cut to customize the length needed. The portals have 7-mm, 15-mm, or 20-mm diameters. The wider portals have an oval cross section to fit within the intercostal spaces without compressing the intercostal nerves. [Photograph courtesy of Ethicon Endosurgery.] **(B)** Disposable portals (thoracoports) may also have threads to help anchor the portals to the soft tissues of the chest wall. [Photograph courtesy of Auto Suture United States Surgical Corp.] **(C)** Nondisposable flexible or rigid endoscopic portals are also available. [Photograph courtesy of Aesculap, Inc.]

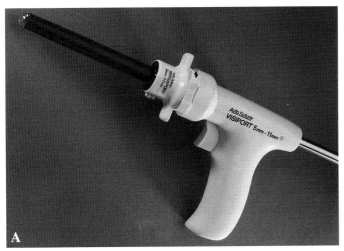

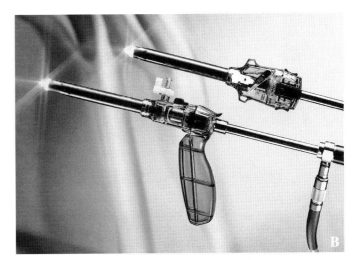

Figure 4–16.   **(A and B)** Optical trocars have a translucent cutting tip that permits endoscopic visualization as the trocar is inserted through the soft tissues. [Photograph A courtesy of Auto Suture, United States Surgical Corp; photograph B courtesy of Ethicon Endosurgery.]

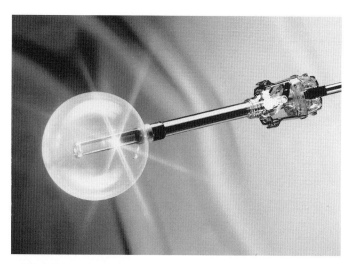

Figure 4–17. Balloon-dilating mechanisms integrated into endoscopic portals allow tissue planes to be dissected. This feature is particularly useful for accessing the retroperitoneal space. [Photograph courtesy of Ethicon Endosurgery.]

faced blades that are spread apart within the chest cavity and provide a wide surface area for gentle retraction of the lung. The lung retractors also can be "angled" or "towed in" if additional retraction is needed. Retractors must be used gently to avoid contusing or lacerating the lung parenchyma. They are always opened, closed, and repositioned under direct endoscopic visualization to avoid injuring the lung tissue.

The use of a lung retractor can be minimized or eliminated by rotating the patient anteriorly intraoperatively, allowing gravity to retract the lung away from the surface of the spine. Often a tool or temporary retractor is needed initially to help position the lung away from the spine. Once dense atelectasis is achieved, the retractor is removed and gravity is used for retraction.

The soft-tissue tools that are most useful for pleural, vascular, and soft-tissue dissection for exposure of the spine include microscissors with integrated cautery, fine Debakey tissue forceps, right-angle tissue clamps, pleural dissectors, suction, bipolar and monopolar cautery devices, cotton-tipped dissectors, Allis clamps, and Babcock forceps.

Endoscopic scissors are available in several sizes and configurations (Figs. 4–18A, 4–19A, and 4–21). They

Lung retractors help mobilize the lung away from the surface of the spine. Several types of lung retractors are available (Fig. 4–20). They usually have blunt-tipped, broad-sur-

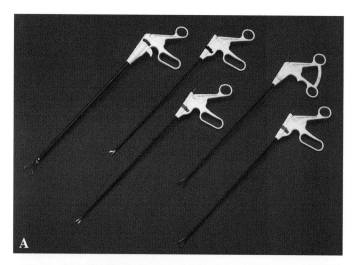

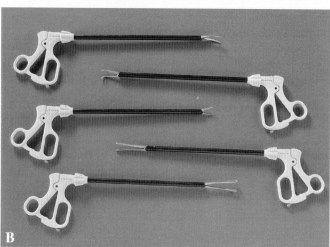

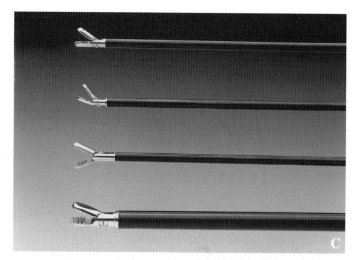

Figure 4–18. Endoscopic soft-tissue dissection tools have rotating shafts to alter the position of the tip without requiring the surgeon to reposition his or her hands. **(A, *left to right*)** Grasping forceps, scissors, and several types of fine tissue forceps. [Photograph courtesy of United States Surgical Corp.] **(B, *top to bottom*)** Curved forceps, angled forceps, Debakey forceps, lung grasping forceps, and ringed forceps. [Photograph courtesy of Ethicon Endosurgery.] **(C)** Nondisposable soft-tissue graspers. [Photograph courtesy of Aesculap, Inc.]

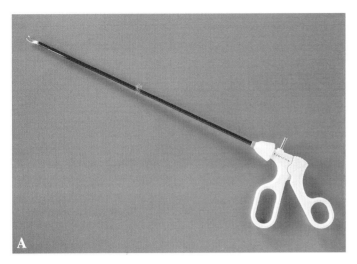

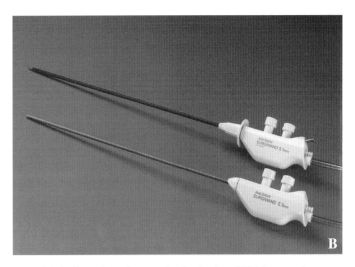

Figure 4–19. Multipurpose soft-tissue dissection tools that integrate multiple functions into a single device. **(A)** Monopolar cautery scissors allow tissue to be cauterized and cut sequentially without changing tools. [Photograph courtesy of Ethicon Endosurgery]. **(B)** Suction, irrigation, and cautery are integrated into this tool. The cautery tip of the upper tool can be extended beyond the tip of the suction. The cautery tip is retracted back into the suction sheath when it is not used. [Photograph courtesy of Auto Suture, United States Surgical Corp.]

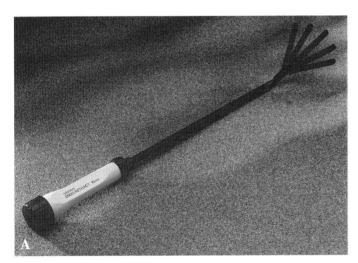

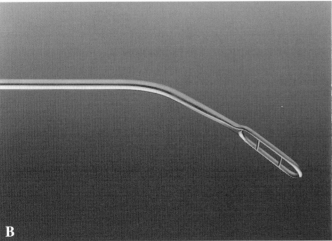

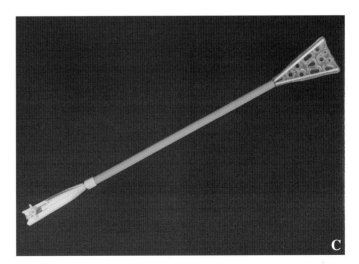

Figure 4–20. **(A)** A disposable fan retractor can be used to retract the lung or diaphragm in the chest. In the abdomen, this retractor can be used on the viscera. [Photograph courtesy of Auto Suture, United States Surgical Corp.] **(B)** A nondisposable lung retractor can be used to hold the lung gently away from the surface of the spine. [Photograph courtesy of Aesculap, Inc.] **(C)** An inflatable soft fan retractor can be used to minimize retraction injury to tissue. [Photograph courtesy of Ethicon, Endosurgery.]

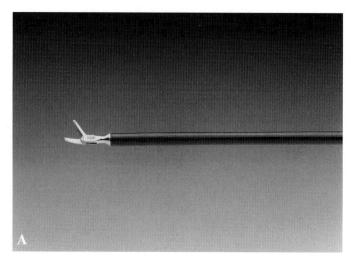
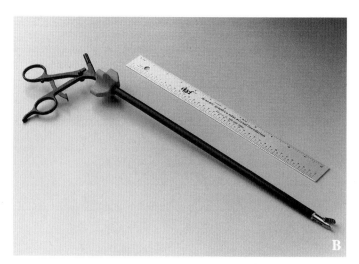

Figure 4–21. **(A)** Curved nondisposable endoscopic microscissors. **(B)** A locking mechanism, a rotating shaft, and ring grips are commonly used for endoscopic soft tissue tools. [Photographs courtesy of Aesculap, Inc.]

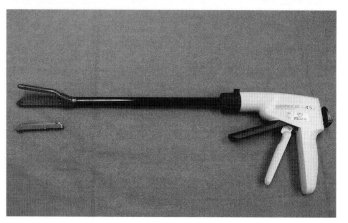

Figure 4–22. Endoscopic lung stapler. [Photograph courtesy of Ethicon Endosurgery.]

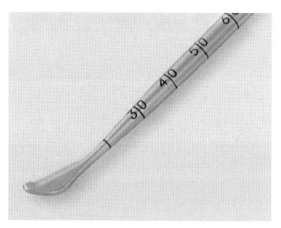

Figure 4–23. This pleural dissector has a dull distal edge. The cutting surface is located on the dorsal surface. The tool is used to elevate the parietal pleura from the surface of the spine and ribs, elevating and separating the pleura from the segmental vessels and cutting the pleura to expose the spine. [Photograph courtesy of Sofamor Danek.]

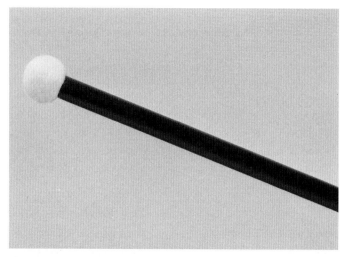

Figure 4–24. Cotton-tipped endoscopic dissectors are used to apply bone wax, dissect tissues planes bluntly, retract tissue, or tamponade small blood vessels gently. [Photograph courtesy of Ethicon Endosurgery.]

usually have integrated cautery so the blades can cauterize or cut tissue sequentially or simultaneously.

Adhesions of the lung may need to be detached to expose the spine. Adhesions can be removed by sharp dissection with scissors and cauterization, sometimes combined with blunt dissection and gentle retraction of the lung. Entry into the lung parenchyma is avoided; otherwise, an air leak will occur. If an intraoperative lung laceration is encountered, it may be closed with an endoscopic lung stapler (Fig. 4–22).

Pleural dissectors are hooked or curved tools used to incise and mobilize the pleura away from the segmental vessels, spine, and chest wall (Fig. 4–23). These dissectors are used to lift the parietal pleura away from the spine and incise the pleura rapidly, while sparing the underlying vessels. Cotton-tipped dissectors (i.e., cherry and peanut dissectors, Fig. 4–24) can be used for the blunt dissection of soft tissue, gentle tamponade of small bleeding vessels, retraction of tissue, or the application of bone wax to bone surfaces.

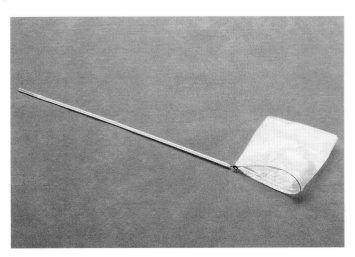

Figure 4–25. An endoscopic specimen basket is used to remove tumors from the chest, minimizing spillage or contamination. This device can also be used to remove debris from the chest. [Photograph courtesy of Auto Suture, United States Surgical Corp.]

Fine tissue forceps, right-angle dissectors, and curved microscissors also are useful for opening the pleura and isolating the segmental arteries and veins. Once the segmental artery and vein have been isolated individually, they can be ligated with hemoclips for security before the vessels are transected. The surgeon usually dissects the pleura and vessels using a forceps in the nondominant hand and a scissor in the dominant hand.

Suction and irrigation tools are very important components of endoscopic surgery. Suction devices must generate a sufficient vacuum to rapidly clear the operative field of blood. When moderate amounts of blood cover the dissected surfaces, the blood absorbs light, darkening and hence degrading the quality of the endoscopic image. Long Frazier-tipped suction tools, disposable pediatric Yankhauer suctions tools, and endoscopic suction tools that combine suction, irrigation, and cauterization mechanisms are useful for thoracoscopic spinal surgery. Strong, pressurized irrigation devices are also needed. Pressurized intravenous bags and pressurized sterile intravenous or prostatic irrigation tubes are used to deliver warm, sterile, pressurized irrigation. A forceful stream of irrigation is required to clear the endoscopic field of debris and blood. Pressurized irrigation also can be provided using a 50-ml syringe with a long, rigid, sterile plastic catheter. The syringe and catheter can be used to inject a forceful stream of fluid manually onto the surgical field. A central venous pressure introducer sheath provides an excellent tip for this application.

Other useful endoscopic tools include specimen pouches, suturing tools, dural closure clips, and loop ligatures. Stented endoscopic specimen bags can be used to remove debris or tumors from the chest cavity without spilling the tumor into the chest or seeding the chest wall (Fig. 4–25). The pleura or the dura may be closed endoscopically with suture or tissue closure clips (Fig. 4–26). The nerve root sleeves or blood vessels can be ligated with hemoclips or an

endoscopic suture loop (Endoloop, Ethicon Endosurgery, Somerville, NJ; Fig. 4–27). If the nerve root must be transected, the ligature may be placed on the dural sleeve of the proximal thoracic nerve root to prevent a cerebrospinal fluid (CSF) leak. The ligature also can be used to ligate medium- and large-sized blood vessels as well as to reinforce a hemoclip to ensure secure hemostasis.

Hemostatic Tools and Techniques

Endoscopic hemostatic techniques are identical to methods used in conventional open surgery. Hemostasis can be achieved with monopolar or bipolar cauterization (Fig. 4–28) or by the application of hemoclips, bone wax, Gelfoam® (Upjohn, Kalamazoo, MI), Endoavitene®, Nu-Knit™ (Johnson & Johnson, Arlington, TX), or cottonoid patties.

Endoscopic straight or right-angled vascular clip appliers are available for ligation of small and medium-sized blood vessels (Fig. 4–29). Disposable and reusable clip appliers are available. The disposable clip appliers contain multiple clips preloaded in the shaft of the tool. In that way, several clips can be applied without removing, reloading, and reinserting the tool into the thorax. When the segmental spinal vessels are secured, proximal and distal vascular clips are applied to achieve hemostasis, and the vessels are divided between the clips. The segmental spinal vessels communicate directly with the aorta and the azygos venous system. There are no intervening structures to reduce vascular pressure. Therefore, secure hemostasis of these vessels is mandatory. Cauterization of the segmental vessels without applying hemoclips should be avoided because there is a risk of delayed hemorrhage from the vessel.

Bone bleeding can be controlled with small pieces of bone wax that are applied with an endoscopic peanut or cherry dissector.

Epidural hemostasis is achieved with bipolar coagulation or with small pieces of hemostatic agents applied gently and precisely with $\frac{1}{2} \times \frac{1}{2}$-inch or $\frac{1}{2} \times 1$-inch cottonoid patties. The end of the string of the cottonoid should be grasped with a hemostat outside the chest to prevent its loss within the thorax. Monopolar cauterization can cause neurological injury and should be used sparingly near the spine and avoided near the dura, nerve roots, and sympathetic chain. Endoscopic avitene is available. A large, rolled piece of compressed avitene is delivered to the surgical site using a hollow cylinder with a plunger. Usually, we avoid this technique for epidural hemostasis because too much avitene is delivered and the dura inadvertently could become compressed. We prefer to deliver small pieces of hemostatic materials to the epidural space with small cottonoids, identical to the technique used for epidural hemostasis in open surgery.

The surgeon must *always* be prepared to obtain immediate hemostasis if a complication, such as an injury to a great vessel, occurs. A tightly rolled 4 × 4 sponge on a long clamp (sponge stick) and a thoracotomy tray *should* be available and open in the sterile field. If a rapid, massive

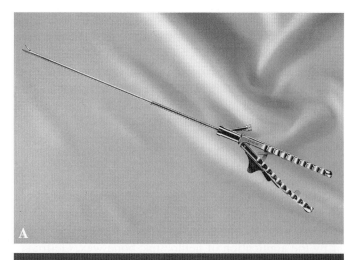

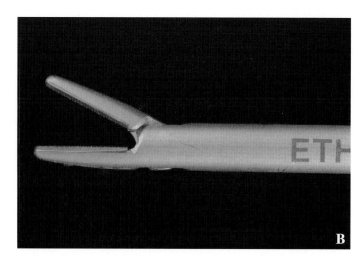

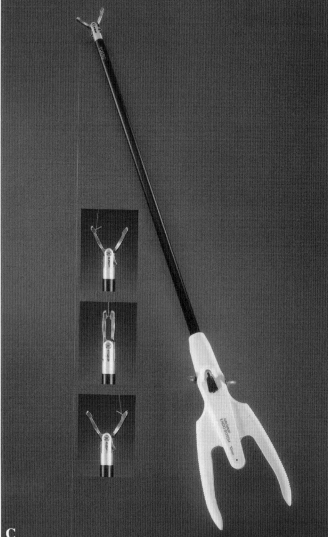

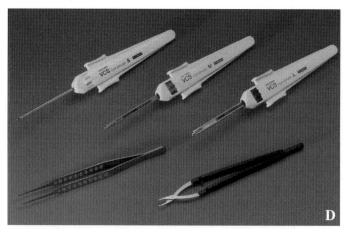

Figure 4–26. Endoscopic suturing tools. **(A)** A fine-tipped microsurgical endoscopic needle-holder may be used for either a dural or pleural closure, if needed. **(B)** Close-up of tips of the needle-holder. [Photographs A and B courtesy of Ethicon Endosurgery.] **(C)** The Autosuture Endostitch Device (Auto Suture, United States Surgical Corp., Norwalk, CT) is useful for suturing the pleura or the diaphragm. The tip is too large to permit dural suturing. The needle is passed back and forth between the tip of the holder (*inset*) to suture tissue like an automated sewing machine. **(D)** Vascular closure clips on long appliers can be used to close the dura endoscopically. [Photographs C and D courtesy of Auto Suture, United States Surgical Corp.]

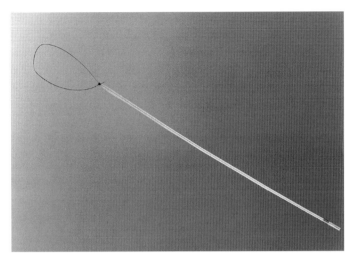

Figure 4–27. An endoloop suture ligature can be used to ligate blood vessels, a nerve root sleeve, or other soft tissue. [Photograph courtesy of Ethicon Endosurgery.]

hemorrhage were to occur, the endoscope would be repositioned from the depths of the operating field. The tip would be moved superficially near the chest wall so that the lens would not become covered with blood. The sponge stick would be inserted through a portal and used to tamponade the bleeding vessel *gently* until a thoracotomy could be performed and secure hemostasis achieved. Routine intraoperative hemostasis is easily obtained with endoscopic techniques. It is, however, important to be prepared for an immediate thoracotomy if a major vascular complication were to occur.

Ultrasonic Scalpel

The ultrasonic scalpel (Harmonic scalpel; Ethicon Endosurgery, Somerville, NJ) is a combined cutting and cauterization tool for soft tissue (Fig. 4–30). The blades

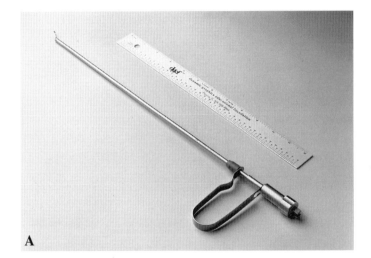

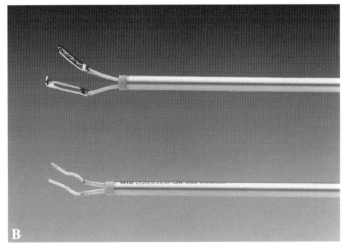

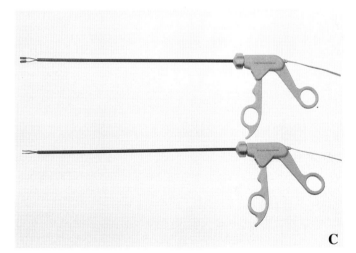

Figure 4–28. Endoscopic bipolar cauterization tools. **(A)** A pistol grip mechanism is used to close the tips of this tool. **(B)** Narrow (*bottom*) or broad-surfaced (*top*) tips are available to coagulate different sized vessels. [Photographs A and B courtesy of Aesculap, Inc.] **(C)** Disposable insulated bipolar forceps. [Photograph courtesy of Ethicon Endosurgery.]

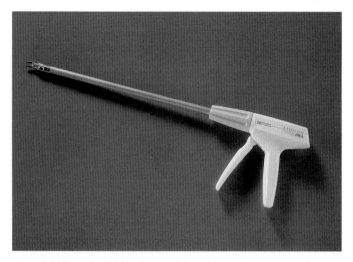

Figure 4–29. Endoscopic vascular clip appliers are used to ligate medium-sized blood vessels for secure hemostasis. Multiple clips may be delivered without removing the clip applier from the thorax. These tools are required for permanent control of the segmental spinal arteries and veins during exposure of the spine. [Photograph courtesy of Ethicon Endosurgery.]

oscillate at 55 kHz and move a distance of 60 to 80 microns. The ultrasonic effect denatures intravascular protein and collagen to seal blood vessels. The depth of penetration of the ultrasonic effect is very shallow. No thermal damage, smoke, or damage to adjacent tissue is created. It can be used for pleural and muscular dissection and for small blood vessels (smaller than 1 mm). It should not be applied directly to the dura or nerve roots. Vessels with diameters wider than 1 mm may be difficult to seal.

Spinal Dissection Tools

The spinal dissection tools used endoscopically are modified versions of spinal tools used for open surgery. They are usually 30- to 40-cm long and have calibrated markings at 1-cm increments. Their tips are slightly curved or angled. Kerrison rongeurs, disc rongeurs, curettes, osteotomes, bone-graft impactors, periosteal elevators, rib dissectors, Penfield instruments, and microsurgical spinal cord and dural dissection tools are all available (Figs. 4–31, 4–32, and 4–33).

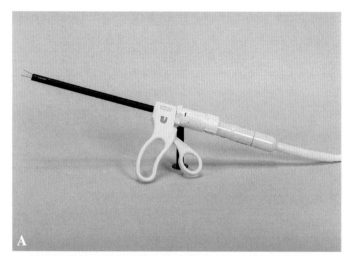

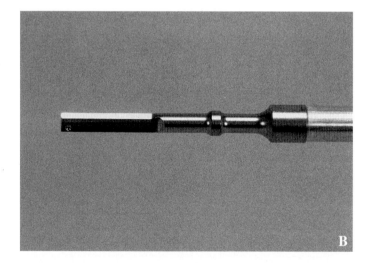

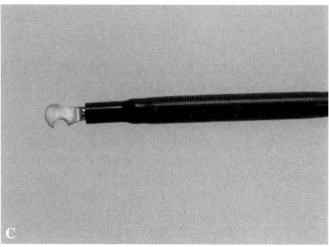

Figure 4–30. **(A)** Harmonic scalpel ultrasonic cauterization and cutting tool. **(B)** A straight cutting blade and **(C)** a hook blade are used. The blunt surfaces of the tips are used to cauterize blood vessels. The sharp surfaces of the blades are used to cut tissue.

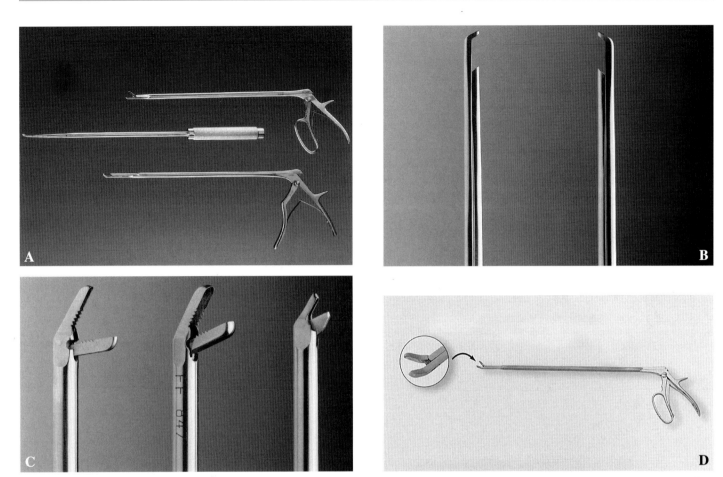

Figure 4–31. **(A)** Thoracoscopic spinal dissection tools are modified from conventional spinal dissection tools. (*Top to bottom*): Disc rongeur, periosteal elevator, and Kerrison rongeur. [Photograph courtesy of United States Surgical Corp.] **(B)** Forward- (*top*) and reverse-biting (*bottom*) angled Kerrison rongeurs are useful for microsurgical bone dissection. The footplates are narrow to allow them to be inserted under the pedicles without narrowing the spinal canal. **(C)** Angled bone and disc rongeurs are available in a variety of sizes. [Photographs B and C courtesy of Aesculap, Inc.] **(D)** The angled tips allow clear visualization of the tips during dissection. [Photograph courtesy of Sofamor Danek.]

Rib dissectors and rib cutting tools are used to free the ligamentous attachments, transect and remove the proximal 2 cm of the rib and rib head, and expose the pedicle and disc space (Fig. 4–34).

Long drill bits are needed for endoscopic bone dissection. High-speed pneumatic drill systems are preferred for endoscopic drilling. The Midas Rex® drill system (Midas Rex Pneumatic Tools, Inc., Fort Worth TX) has bits that are 25-cm (R- or L-attachments) or 40-cm long (Rx attachment), both of which are useful for thoracoscopic spine work (Fig. 4–35). These attachments have a long, protective sheath that prevents injury to the lung and paraspinal soft tissue. A telescoping, adjustable sheath allows the surgeon to vary the length of the exposed drill tip to protect the soft tissues of the thorax. A pistol grip handle is attached to the proximal drill

shaft for precise stabilization of the drill. Secure three-point control of the drill is achieved by grasping the pistol grip and handpiece with both hands and further stabilizing the shaft of the drill against the chest wall within the portal. These maneuvers provide accurate and fine control of the drill tip.

Various drill bits are available for endoscopic use (Fig. 4–36). Coarse diamond burrs are useful for endoscopic drilling of the vertebral body. The coarse diamond burrs create a bone dust slurry that fills the interstices of the cancellous bone and reduces bone bleeding without generating excessive debris within the chest cavity. Foot-plated attachments are useful for transecting ribs. Ball-shaped bits, cylinder-shaped bits, and small cutting burrs are useful for corpectomy and spinal microsurgical bone dissection.

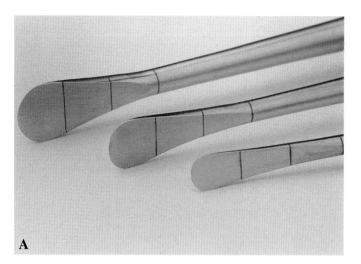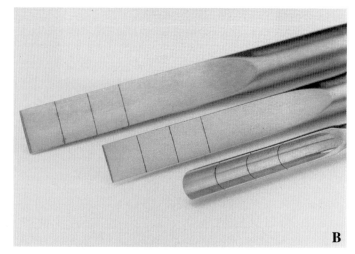

Figure 4–32. **(A)** Endoscopic Cobb periosteal elevators are used to dissect soft tissue from the bone surfaces. **(B)** Endoscopic osteotomes and bone gouges are used to cut through bone sharply. [Photographs courtesy of Spine Tech.]

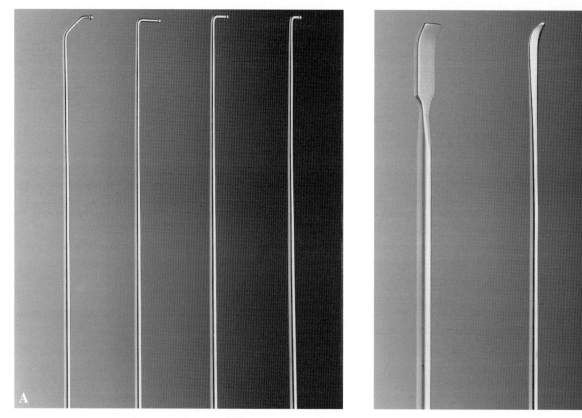

Figure 4–33. Microsurgical spinal dissection tools are designed for working in the epidural space to decompress the spinal cord and spinal nerves. The tips are small and have a low profile to minimize encroaching on the spinal cord. The tips are angled to allow clear visualization. The calibrations facilitate judging the depth of dissection intraoperatively. **(A)** Microsurgical nerve hooks. **(B)** Ligament and disc dissection tools. [Photographs A and B courtesy of Aesculap, Inc.]

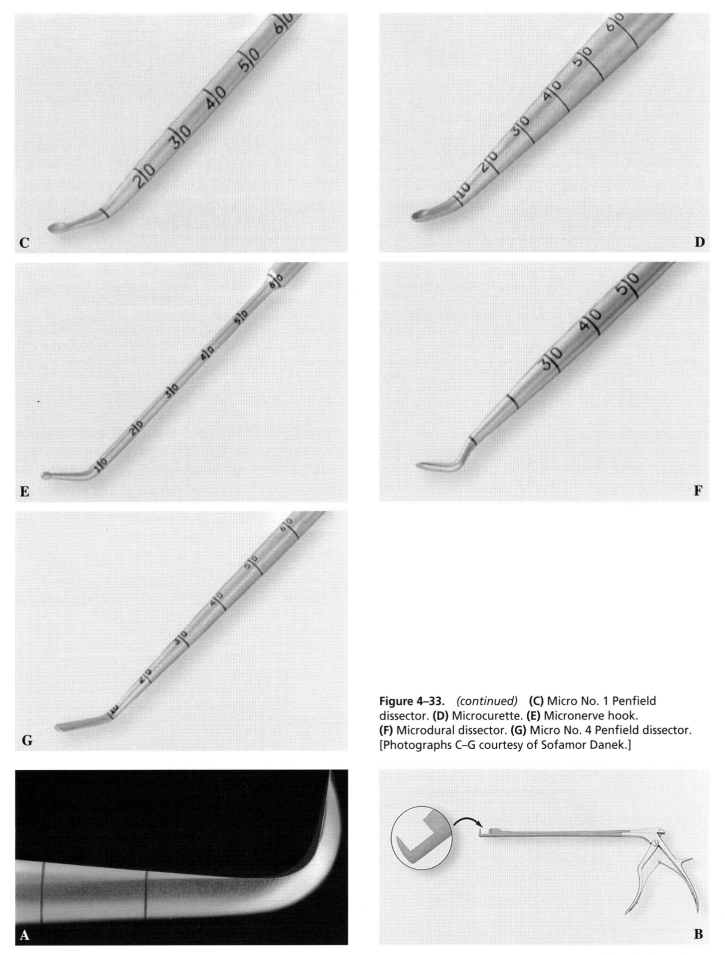

Figure 4–33. *(continued)* **(C)** Micro No. 1 Penfield dissector. **(D)** Microcurette. **(E)** Micronerve hook. **(F)** Microdural dissector. **(G)** Micro No. 4 Penfield dissector. [Photographs C–G courtesy of Sofamor Danek.]

Figure 4–34. **(A)** A right-angled periosteal rib dissector is used to transect the costotransverse ligaments and detach the soft tissues from the lateral surfaces of the ribs. **(B)** The rib cutter is used to transect the rib so the distal rib and rib head can be removed as a single piece. [Photographs courtesy of Sofamor Danek.]

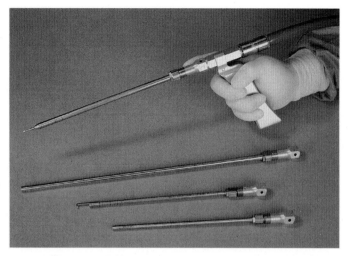

Figure 4–35. The Midas Rex® pneumatic drill system (Midas Rex® Pneumatic Tools, Inc., Fort Worth, TX) has bits that are 25 cm and 40 cm long for endoscopic use. The pistol grip facilitates precise stabilization of the drill. A telescoping protective tissue sheath can be adjusted to vary the length of the stem of the drill bit that is exposed. [Photograph courtesy of Midas Rex Pneumatic Tools, Inc.]

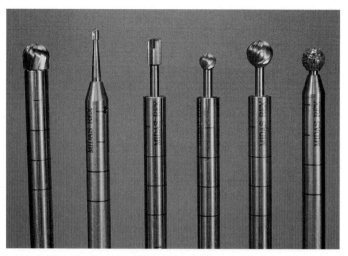

Figure 4–36. The telescoping sheaths can be adjusted to vary the amount of stem exposed. This feature allows the surgeon to protect the adjacent soft tissues during endoscopic bone dissection. Various bits are available for bone dissection. (*Left to right*) R-195 bit, R-8 bit, R-12 bit, R-33 bit, R-32 bit, and the coarse diamond R-382 DXC bit. [Photograph courtesy of Midas Rex Pneumatic Tools, Inc.]

CONCLUSIONS

A wide variety of tools and equipment is required for endoscopic access and dissection of the spine. Technological advances and modifications of standard spine dissection tools have made thoracoscopic spine surgery feasible, permitting extensive decompression and reconstruction of the spine.

RECOMMENDED READINGS

1. Krasna MJ, Mack MJ: Equipment and instrumentation. In Krasna MJ, Mack MJ, eds: *Atlas of Thoracoscopic Surgery*. St. Louis: Quality Medical Publishing; 1994:19–34.
2. Talamini MA, Gadacz TR: Laparoscopic equipment and instrumentation. In Zucker KA, Bailey RW, Reddick EJ, eds: *Surgical Laparoscopy Update*. St. Louis: Quality Medical Publishing; 1993:23–55.
3. Regan JJ: Equipment and instrumentation for endoscopic spine surgery. In Regan JJ, McAfee PC, Mack MJ, eds: *Atlas of Endoscopic Spine Surgery*. St. Louis: Quality Medical Publishing; 1995:69–81.
4. Allen MS, Trastek VF, Daly RC, et al: Equipment for thoracoscopy. *Ann Thorac Surg* 1993; 56(3):620–623.
5. Allen MS, Trastek VF, Deschamps C, et al: Equipment for thoracoscopic surgery. In Kaiser LR, Daniel TM, eds: *Thoracoscopic Surgery*. Boston: Little Brown; 1993:47–57.
6. Semm R: *Operative Manual for Endoscopic Abdominal Surgery*. Chicago: Yearbook; 1987:48–129.
7. Aronoff RJ, Mack MJ: Equipment and instrumentation for thoracoscopy and laparoscopy. In Regan JJ, McAfee PC, Mack MJ, eds: *Atlas of Endoscopic Spine Surgery*. St. Louis: Quality Medical Publishing; 1995:35–48.
8. Kirsch WM, Zhu YH, Gaskill D, et al: Tissue reconstruction with nonpenetrating arcuate-legged clips. Potential endoscopic applications. *J Reprod Med* 1992; 37(7):581–586.
9. Landreneau RJ, Mack MJ, Hazelrigg SR, et al: Video-assisted thoracic surgery: Basic technical concepts and intercostal approach strategies. *Ann Thorac Surg* 1992; 54:800–807.
10. Kavoussi LR, Moore RG, Adams JB, et al: Comparison of robotic versus human laparoscopic camera control. *J Urol* 1995; 154(6):2134–2136.

CHAPTER **5**

Thoracoscopic Perspectives of Thoracic and Mediastinal Anatomy

Randall K. Wolf, M.D., Toshiya Ohtsuka, M.D., and Alvin H. Crawford, M.D.

This chapter reviews intraoperative endoscopic views of thoracic and mediastinal structures, focusing on the anatomy of the paraspinal soft tissue. Knowledge of this anatomy is required for the safe practice of thoracoscopic spinal surgery. All pictures and the accompanying videotape were taken during surgery with a rigid 30°-angled endoscope. The endoscope was introduced through a portal placed laterally in an intercostal space, just above the diaphragm, to provide a panoramic view of the thorax.

The anatomy of the thorax is viewed in four regions: the thoracic outlet, the upper thorax, the middle thorax, and the lower thorax. The anatomical components of each region visualized thoracoscopically are shown in intraoperative photographs obtained during thoracoscopic surgical proce-

dures. A few common thoracoscopic surgical procedures related to the thoracic spine are also used to demonstrate the anatomy.

RIGHT THORACIC OUTLET

At the right thoracic outlet, the right subclavian artery and vein are seen after the first rib has been resected (Fig. 5–1). The subclavian artery is partially covered by the adjacent subclavian vein; it exits the chest cavity beyond the first rib posteriorly and courses parallel to the subclavian vein. From anteriorly to posteriorly, the subclavian vein, subclavian artery, and brachial plexus lie within a groove on the

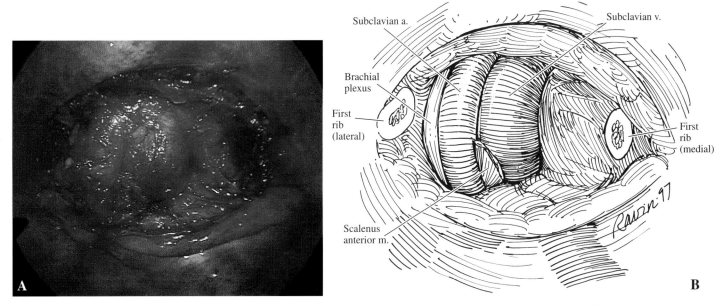

Figure 5–1. **(A)** Thoracoscopic view and **(B)** corresponding illustration of the right thoracic outlet after the first rib has been resected.

first rib. These structures are revealed after the first rib was resected to treat thoracic outlet syndrome.

RIGHT UPPER THORAX

In the right upper thorax, the large right superior intercostal vein is visible on the surface of the vertebral bodies (Fig. 5–2). It receives drainage from the second and third intercostal veins and empties into the azygos arch. The azygos arch is formed at the level of the T4 vertebra over the root of the lung and empties medially into the superior vena cava. The supreme (first) intercostal vein, positioned lateral to the vagus nerve, is usually not visible and empties directly into the right brachiocephalic vein. Typically, the second rib is the first rib structure visible endoscopically when the upper thorax is viewed. The first rib can be palpated, but the first rib and rib head are seldom readily visible because they are covered by apical fat, the brachiocephalic vessels, and the stellate ganglion. This anatomic perspective is important for localizing the level of spinal pathology in the thoracic spine. The ribs can be identified and sequentially counted internally to confirm the spinal localization.

The sympathetic chain overlays the heads of the ribs and the segmental blood vessels, just beneath the surface of the parietal pleura. The segmental arteries and veins course over the middle of the vertebral bodies and join the intercostal nerve to run along the inferior surface of each rib. The disc spaces are positioned midway between the segmental vessels, adjacent to the heads of the ribs.

In a right apical view (Fig. 5–3), the right vagus nerve enters the thorax adjacent to the anterior surface of the subclavian artery and gives rise to the right recurrent laryngeal nerve. The right recurrent laryngeal nerve hooks beneath the right subclavian artery and is seldom visible. The vagus nerve runs posteroinferiorly on the right surface of the trachea, gives rise to its cardiac and pulmonary branches, and runs adjacent to the esophagus where it forms a plexus around the esophagus. The right vagus nerve courses medi-

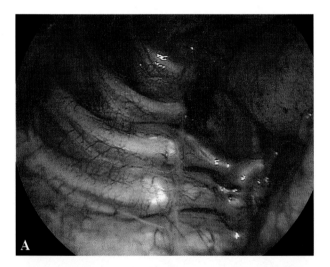

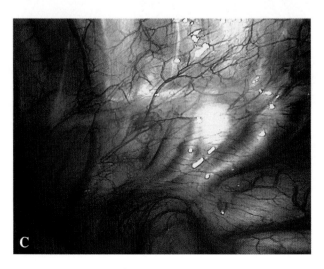

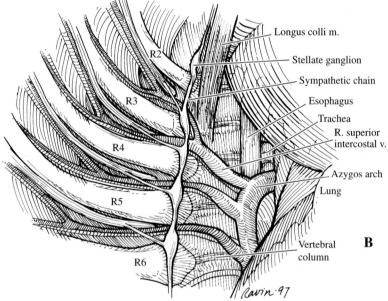

Figure 5–2. **(A)** Thoracoscopic view and **(B)** corresponding illustration of the paraspinal anatomy in the right upper thorax. **(C)** Another perspective of the superior intercostal veins draining into the azygos arch in the right upper thorax.

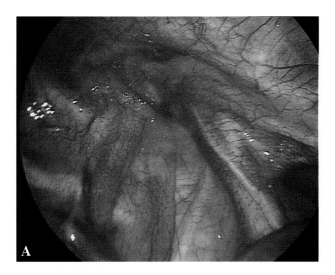

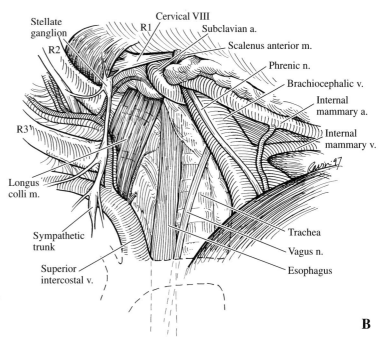

Figure 5–3. **(A)** Thoracoscopic view and **(B)** corresponding illustration of the right thoracic apex and upper mediastinum.

ally to the azygos vein. The long, slender phrenic nerve is visible lateral to the brachiocephalic vein and the superior vena cava. It runs inferiorly adjacent to the pericardium, accompanying the pericardiacophrenic vessels to supply the diaphragm. The trachea and esophagus are ventral to the spine. The sympathetic trunk and ganglia cross the rib heads longitudinally. They are visible on the rib heads superficial to the intercostal vessels and nerves.

Typically, the highest sympathetic ganglion is fused with the inferior cervical ganglion to form the stellate ganglion. The stellate ganglion is readily visualized with a magnifying thoracoscope: It is adjacent to the head of the first rib, and its caudal border is adjacent to the inferior border of the first rib. The borders of the stellate ganglion are important surgical landmarks for performing a thoracic sympathectomy. Thoracoscopic sympathectomy can be used to treat palmar hyperhidrosis, reflex sympathetic dystrophy, and various vascular disorders of the upper extremity. The stellate ganglion is preserved surgically to avoid causing Horner's syndrome.

RIGHT MIDDLE THORAX

In the right middle thorax, the azygos vein, which drains the fourth through twelfth intercostal veins, courses rostrally on the right anterior surface of the vertebral bodies and arches medially to empty into the superior vena cava (Fig. 5–4). The intercostal arteries (except for the most superior arteries) arise from the descending aorta and course adjacent and parallel to the intercostal veins, transversely

across the middle of the vertebral bodies. From rostral to caudal, the vein, artery, and nerve lie in the costal groove just beneath the inferior edge of the rib. To avoid injuring these neurovascular structures, thoracoscopic portals should be inserted through the chest wall close to the upper margins of the ribs. If the ribs must be resected, the neurovascular bundles are preserved by incising and dissecting the periosteum from the surface of the ribs. The greater splanchnic nerve, which is formed by branches from the fifth to ninth sympathetic ganglia, is visible, coursing caudally and ventrally across the vertebral bodies to pass through the crus of the diaphragm. The esophagus, encircled with the vagus trunks and the esophageal plexus, is ventromedial to the azygos vein.

The paraspinal tissues (e.g., the sympathetic chain, splanchnic nerves, segmental arteries and veins) must either be mobilized and preserved or transected to expose the vertebral bodies and discs (Fig. 5–5). The segmented vascular bundles, consisting of the intercostal artery and vein, are isolated, cauterized, ligated, and transected over the vertebrae that need to be exposed. The parietal pleural incisions may be connected longitudinally across the vertebral bodies and extended laterally and medially if needed. For a wide exposure of the surface of the spine over more than one level, the parietal pleura is mobilized, multiple segmental vessels are ligated, and the pleura is gently retracted medially along with the major blood vessels (i.e., the aorta or azygos vein), the ligated vascular bundles, and the esophagus. The entire ventral surface of the vertebral bodies and discs can be exposed with this wide mobilization (Fig. 5–6).

The thoracic duct or its tributaries are transparent and may be glimpsed on the right posterior side of the retracted

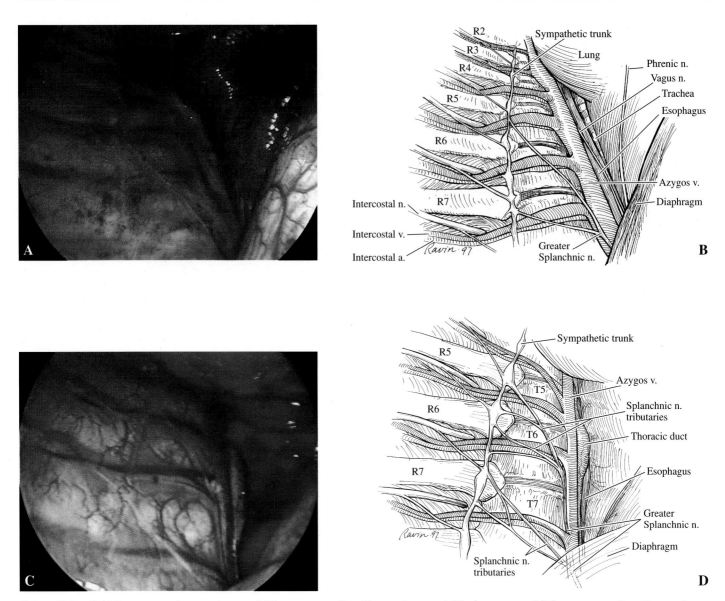

Figure 5–4. **(A)** Thoracoscopic overview and **(B)** corresponding illustration, and **(C)** close-up and **(D)** corresponding illustration of the paraspinal anatomy in the right middle thorax.

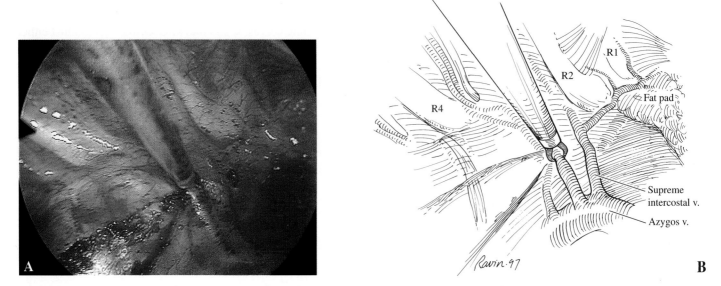

Figure 5–5. **(A)** Thoracoscopic surgical view and **(B)** corresponding illustration during a procedure for scoliosis showing control of the segmental vascular bundles on the surface of the spine by bipolar electrocauterization.

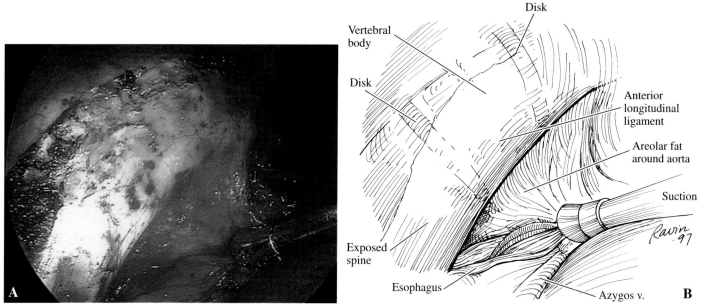

Figure 5–6. **(A)** Thoracoscopic view and **(B)** corresponding illustration showing the exposed scoliotic spine during a right-sided approach after the pleura has been dissected and the esophagus and azygos vein have been mobilized and retracted. The descending aorta is visible on the contralateral surface of the spine. The entire ventral surface and right lateral surfaces of the spine are exposed. The entire anterior longitudinal ligament and multiple disc spaces are exposed for an anterior release.

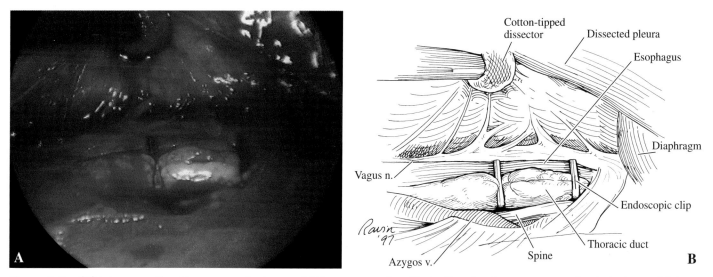

Figure 5–7. **(A)** Intraoperative thoracoscopic view and **(B)** corresponding illustration for the treatment of a chylothorax (right-sided approach). The thoracic duct was ligated with endoscopic clips.

esophagus, medial to the azygos vein (Fig. 5–7). This lymphatic duct enters the thorax through the aortic hiatus of the diaphragm and ascends between the aorta and azygos vein. The thoracic duct usually courses rostrally on the right side of the posterior mediastinum in the lower thorax and crosses the spine anterior to the T5 vertebral body. It continues rostrally on the left side of the esophagus, behind the aorta and subclavian artery, in the superior mediastinum. The thoracic duct empties into the left subclavian vein near the junction of the left internal jugular and subclavian veins.

Embryologically, the thoracic duct develops from paired lymphatic trunks with numerous cross-anastomoses. In 60 to 70% of cases, it runs as described above and enters the left subclavian vein. However, because of its primitive paired bilateral configuration on the surface of the spine, its course also has many normal variations.[1] The most common anomaly is a doubling of the lower part of the thoracic duct from persistent right and left trunks, below the crossing at the fourth to sixth thoracic vertebrae. The vestigial rostral thoracic duct on the right side of the esophagus also may persist. Injury to the thoracic duct or its branches must be avoided or recognized during surgery to prevent a postoperative chylothorax. An injury can be treated thoracoscopically by clipping or ligating the main thoracic duct or its tributaries (Fig. 5–7).

RIGHT LOWER THORAX

The diaphragm, which is shaped like a dome, can be carefully retracted caudally with an endoscopic fan retractor to expose the costodiaphragmatic recess for visualization of the lowest segments of the thoracic spine (Fig. 5–8). Within the thorax, the thoracolumbar junction can be visualized endoscopically as low as the T12–L1 disc space and the L1 vertebral body. The pleural reflection (the pulmonary ligament) and the right crus of the diaphragm can be incised posteriorly to gain caudal exposure of the L1 vertebrae (Fig. 5–9). The greater splanchnic nerve is formed by branches from the fifth through ninth sympathetic ganglia. The nerve courses caudally just lateral to the azygos vein, pierces the crus of the diaphragm, and ends in the celiac ganglion (Figs. 5–4, 5–9, and 5–11). The lesser splanchnic nerve is formed by branches from the tenth and eleventh sympathetic ganglia (Fig. 5–9). Together with the greater splanchnic nerve, it pierces the crus of the diaphragm and courses to the celiac ganglia. The eleventh and twelfth ribs, respectively, articulate with the eleventh and twelfth vertebrae *caudal* to the disc spaces, unlike the other ribs, which articulate with the vertebrae *adjacent* to the disc spaces.

LEFT UPPER THORAX

Anatomically, the two hemithoraces differ. On the left side, the aorta, arch vessels, thoracic outlet, recurrent laryngeal nerve, venous structures, and thoracic duct anatomy are unique. The aortic arch is lateral to the trachea and esophagus. The left common carotid artery and the left subclavian artery arise directly from the aortic arch on the left. Distal to the arch, the descending aorta runs caudally, ventrolateral to the thoracic spine. The left superior intercostal vein (also called the highest intercostal vein) crosses obliquely anterior to the aortic arch to empty into the left brachiocephalic vein (Fig. 5–10).

The left vagus nerve courses caudally between the left common carotid and subclavian arteries and reaches the lateral side of the aortic arch deep to the superior intercostal vein. The left vagus nerve gives rise to the left recurrent laryngeal nerve, which hooks beneath the aortic arch and runs between the trachea and esophagus. The left phrenic nerve runs caudally in front of the vagus nerve and crosses the left internal mammary artery either anteriorly or posteriorly and the superior intercostal vein superficially. It runs along the pericardium and supplies the diaphragm.

LEFT MIDDLE THORAX

The aorta and hemiazygos veins are positioned more laterally adjacent to the spine than the right azygos vein

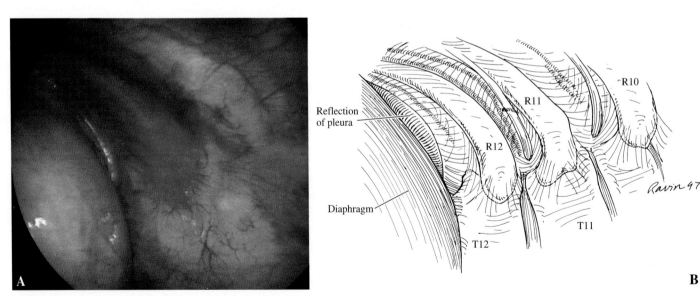

Figure 5–8. **(A)** Thoracoscopic view and **(B)** corresponding illustration of the paraspinal anatomy in the right lower thorax. The diaphragm can be retracted to expose the thoracolumbar junction.

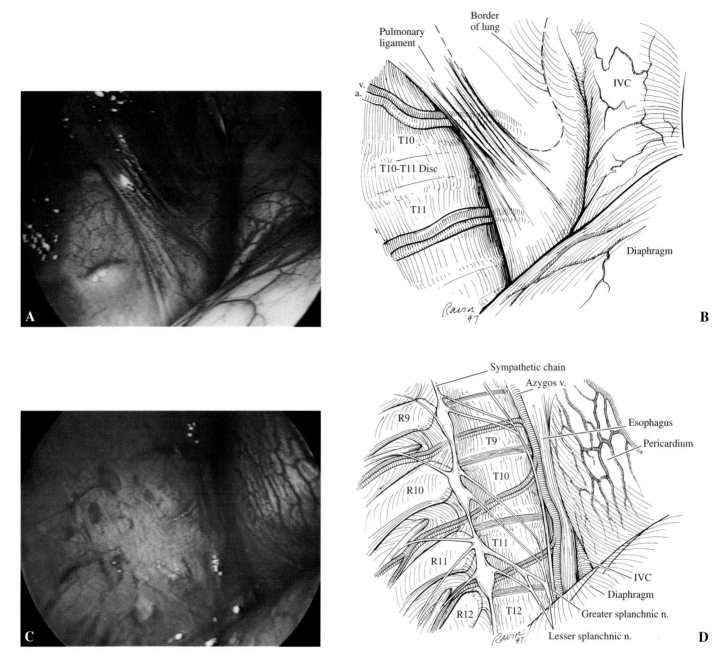

Figure 5–9. Thoracoscopic views of the right costovertebral angle showing the pulmonary ligament and inferior vena cava (IVC). In this **(A)** intraoperative view and **(B)** corresponding illustration, the pulmonary ligament represents the transition between the parietal and visceral pleural surfaces adjacent to the diaphragm posteroinferiorly. **(C)** Intraoperative view and **(D)** corresponding illustration after the pulmonary ligament has been cut to expose the surfaces of the lower thoracic vertebrae.

(Fig. 5–11). On the left surface of the spine, the hemiazygos veins are posterolateral to the aorta. The inferior hemiazygos vein drains the lower thoracic segmental veins (eighth through twelfth) and upper lumbar veins. The superior hemiazygos vein drains the middle thoracic (fourth through eighth) segmental veins. Both the superior and inferior hemiazygos veins cross the midline and drain into the azygos vein.

If wide ventral exposure of the spine is needed, the aorta and hemiazygos vein can be mobilized ventrally (by ligat-ing the segmental vessels and mobilizing the pleura). The surface area of the spine is usually greatest on the right side because of the relative position of the blood vessels adjacent to the spine. Consequently, if a midline pathology involves the spine or spinal cord, a right-sided thoracoscopic approach may be preferred. If the pathology is eccentric to the left, a left-sided approach is used.

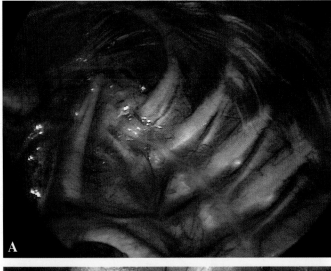

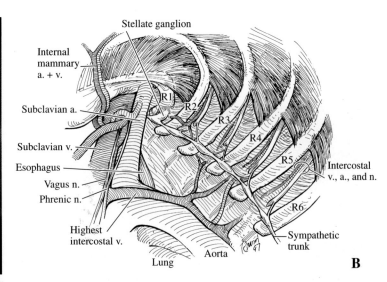

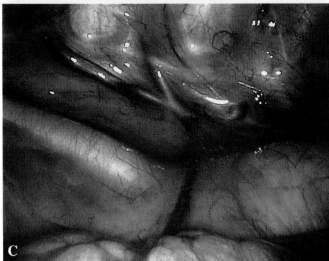

Figure 5–10. **(A)** Thoracoscopic view and **(B)** corresponding illustration of the left upper thoracic cavity. **(C)** Another surgical view of the aortic arch, subclavian artery, and the highest intercostal vein in the left upper thoracic cavity.

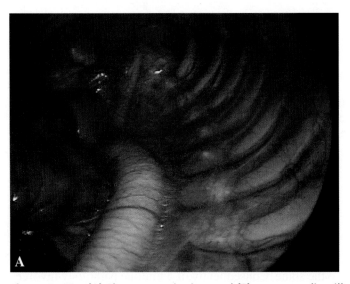

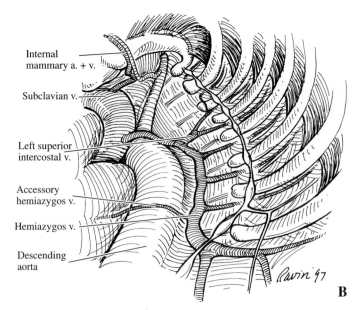

Figure 5–11. **(A)** Thoracoscopic view and **(B)** corresponding illustration of the left middle and lower thoracic cavity.

REFERENCES

1. Davis, HK: A statistical study of the thoracic duct in man. *Am J Anat* 1915; 17:211–244.

CHAPTER **6**

Surgical Anatomy of the Thoracic Spine

T. Glenn Pait, M.D., Ugur Türe, M.D., Kenan I. Arnautović, M.D., and Ron M. Tribell

The vertebral column functions as a supporting pillar and a bony envelope for the protection of the spinal cord and nerve roots. This bony framework consists of a series of bones called vertebrae, closely connected by means of fibrous and elastic structures. These elements allow motion between any two adjacent members of this bony series and provide the column, as a whole, with a rather high degree of flexibility. Stability to the vertebral column is secured through the individual bony elements as well as by means of ligamentous connections and muscular control.

There are 33 vertebrae. In most cases, the upper 24 remain separate and are distinguished as movable or true vertebrae.[1-3] The lower five vertebrae are consolidated and form a mass commonly known as the sacrum. The terminal part of the spine is composed of four rudimentary vertebrae that become united and form the coccyx. The sacrum and the coccyx lose their mobility and are known as fixed or false vertebrae.[1-3]

The active, or true, vertebrae are located in the cervical, thoracic, and lumbar spine.[1-3] The vertebrae all have certain features in common, and they all have two essential parts: a body ventrally and an arch dorsally. The body of the vertebrae is a weight-supporting pillar. The bony arch of the vertebrae is composed of the pedicles, lamina, spinous processes, and projecting processes such as the transverse and costal processes. Together with the vertebral body, the arch encloses the vertebral foramen and serves to protect the spinal cord and the roots of the spinal nerves. This is the function of all the vertebrae.

Even though the thoracic spine is composed of the same basic bony elements, its location and association with the costal processes (ribs) increase its complexity. Consequently, it is often poorly understood. The thoracic spine is mechanically stronger and less mobile than other active regions of the spinal column.[4] The blood supply for the thoracic spinal cord is precarious and therefore less reliable,

and it can be unforgiving. These are sufficient reasons to give this part of the spine its due respect. Only by understanding its complex anatomy can surgeons treat this region of the spine successfully. In this chapter, the anatomy is separated into three separate entities to facilitate the reader's understanding of the complex thoracic spine: (1) bony architecture, (2) articulations and ligaments, and (3) neurovascular elements.

BONY ARCHITECTURE

There are 12 thoracic vertebrae. Their size gradually increases rostrally to caudally. This increase in size accommodates the increasing load carried from head to sacrum.[1-4] All the thoracic vertebrae are distinguished by either a costotransverse and/or costovertebral complex (Figs. 6–1 and 6–2). Ventrolateral outgrowths of the body of each vertebra constitute the costal processes.[2] The costal processes in the thoracic spine develop into the ribs. The costal processes (ribs) articulate with the vertebral bodies by costal facets (costotransverse and costovertebral), which are located on the sides of the bodies (Fig. 6–3).[1,5] Such articulations are found on the transverse processes and the vertebral bodies of all thoracic vertebrae except the last two or three bodies.[1-3] At T11 and T12, there is no costotransverse articulation—only a costovertebral articulation.[1-3] The costotransverse-costovertebral complex articulates, respectively, with the tubercles and the head of the rib (costa) (Figs. 6–1 and 6–2).

The body of the vertebra is a short, cylindrical column of bone with cranial and caudal surfaces, which are rough and broad for attachment of the intervertebral fibrocartilaginous disc (Fig. 6–4). The anteroposterior diameter of a typical thoracic vertebra is slightly greater than its transverse dimension (Fig. 6–5).[1-3] Craniocaudally, the ventral and lateral surfaces

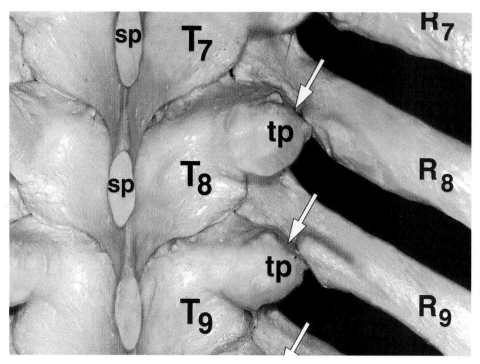

Figure 6–1. Dorsal view of the midthoracic spine. sp = spinous process, tp = transverse process, T = vertebra, and R = rib. Arrows point to the costotransverse articulation.

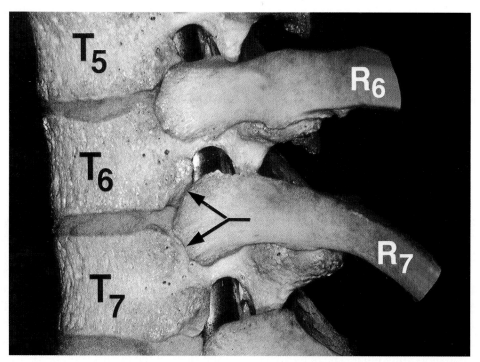

Figure 6–2. Lateral view of the midthoracic spine (left side). Arrows point to the costovertebral articulation. R = rib, T = vertebra.

are concave. In fact, when viewed from the side, this concavity is like a valley that rises to a prominence, which borders the interspace (Fig. 6–4). The segmental arteries and veins course through the valley of the bony vertebral body. Therefore, when segmental vessels are identified, one is in the middle of the vertebral body (Fig. 6–6). Dorsally, the vertebral body is concave from side to side. Usually, large foramina are located on the dorsal surface for the passage of vascular structures to and from the spongy interior (Fig. 6–7).[5] Facets are located at the junction where the posterior elements (arch of the vertebra) join the vertebral body. A typ-

ical body will have two facets: a larger cranial (superior) and a smaller caudal (inferior) facet. The cranial facets are either circular or semicircular. The shape of the caudal facets is semilunar. These facets are the docking sites of the head of the rib (costal process) (Fig. 6–3).

The arch of the vertebra is a protective bony roof, which is formed by two laminae and two pedicles. The arch supports seven processes—one spinous, two transverse, two superior, and two inferior processes (Figs. 6–8 and 6–9). The pedicles are short columns of bone that arise from the dorsal surface of the vertebral body and project dorsally.

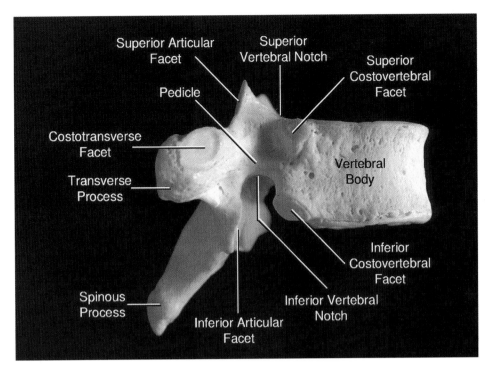

Figure 6–3.   Lateral view of a thoracic vertebral body. The costotransverse, costovertebral, superior articular, and inferior articular facets are well defined.

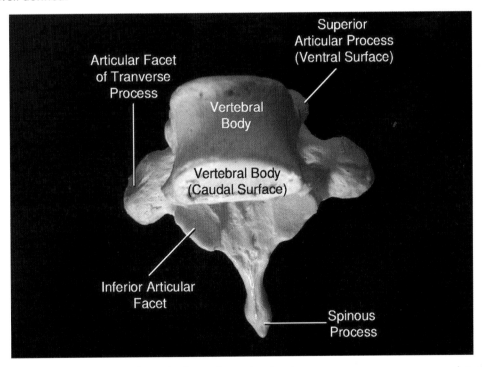

Figure 6–4.   Ventral view of a thoracic vertebra. The laterally projecting transverse processes are appreciated. The inferior articular facets are well defined.

The pedicle has a cranial and a caudal border. Each border is indented with a concavity known as the vertebral notch. The cranial border is the superior vertebral notch; the caudal border is the inferior vertebral notch and the larger of the two notches (Fig. 6–3).[1–3] When two vertebrae are in position, the notches form an intervertebral foramen through which the spinal nerves and the vascular elements course (Figs. 6–2 and 6–10). The dorsal bony arch is completed by two wide symmetrical plates of bone—the laminae. When articulated, the laminae overlap and are sloped.

The spinous process arises from the center of the arch, projects dorsally and caudally, and ends at a small tubercle. This long, thin projection of bone is the attachment for many muscles as well as the supraspinous and interspinous ligaments (Figs. 6–3 and 6–4). The transverse processes are two stout pillars situated at the junction of the laminae and pedicles, and they extend laterally and dorsally. The transverse processes terminate laterally at the costal facets, adding support to the ribs (costal processes). They are also attachments for powerful muscles (Figs. 6–3, 6–4, and 6–8).

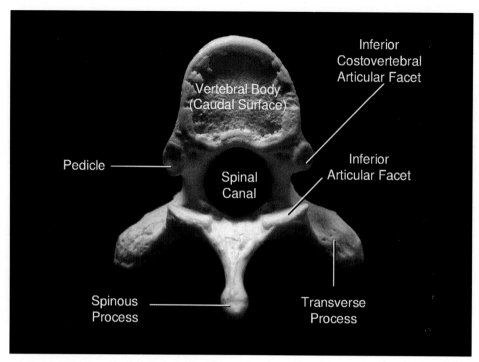

Figure 6–5. The axial configuration of a typical thoracic vertebra.

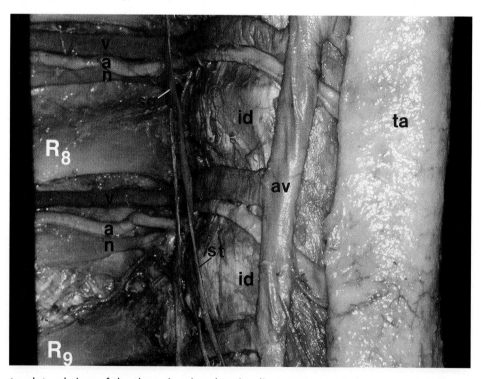

Figure 6–6. Right anterolateral view of the thoracic spine showing ligaments, arteries, veins, and nerves coursing in and around the costotransverse vertebral complexes. a = intervertebral artery, av = azygos vein, id = intervertebral disc, n = nerve, R = rib, ta = thoracic aorta, v = intervertebral vein, sg = sympathetic ganglion, and st = sympathetic trunk.

There are four articular processes: two superior and two inferior. The superior processes are directed cranially, dorsally, and slightly laterally. The inferior articular processes are projected caudally, ventrally, and medially. These thin, flat shelves of bone bear the superior and inferior articular facets (Figs. 6–3, 6–4, and 6–8).

The true intervertebral foramen is bounded ventrally by the vertebral body and the intervertebral disc, dorsally by the articular processes, and cranially and caudally by the pedicles (Fig. 6–11). When viewed laterally, the rib head (costal process) creates a false foramen. The superior vertebral notch is hidden from sight by the rib, which appears to form the caudal wall of the foramen (Fig. 6–12). The rib head, with its facet, must be removed to appreciate the true foramen, to access the pedicle and spinal canal, and to provide a flat surface for any type of instrumentation (Fig. 6–11).

The previous description is that of a so-called typical thoracic vertebra; however, several vertebrae in this column differ from this typical description. The exceptions are the first, ninth, tenth, eleventh, and twelfth vertebrae (Fig. 6–13).[1,5,6]

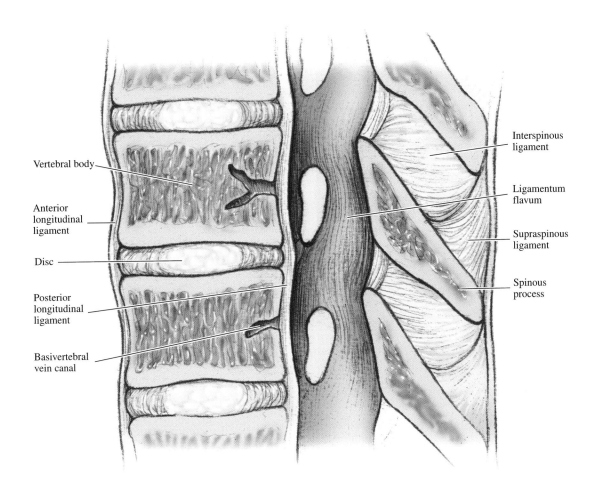

Vertebral body

Anterior
longitudinal
ligament

Disc

Posterior
longitudinal
ligament

Basivertebral
vein canal

Interspinous
ligament

Ligamentum
flavum

Supraspinous
ligament

Spinous
process

Figure 6–7. Illustration demonstrating ligamentous structures, disc space, and basivertebral vascular channels.

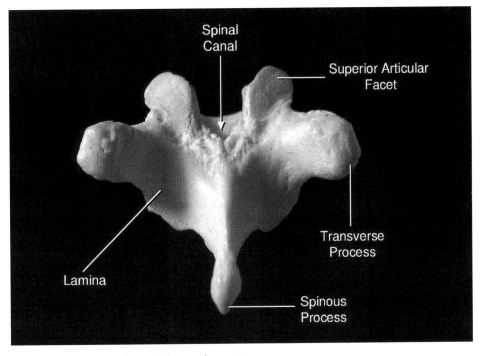

Spinal
Canal

Superior Articular
Facet

Transverse
Process

Lamina

Spinous
Process

Figure 6–8. Dorsal view of the posterior thoracic bony elements.

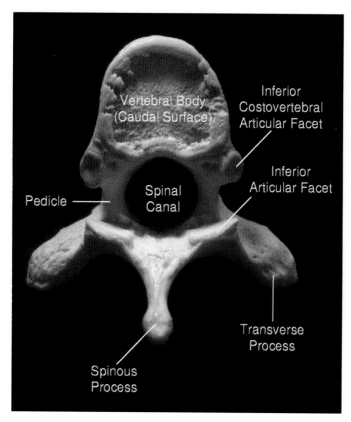

Figure 6–9. Caudal view of a typical thoracic vertebra.

The first thoracic vertebra is a transitional vertebra. Its body closely resembles that of a cervical vertebra. The ventral surface of the body is flat, and its transverse diameter is greater than its anteroposterior diameter. Its spinous process is stout and thick and often more prominent than that of the seventh cervical. A large costal facet is present on each side to receive the rib (Fig. 6–13).[1-3] The ninth thoracic vertebra resembles a typical thoracic vertebra, except that it seldom possesses a caudal facet; therefore, it does not articulate with the tenth rib (Fig. 6–13).[1-3] The tenth thoracic vertebra is similar to the ninth vertebra in that it, too, lacks a caudal facet. It contains a large singular facet for articulation with only the tenth rib. It is the last vertebra to have both costotransverse and costovertebral articulations (Fig. 6–13).[1-3] The eleventh thoracic vertebra forms joints only at the costovertebral site. The eleventh rib communicates only with the eleventh vertebral body. Its transverse process is small and lacks a costotransverse process (Fig. 6–13).[1-3] The twelfth thoracic vertebra is similar to the eleventh vertebra. The only true difference is that its costovertebral articulation is located more caudally. Both the eleventh and twelfth thoracic vertebrae are larger than other thoracic vertebral bodies and approximate the configuration of the lumbar vertebrae (Fig. 6–13).[1,5]

It is important to remember the location and numbering of the ribs when lesions of the thoracic spine must be managed. The first rib communicates with the first vertebral body. The second rib articulates with the body of the second vertebra. The third rib articulates with the second and third vertebral bodies. The fourth rib, located between the third and fourth vertebral bodies, can serve as a guide to the third and fourth intervertebral disc space. This pattern continues until the tenth vertebral body. The tenth, eleventh, and twelfth ribs articulate only with the vertebral body of the

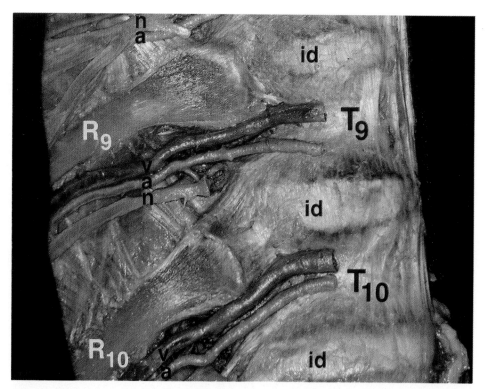

Figure 6–10. Neurovascular elements have been transected at the midvertebral body (right side). Neurovascular elements can be appreciated coursing through the intervertebral foramen at T9. v = intervertebral vein, a = intervertebral artery, n = nerve, id = intervertebral disc, and R = rib.

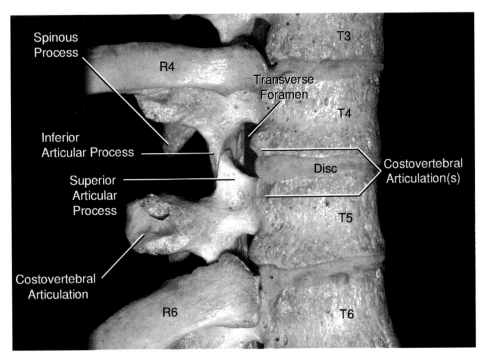

Figure 6–11. The neural foramen (right side) can be appreciated after the fifth costal process (rib) has been removed. R = rib, T = vertebra.

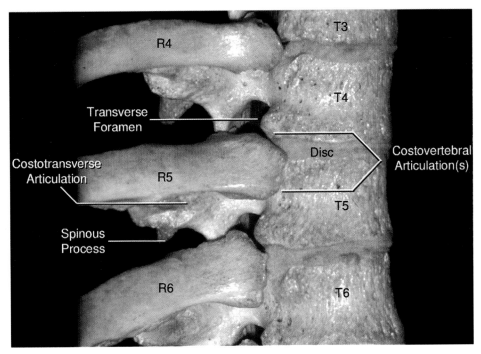

Figure 6–12. Lateral view of the thoracic spine (right side) depicting the costal process and rib head, which obscure the visibility of the neural foramen and pedicle. R = rib, T = vertebra.

same number. The tenth, eleventh and twelfth ribs do not cover an interspace; they articulate only with their respective vertebral body (Fig. 6–13).[7]

ARTICULATIONS AND LIGAMENTS

Articulations between the Vertebral Bodies

Three elements provide the articulations between the thoracic vertebral bodies: (1) the anterior longitudinal liga-ment, (2) the posterior longitudinal ligament, and (3) the intervertebral disc (Fig. 6–7).

The anterior longitudinal ligament is a broad and strong band of fibers that extends along the anterior surfaces of the bodies of the vertebrae, from the axis to the sacrum. It is a bit narrower, but thicker, in its passage over the vertebral bodies than over the intervertebral discs. It consists of dense longitudinal fibers that adhere intimately to the interverte-bral discs and the prominent margins of the vertebrae, but it is not attached firmly to the middle parts of the vertebral bodies.[1,5,7,8]

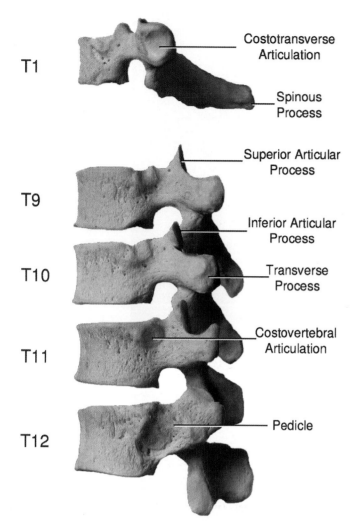

Figure 6–13. Vertebrae that are exceptions to the typical thoracic patterns: T1, T9, T10, T11, and T12 (left side).

Articulations between the Vertebral Arches

Five elements provide the articulations of the vertebral arches: (1) the articular capsules, (2) the ligamentum flavum, (3) the supraspinous ligaments, (4) the interspinous ligaments, and (5) the intertransverse ligaments (Fig. 6–7).[1,5,9–11]

The articular capsules are thin, loose, and attached to margins of the articular processes of adjacent vertebrae (Fig. 6–7).

The ligamentum flavum connects the laminae of adjacent vertebrae. Each ligamentum flavum consists of yellow elastic tissue. The almost perpendicular fibers are attached to the ventral surface of the lamina above and to the dorsal surface and superior margin of the lamina below (like the tiles on a rooftop). Their marked elasticity permits separation of the laminae during flexion of the vertebral column and also serves to preserve upright posture (Fig. 6–7).

The supraspinous ligament is a strong fibrous cord that connects the apices of the spinous processes from the seventh cervical vertebra to the sacrum. At its points of attachment to the tips of the spinous processes, fibrocartilage is developed in the ligament (Fig. 6–7).

The thin and membranous interspinous ligaments interconnect adjoining spinous processes. Their attachment extends from the root to the apex of each spinous process. Consequently, they meet the ligamenta flava ventrally and the supraspinous ligament dorsally. They are narrow and elongated in the thoracic region, broad and thick in the lumbar region, and only slightly developed in the neck (Fig. 6–7).

The intertransverse ligaments are interposed between the transverse processes. In the thoracic region they are rounded cords intimately connected with the deep muscles of the back (Fig. 6–7).

The posterior longitudinal ligament extends along the dorsal surfaces of the bodies of the vertebrae from the axis to the sacrum. It lies within the vertebral canal. It is broader rostrally than caudally and thicker in the thoracic region than in the cervical and lumbar regions. The ligament is composed of longitudinal fibers that are more dense and compact than those of the anterior ligament.[1,5,7,8]

The intervertebral discs are interposed between the adjacent surfaces of the vertebral bodies from the axis to the sacrum, forming their chief bonds of connection. The thickness of the discs in the thoracic region is almost uniform, and the anterior concavity of this part of the column almost entirely reflects the shape of the vertebral bodies. The intervertebral discs are adherent to thin layers of hyaline cartilage, which cover the superior and inferior surfaces of the bodies of the vertebrae. The rounded border of the intervertebral discs is firmly attached to the anterior and posterior longitudinal ligaments. In the thoracic region the discs are joined laterally, by means of interarticular ligaments, to the heads of those ribs that articulate with the two adjacent vertebrae (Fig. 6–10).[1–3,6,8]

Articulations between the Vertebrae and Ribs

There are two types of articulations between the ribs and thoracic vertebrae: costovertebral and costotransverse.[1,5,9–11] The costovertebral articulation is the articulation between the head of the rib (costa) and the vertebral body. This articulation provides additional stability to the thoracic spine motion segments. The articular capsule and the radiate and intraarticular ligaments stabilize this articulation (Fig. 6–14).[4,12] The articular capsule surrounds the joint and is composed of short, strong fibers that connect the head of the rib with the circumference of the articular cavity formed by the intervertebral disc and the adjacent vertebrae. The capsule is most distinct at the superior and inferior parts of the articulation (Fig. 6–14). The radiate ligament connects the anterior part of the head of each rib with the side of the bodies of two vertebra and with the intervertebral disc between them. The radiate ligaments along the spinal column are in relationship anteriorly to the thoracic ganglia of the sympathetic trunk, the pleura, and, on the right side, the azygos vein. Immediately behind the radiate ligaments at

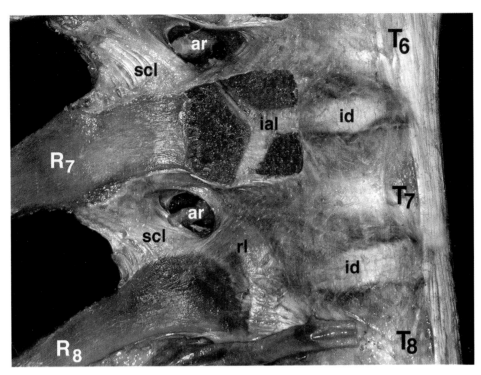

Figure 6–14. Lateral view of the thoracic spine (right side) demonstrating the ligamentous complex. ar = anterior ramus of the intercostal nerve, ial = interarticular ligament, id = intervertebral disc, rl = radiate ligament, scl = superior costotransverse ligament, and R = rib, T = vertebra.

each level are the intraarticular ligaments and the synovial membranes (Fig. 6–14).

The intraarticular ligament is situated in the interior of the joint. It consists of a short, flat band of fibers, attached by one extremity to the crest separating the two articular facets on the head of the rib and by the other to the intervertebral disc (Fig. 6–14). The interarticular crest is closely bound with the intervertebral disc through the intraarticular ligament. The rib belongs to the body of the vertebrae below. In the joints of the first, tenth, eleventh, and twelfth ribs, the intraarticular ligament does not exist because there is only one cavity and one synovial membrane at each of these articulations.

The costotransverse articulation is situated between the neck and the tubercle of the rib (costa) and the transverse process of the thoracic spine (Fig. 6–1). The T11 and T12 transverse processes do not articulate with the corresponding ribs (Fig. 6–13). The thoracic transverse processes are much stronger than in the lumbar region because they have to buttress the ribs. They are also stouter and extend more laterally in the upper thoracic spine. Their mass and length diminish down to the lumbar region, reflecting the need for strong attachments for the powerful arm muscles. Facets on the transverse processes (which articulate with the tubercle of the ribs) are not uniform, and their arrangement and structure reflect the different mechanical characteristics of the corresponding rib.

The ligaments that connect these gliding articulations are the superior costotransverse ligament (the internal and external costotransverse ligament), the lateral costotrans-

verse ligament, and the costotransverse ligament (Fig. 6–15).[4,12] The superior costotransverse ligament splits laterally into two sheets (internal and external) between which lie the levator costae and external intercostal muscles. The dorsal ramus of the thoracic nerve passes posterior to this ligament and the ventral ramus (the intercostal nerve) passes anterior. The lateral costotransverse ligament is quite strong and articulates with the dorsal surface of the transverse process and its corresponding rib (Fig. 6–15). The costotransverse ligament passes between the anterior aspect of a transverse process and the posterior aspect of the neck of its own rib.

NEUROVASCULAR ELEMENTS

Arteries

In contrast to the cervical vertebrae, each thoracic vertebra is supplied by right- and left-sided branches of the aorta. There are 11 intercostal arteries and one subcostal artery along each side. Approximately 10 pairs of intercostal arteries arise from the posterior aorta. The first intercostal space and, occasionally, the second one are supplied by branches of the subclavian artery. At the anterior costotransverse foramen, each artery divides into two branches, an anterior and a posterior (Figs. 6–6 and 6–10). The posterior branch passes posteriorly to the anterior costotransverse foramen and gives rise to a spinal branch, which supplies the vertebrae, the spinal cord, and its membranes. The anterior branch supplies the wall of the thorax and is accompanied

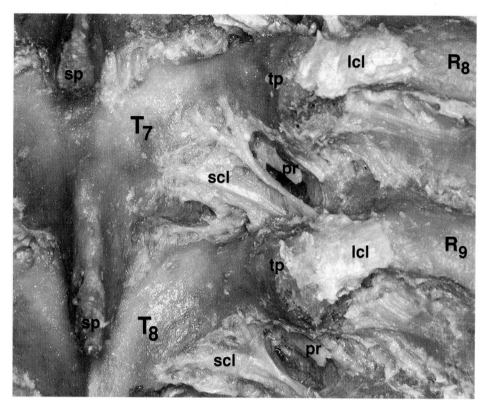

Figure 6–15. Dorsal view of the thoracic spine (right side). Ligaments and nerves are in the costotransverse vertebral complexes on the right side. lcl = lateral costotransverse ligament, pr = posterior ramus of the spinal nerve, scl = superior costotransverse ligament, sp = spinous process, tp = transverse process, and R = rib, T = vertebra.

by an intercostal vein and nerve (Figs. 6–6 and 6–10).[1–3,7,8,11,13–17] The artery of Adamkiewicz, also known as the arteria radicularis anterior magna, usually enters the vertebral canal between T7 and L4, with a predilection for T9 to T11. It is a unilateral artery and occurs in the left side in 80% of the specimens studied.

Veins

The azygos vein receives intercostal veins from the lower eight intercostal spaces on the right side (Fig. 6–6). Veins from the second and third intercostal spaces drain into the right superior intercostal vein, which terminates in the azygos vein. The venous return from the first intercostal space drains into the right brachiocephalic vein. The azygos vein also receives the hemiazygos veins. The hemiazygos and accessory hemiazygos veins drain the lower 8 posterior intercostal spaces on the left side. The second and third intercostal spaces on the left are drained by the left superior intercostal vein, which crosses the aortic arch to end in the left brachiocephalic vein. The first left intercostal space drains into the corresponding brachiocephalic vein. At the anterior costotransverse foramen, each vein receives an anterior and posterior tributary (Fig. 6–6). The posterior tributary anastomoses with the vertebral venous system and passes through the anterior costotransverse foramen. The anterior tributary originates from the intercostal space and merges into a common trunk (Fig. 6–6).[1,5,7,10–12,14–16]

Nerves

The spinal nerves arise from the thoracic spinal cord. They give rise to the anterior ramus, which is the intercostal nerve, and the posterior ramus (Fig. 6–16). The posterior ramus passes posteriorly to the posterior costotransverse foramen and innervates the paraspinal muscles and adjacent skin (Fig. 6–16). The anterior ramus, or the intercostal nerve, passes through the anterior costotransverse foramen and innervates the wall of the thorax and upper abdomen (Figs. 6–6 and 6–10). It is connected to the adjoining ganglia of the sympathetic trunk by one or two filaments at the anterior costotransverse foramen (Fig. 6–6). The thoracic part of the sympathetic trunk is located on the anterior surface of the head of the rib. In continuity with the cervical and abdominal parts, the thoracic sympathetic trunk consists of a series of interconnected enlargements (ganglia) that occur at intervals along its length (Fig. 6–6).[1,5,7,10–12,14–16]

CONCLUSION

The anatomy of the thoracic spine is like that of any other part of the human form—it is complex. However, if this complex anatomy is divided into its individual bony, ligamentous, and neurovascular parts, it is easily understood. This anatomy must be understood to achieve good surgical outcomes. Anatomy is indeed the surgeon's roadway to success.

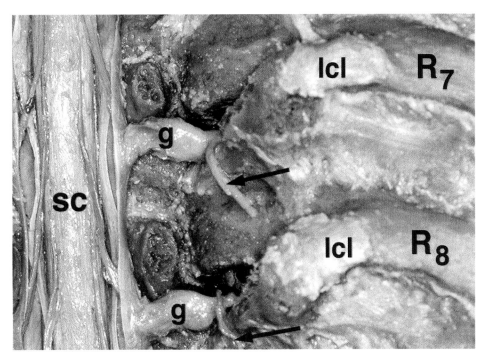

Figure 6–16. Dorsal view of thoracic spine (right side). Laminectomies have been performed, pedicles drilled away, the ganglion exposed, the dura opened, and the spinal cord with nerve roots exposed. Arrows point to the posterior rami of the spinal nerves. g = ganglion, lcl = lateral costotransverse ligament, sc = spinal cord, and R = rib.

ACKNOWLEDGMENTS

The authors wish to thank Patrick Tank, Ph.D., for his help in providing anatomical specimens. We are grateful for the talents of Betty Patterson in preparing this chapter. We are indebted to Alice Fratus for her tolerance and support during the many changes and corrections of the illustrations.

REFERENCES

1. Clemente CD: *Gray's Anatomy*, 30th American ed. Baltimore: Williams & Wilkins; 1984:114–422.
2. Williams PL, Bannister LH, Berry MM, et al: *Gray's Anatomy*. London: Churchill Livingstone; 1995:522–543.
3. Terry RJ: Osteology. *Morris' Human Anatomy*. Philadelphia: Blakiston; 1947:77–265.
4. White AA, III, Panjabi MM: The problem of clinical instability in the human spine: A systematic approach. In White AA, III, Panjabi MM, eds: *Clinical Biomechanics of the Spine*. Philadelphia: J Lippincott; 1978:236–251.
5. Arey LB: *Developmental Anatomy*, 5th ed. Philadelphia: W.B. Saunders; 1946:363–389.
6. Romanes GJ: *Cunningham's Textbook of Anatomy*, 12th ed. Oxford: Oxford University Press; 1981:220–227.
7. Grieve GP: *Common Vertebral Joint Problems*. New York: Churchill Livingstone; 1981:33–50.
8. Ferner H, Staubesand J: *Sobotta Atlas of Human Anatomy*. Baltimore: Urban & Schwarzenberg; 1983.
9. Breathnach AS: *Frazer's Anatomy of the Human Skeleton*, 6th ed. Boston: Little, Brown; 1965.
10. Toldt C: *An Atlas of Human Anatomy for Students and Physicians*, 2nd ed. New York: Macmillan, 1948.
11. Ferner H: *Pernkopf Atlas of Topographical and Applied Human Anatomy*. Baltimore: Urban & Schwarzenberg; 1980.
12. Jiang H, Raso JV, Moreau MJ, et al: Quantitative morphology of the lateral ligaments of the spine. Assessment of their importance in maintaining lateral stability. *Spine* 1994; 19(23):2676–2682.
13. Platzer W: *Pernkopf Anatomie*. Munich: Urban & Schwarzenberg; 1987.
14. Luyendijk W, Cohn B, Rejger V, et al: The great radicular artery of Adamkiewicz in man. Demonstration of a possibility to predict its functional territory. *Acta Neurochir (Wien)* 1988; 95(3–4):143–146.
15. Rodriguez-Baeza A, Muset-Lara A, Rodriguez-Pazos M, et al: The arterial supply of the human spinal cord: A new approach to the arteria radicularis magna of Adamkiewicz. *Acta Neurochir (Wien)* 1991; 109(1–2):57–62.
16. Dommisse GF: The blood supply of the spinal cord. A critical vascular zone in spinal surgery. *J Bone Joint Surg Br* 1974; 56(2):225–235.
17. Crock HV: *An Atlas of Vascular Anatomy of the Skeleton and Spinal Cord*. St. Louis: Mosby; 1996.

CHAPTER 7

Microanatomy of Thoracic Spine Foramina and Ligaments

Gökhan Akdemir, M.D., Mukesh Misra, M.D., Manuel Dujovny, M.D., and M. Serdar Alp, M.D.

Knowledge of the anatomical details of any part of the human body is an imperative part of surgeons' initial training if they are to develop good surgical skills. The spine is no exception. A detailed anatomical knowledge of the thoracic spine facilitates surgery, especially spinal endoscopy, internal fixation and spinal instrumentation techniques, and corrections of spinal deformities. These procedures are difficult, particularly in the thoracic region where the anatomy is complex and access is challenging.

Consequently, we performed a detailed anatomical study of the thoracic spine. At each level, we assessed the shape and measured the size of the thoracic vertebrae. The size of the thoracic vertebral bodies, height of the pedicle, dimensions of the foramina, and the intercostal distance between the vertebral foramina were also measured. In addition, we studied the thoracic intraforaminal ligaments and other contents of the thoracic spinal canal. As endoscopic techniques, spinal instrumentation, and stereotactic approaches to this area rapidly develop, a clear understanding of the related anatomy is crucial. The results of this study may also be useful for generating geometric models of the thoracic vertebrae that could lead to further improvements in surgical techniques.

MATERIALS AND METHODS

Thoracic foraminal anatomy was measured in 11 previously prepared, whole cadavers (five females, six males) whose ages ranged from 16 to 71 years. The thoracic spinal columns were separated from the cervical and the sacral segments en bloc with an electric band saw. The paraspinal muscles and their attachments were removed by sharp and meticulous dissection, and the thoracic spine was examined under a Zeiss OPMI surgical microscope (Carl Zeiss Inc.,

New York, NY). A Minolta X370 camera (Minolta Camera Co., Higashi-ku, Osaka, Japan) was attached to the surgical microscope for photographic documentation and video recording. The video pictures were developed in a Sony developer (Sony Inc., Japan).

After the cadavers were prepared, the height and width of the vertebrae were measured. Then, the height of both the right and left pedicles was measured. Next, the foramen-to-pedicle height and the intercostal distance between foramina were measured on both sides. The foramen-to-body height was the ratio of the height of the vertebral foramen on both sides compared to the height of the vertebral body. The foraminal contents were identified and studied in detail. The various foraminal ligaments were outlined and identified at all thoracic spinal levels. The neurovascular bundle and the other foraminal contents were individually identified and studied.

GROSS AND MICROANATOMICAL RESULTS

The thoracic spine consists of 12 vertebrae. It has a ventral curve that develops in utero and is maintained, although somewhat modified, throughout life (Fig. 7–1). Anteriorly, the vertebral bodies are primarily load-bearing. Posteriorly, the arches act to resist tension. The anteroposterior diameter of the vertebral bodies gradually increases from T1 to T12, whereas the transverse width decreases from T1 to T3 and then progressively increases down to T12.[1,2] Normally, the vertical height of the thoracic vertebral bodies is 2 to 3 mm less anteriorly than posteriorly, which partially contributes to thoracic kyphosis.

The mean height of the thoracic vertebral bodies was 19.3 mm, and the mean width was 28.8 mm. However, both

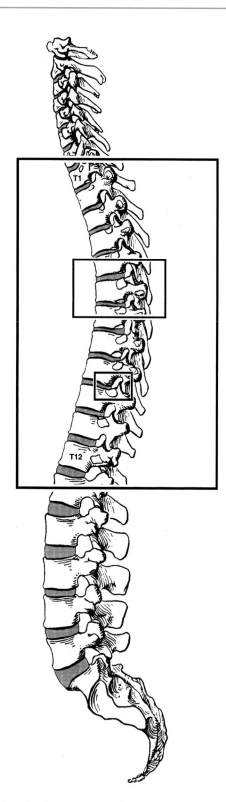

Figure 7–1. The human spine showing the thoracic region evaluated in this study (large box). The medium box highlights the dimensions of a single thoracic vertebra; the small box highlights the dimensions of a vertebral foramen.

parameters increased steadily from T1 to T12 vertebra, a trend easily defined by moving from one thoracic level to the next in descending order (Fig. 7–2). The sides of the vertebral bodies are somewhat concave. In the thoracic spine, the laminae are broad and overlap heavily. The body of the midthoracic vertebra is heart-shaped, and the size of its length and width is intermediate. Often, a flattening of

the left side of the vertebral body indicates its contact with the descending aorta. In the midthoracic region, the heads of the ribs form a joint that spans the intervertebral disc. Consequently, the inferior lip of one vertebral body and the corresponding site of the superior lip of the next inferior element share in the formation of a single articular facet for the rib head. Thus, the typical thoracic vertebra bears two hemifacets on each side of its body.

The pedicles project posteriorly from the superior aspect of the vertebral body. Extending dorsomedially from the pedicles are the laminae, which fuse in the midline to form the dorsal wall of the spinal canal.[3]

The mean height of the thoracic pedicles is displayed in Figure 7–3. The mean height from foramen to pedicle was 35 mm. The height was slightly larger on the left side (Fig. 7–4).

On both sides, the intercostal distance between foramina decreased in the midthoracic spine. The distance was greatest in the lower thoracic vertebrae (Fig. 7–5). The mean foramen-vertebral body height was about 34.9 mm, and it tended to increase from T1 to T12 (Fig. 7–6). The foraminal size at each level varied greatly. The mean cross-sectional area of the thoracic intervertebral foramina was largest at the thoracolumbar junction (T12–L1) and smallest at the level of T1–T2. The mean height and width of the neural foramina were about 12.5 mm and 6.5 mm, respectively. There was no gross difference between the two sides (Figs. 7–7 and 7–8).

The shape of each thoracic vertebra was also outlined. Three foraminal shapes were identified: teardrop, auricular, and oval-round. The shapes of the foramina were also examined on radiographs of the spine. Of the 264 foramina examined, 26.6% were round or oval, 58% were auricular, and 17.4% were teardrop shaped (Fig. 7–9).

The articular processes arise from both the superior and inferior surfaces of the laminae. The articulating facets are situated on the posterior surface articular process and the ventral surface of the inferior process. From T1 to T10, the facets are in the coronal plane, thus providing significant resistance to anterior translation. At T11 and T12, the orientation of the facets begins to change to simulate the lumbar pattern (oblique sagittal orientation), where they limit rotation and have less effect on anterior translation.[3,4]

Few detailed studies are available for comparative investigations. Scoles et al.[5] studied the segments of the vertebral body, pedicle, and foramen in the thoracolumbar spine, and Berry et al.[6] performed a morphometric analysis of selected thoracic and lumbar vertebrae (Table 7–1). Bailey et al.[7] studied the anatomic relationship of the cervicothoracic junction and included the area from the upper three thoracic vertebrae. Measurements of the upper three thoracic vertebral bodies, pedicles, and foramina are comparable in each of the studies.

Thoracic Radicular Canal

The term *thoracic radicular canal* refers to the portion of the spinal canal surrounding the thoracic spinal nerve root

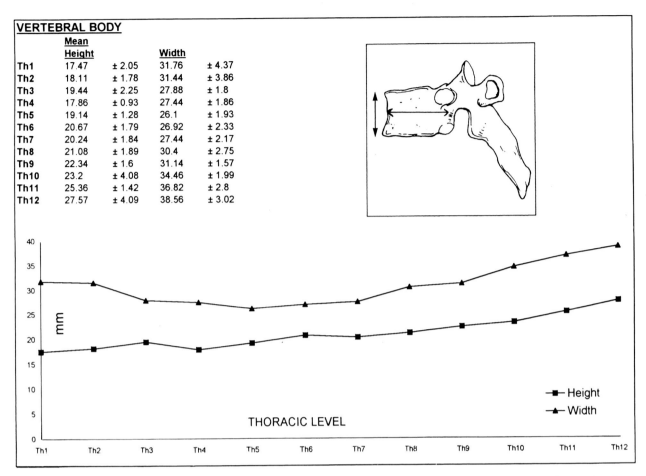

VERTEBRAL BODY

	Mean Height		Width	
Th1	17.47	± 2.05	31.76	± 4.37
Th2	18.11	± 1.78	31.44	± 3.86
Th3	19.44	± 2.25	27.88	± 1.8
Th4	17.86	± 0.93	27.44	± 1.86
Th5	19.14	± 1.28	26.1	± 1.93
Th6	20.67	± 1.79	26.92	± 2.33
Th7	20.24	± 1.84	27.44	± 2.17
Th8	21.08	± 1.89	30.4	± 2.75
Th9	22.34	± 1.6	31.14	± 1.57
Th10	23.2	± 4.08	34.46	± 1.99
Th11	25.36	± 1.42	36.82	± 2.8
Th12	27.57	± 4.09	38.56	± 3.02

Figure 7–2.   The mean height and width of the vertebral bodies as a function of thoracic level. The insert shows the dimensions measured.

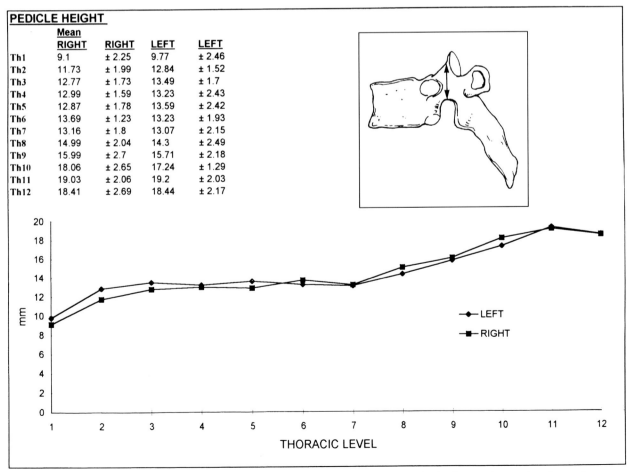

PEDICLE HEIGHT

	Mean RIGHT	RIGHT	LEFT	LEFT
Th1	9.1	± 2.25	9.77	± 2.46
Th2	11.73	± 1.99	12.84	± 1.52
Th3	12.77	± 1.73	13.49	± 1.7
Th4	12.99	± 1.59	13.23	± 2.43
Th5	12.87	± 1.78	13.59	± 2.42
Th6	13.69	± 1.23	13.23	± 1.93
Th7	13.16	± 1.8	13.07	± 2.15
Th8	14.99	± 2.04	14.3	± 2.49
Th9	15.99	± 2.7	15.71	± 2.18
Th10	18.06	± 2.65	17.24	± 1.29
Th11	19.03	± 2.06	19.2	± 2.03
Th12	18.41	± 2.69	18.44	± 2.17

Figure 7–3.   The mean right and left pedicular height as a function of thoracic level. The insert shows the dimension measured.

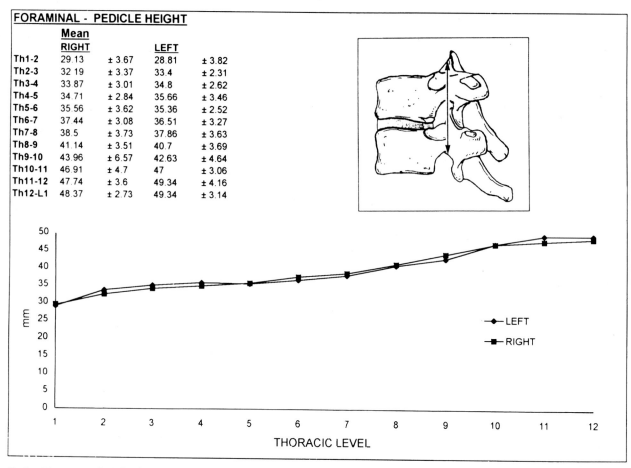

Figure 7–4. The mean height from the foramen to the pedicle on both the right and left sides as a function of thoracic level. The insert shows the dimension measured.

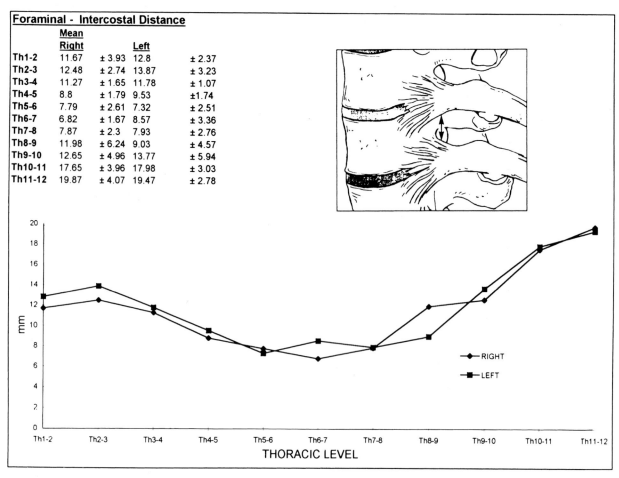

Figure 7–5. The mean intercostal distance between foramina as a function of thoracic level. The insert shows the dimension measured.

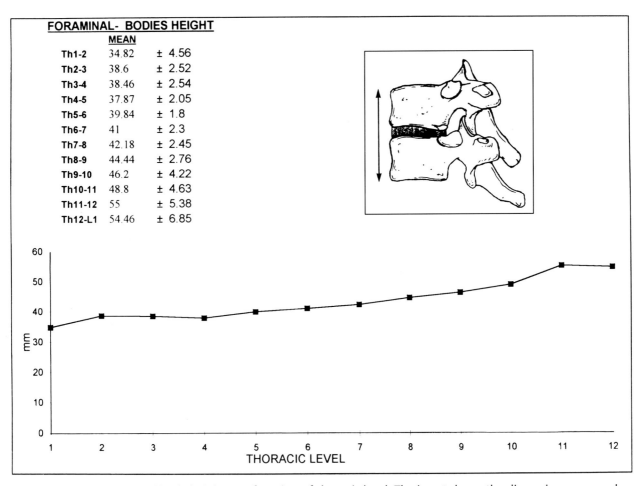

FORAMINAL- BODIES HEIGHT	MEAN	
Th1-2	34.82	± 4.56
Th2-3	38.6	± 2.52
Th3-4	38.46	± 2.54
Th4-5	37.87	± 2.05
Th5-6	39.84	± 1.8
Th6-7	41	± 2.3
Th7-8	42.18	± 2.45
Th8-9	44.44	± 2.76
Th9-10	46.2	± 4.22
Th10-11	48.8	± 4.63
Th11-12	55	± 5.38
Th12-L1	54.46	± 6.85

Figure 7–6. The mean foraminal body height as a function of thoracic level. The insert shows the dimension measured.

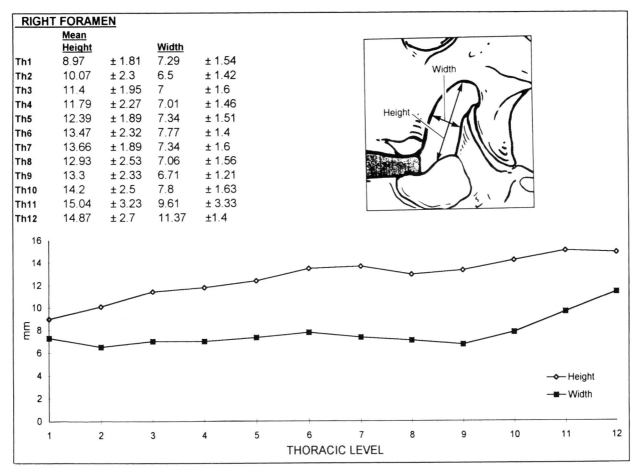

RIGHT FORAMEN	Mean Height		Width	
Th1	8.97	± 1.81	7.29	± 1.54
Th2	10.07	± 2.3	6.5	± 1.42
Th3	11.4	± 1.95	7	± 1.6
Th4	11.79	± 2.27	7.01	± 1.46
Th5	12.39	± 1.89	7.34	± 1.51
Th6	13.47	± 2.32	7.77	± 1.4
Th7	13.66	± 1.89	7.34	± 1.6
Th8	12.93	± 2.53	7.06	± 1.56
Th9	13.3	± 2.33	6.71	± 1.21
Th10	14.2	± 2.5	7.8	± 1.63
Th11	15.04	± 3.23	9.61	± 3.33
Th12	14.87	± 2.7	11.37	±1.4

Figure 7–7. The mean height and width of the right vertebral foramen as a function of thoracic level. The insert shows the dimension measured.

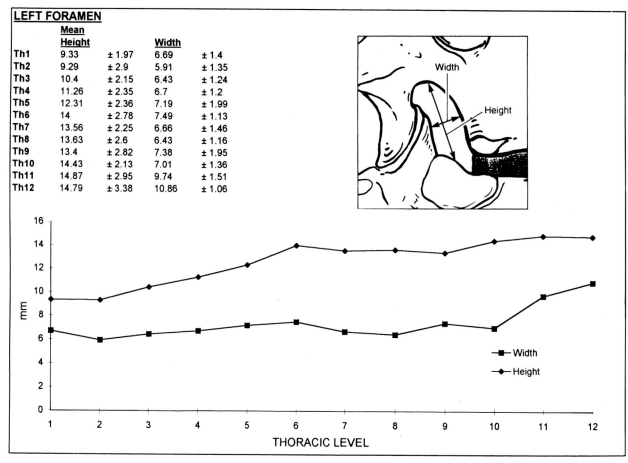

LEFT FORAMEN

	Mean Height		Width	
Th1	9.33	± 1.97	6.69	± 1.4
Th2	9.29	± 2.9	5.91	± 1.35
Th3	10.4	± 2.15	6.43	± 1.24
Th4	11.26	± 2.35	6.7	± 1.2
Th5	12.31	± 2.36	7.19	± 1.99
Th6	14	± 2.78	7.49	± 1.13
Th7	13.56	± 2.25	6.66	± 1.46
Th8	13.63	± 2.6	6.43	± 1.16
Th9	13.4	± 2.82	7.38	± 1.95
Th10	14.43	± 2.13	7.01	± 1.36
Th11	14.87	± 2.95	9.74	± 1.51
Th12	14.79	± 3.38	10.86	± 1.06

Figure 7–8. The mean height and width of the left vertebral foramen as a function of thoracic level. The insert shows the dimension measured.

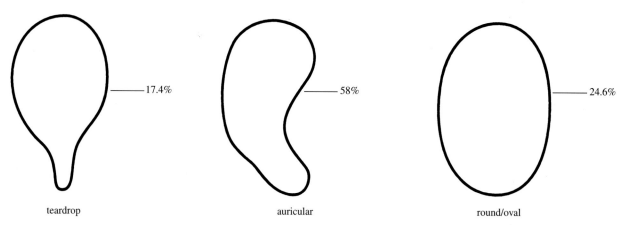

teardrop   ——17.4%

auricular   ——58%

round/oval   ——24.6%

Figure 7–9. Schematic representations of the various shapes of the thoracic vertebral foramina and the frequency with which they occurred in this study.

from its point of emergence through the dural envelope up to its exit from the spinal canal via the intervertebral foramen.[8,9] The radicular canal, resembling a hollow hemicylinder opened toward the midline, can be divided into three parts: the retrodiscal, parapedicular (the lateral recess per se), and the foraminal.[10]

The spinal nerve roots may be compressed by an intervertebral disc herniation and spinal stenosis, leading to a wide range of clinical symptoms. Little, however, is known about the pathophysiology of the nerve tissue involved in

these situations, a fact that is surprising given the extensive literature on the reaction of peripheral nerves to various kinds of trauma.[11–13] The caliber of thoracic nerve roots is much smaller than their corresponding intervertebral foramina, and thus they incompletely fill the foramen. These spinal roots contact the inferior aspect of the *upper* pedicle of the intervertebral foramen during their course through the foramen and thus come to lie above the level of the corresponding intervertebral discs. Each thoracic spinal ganglion is located directly below the corresponding pedicle.

TABLE 7–1   Comparative Measurements of the Thoracic Spine

Vertebral Element		Mean Height (mm)	
Vertebral Body	Present Study		Scoles et al.[5]
T1	17.47 ± 2.05		13.7 − 17.6,* 15.0 − 18.8**
T3	19.44 ± 2.25		15.5 − 19.3,* 16.7 − 20.5**
T6	20.67 ± 1.79		16.0 − 21.4,* 16.9 − 21.9**
T9	22.34 ± 1.60		18.4 − 22.0,* 19.5 − 27.8**
T12	27.57 ± 4.09		22.0 − 27.9,* 23.8 − 28.8**
Pedicle	Present Study		Berry et al.[6]
T2	11.73 ± 1.99,[†] 12.84 ± 1.52[‡]		11.7 ± 1.2,[†] 11.9 ± 1.3[‡]
T7	13.16 ± 1.80,[†] 13.07 ± 2.15[‡]		12.1 ± 1.0,[†] 11.9 ± 1.0[‡]
T12	18.41 ± 2.69,[†] 18.44 ± 2.17[‡]		17.2 ± 1.6,[†] 17.0 ± 1.3[‡]
Pedicle	Present Study		Scoles et al.[5]
T1	9.1 ± 2.25,[†] 9.77 ± 2.46[‡]		6.4 − 10.8,* 7.9 − 10.4**
T4	12.99 ± 1.59,[†] 13.23 ± 2.43[‡]		8.3 − 12.1,* 9.3 − 15.2**
T6	13.69 ± 1.23,[†] 13.23 ± 1.93[‡]		8.3 − 12.1,* 9.3 − 15.2**
T9	15.99 ± 2.7,[†] 15.71 ± 2.18[‡]		9.6 − 14.9,* 10.1 − 16.9**
T12	18.41 ± 2.69,[†] 18.44 ± 2.17[‡]		12.2 − 17.2,* 17.2 − 20.2**

Range in females* and males**; [†] = right; [‡] = left.

The course of the nerve differs according to the thoracic level. The course of the upper thoracic roots is upward. The middle thoracic roots lie in a horizontal plane, and the lower thoracic roots are clearly directed downward within the upper part of the intervertebral foramina.[3]

In the thoracic vertebral canal, the nerve roots are horizontal and emerge from the center of the intervertebral foramina. The spinal nerve runs flattened against the hollow of the gutter. Its anterior and posterior nerve roots join together distal to the spinal ganglion lying at the level of the intervertebral foramen. The foramina are covered laterally by a fascial sheet, which is part of the anterior layer of the thoracolumbar fascia. Usually, there are two oval perforations in the fascia—a distal one for the nerve root and a smaller proximal one for the blood vessels (Fig. 7–10). The overall shape of the radicular canal is that of a medially concave gutter running vertically or slightly obliquely downward and backward. This gutter widens at its lower end along a sagittal arch with an inferior concavity (i.e., the intervertebral foramen).

The intervertebral foramen is bounded rostrally by the inferior vertebral notch of the pedicle of the superior vertebra. The floor is the superior vertebral notch of the pedicle of the inferior vertebra. The anterior border is formed by the posterior aspect of the adjacent vertebral bodies and intervertebral disc, the lateral expansion of the posterior longitudinal ligament, and the anterior longitudinal venous sinus. Posteriorly lie the superior articular process of the inferior vertebra and the inferior articular process of the superior vertebra, covered by the articular capsule into which blends the lateral prolongation of the ligamentum flavum. The dural sleeve with its emerging nerve root is medial and the fascial sheet and psoas muscle are lateral. The foramen contains the nerve root and the sinuvertebral nerve anteroposteriorly as well as scattered sympathetic

fibers. The intervertebral arteries and veins as well as numerous small lymphatic vessels traverse the fatty areolar network that fills the foramen.

In most cases, the transforaminal ligaments grossly diminished the space available for the emerging nerve root. These ligaments were easily distinguished from the fibrous covering. The width and thickness of these strong and unyielding ligaments ranged from 2 to 5 mm. Six types of transforaminal ligaments were noted and were anatomically designated as (1) the superior corporopedicular ligament, (2) the inferior corporopedicular ligament, (3) the superior transforaminal ligament, (4) the midtransforaminal ligament, (5) the inferior transforaminal ligament, and (6) the suspensor radial ligament (Fig. 7–11).

The superior corporopedicular ligament runs from the superior pedicle and vertebral notch obliquely, anteriorly and inferiorly to the posterolateral aspect of the vertebral body and adjacent annulus. The inferior corporopedicular ligament runs from the inferior pedicle and vertebral notch obliquely, superiorly and anteriorly to the posterolateral aspect of the vertebral body and adjacent annulus. The superior transforaminal ligament runs from the articular capsule and posterior vertebral notch obliquely, superiorly to the superior pedicle. The midtransforaminal ligament extends from the articular capsule across the midforamen to the annulus and superior corporopedicular and inferior corporopedicular ligaments. The inferior transforaminal ligament extends from the superior facet, across the superior vertebral notch to the junction of the annulus and vertebral body. In contrast, the suspensor radial ligaments extend around the ligaments to the nerve root.

As early as 1911, Bailey and Casamajor identified radicular compression with a bony origin.[14] In 1934, Mixter and Barr related compression to the rupture of an intervertebral disc.[9] Epstein et al. first emphasized the importance of this

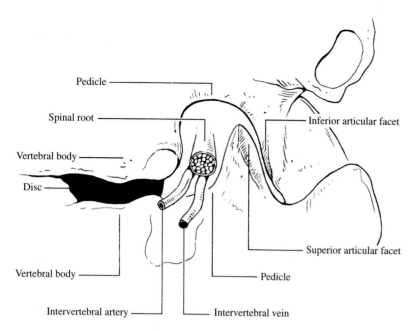

Pedicle

Spinal root

Vertebral body

Disc

Vertebral body

Intervertebral artery — Intervertebral vein

Inferior articular facet

Superior articular facet

Pedicle

Figure 7–10. Cross section of a thoracic spine foramen showing the neurovascular bundle.

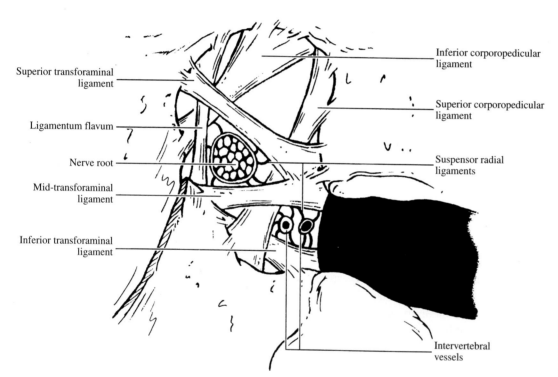

Superior transforaminal ligament

Ligamentum flavum

Nerve root

Mid-transforaminal ligament

Inferior transforaminal ligament

Inferior corporopedicular ligament

Superior corporopedicular ligament

Suspensor radial ligaments

Intervertebral vessels

Figure 7–11. The various intervertebral foraminal ligaments found at all levels of the thoracic spine.

region of the spinal canal by recognizing articular hypertrophy as a main cause of spinal nerve root compression.[10] Golub and Silverman reported the appearance and anatomical location of lumbar transforaminal ligaments analogous to the costovertebral ligaments in the thoracic spine.[15] Rausching illustrated intraforaminal ligaments in a cross-sectional cryomicrotomic study of the lumbar spine, but did not indicate the frequency of the ligaments at each level.[16]

The detailed anatomy of the transforaminal ligaments in the thoracic region has not been described systematically. However, a comparative study on lumbar foraminal ligaments suggests that fibrous ligaments have been identified. Nowicki and Haughton found that the most constant liga-

ment was the fibrous band behind the annulus fibrous.[17] Distinct from the latter, the band originated from one vertebral body and inserted on the next. The ligaments connecting the posterior disc margin and superior articular process were found in 48% of the neural foramina. Three other distinct types of ligaments were found less often.[17]

An earlier study on lumbar transforaminal ligaments by Golub and Silverman was more detailed and elaborate.[15] They easily diminished these transforaminal ligaments from the fibrous tissue. In most of their cases, the transforaminal ligaments grossly diminished the space available for the emerging nerve root. Five major types of transforaminal ligaments were identified and designated according to their anatomical relationship: (1) corporotransverse superior, (2) corporotransverse inferior, (3) superior transforaminal, (4) midtransforaminal, and (5) inferior transforaminal. These lumbar transforaminal ligaments are comparable to those identified in our study of the thoracic region.

CLINICAL AND SURGICAL APPLICATIONS

The primary structural functions of the thoracic spine are to ensure proper pulmonary ventilation and to protect the heart by adaptations of the deformable thoracic cage. The mobility of the thoracic spine is relatively low because of the attachment of the ribs, the decreased height of the discs, and the orientation of the articular surfaces. From T1 to T12, flexion and extension ranges from 4° to 12°, lateral bending from 6° to 9°, and axial rotation from 9° to 2°.

The supple anterior junction of the ribs through the costal cartilage further increases the elasticity of the thorax and strengthens its resistance to deforming pressures applied to the cartilage. Calculations of the stiffness of the entire thoracic spine and the thoracic cage have demonstrated that stiffness increases because of the presence of the ribs and sternum (30% during flexion and axial rotation, 50% during lateral bending, and 110% during flexion and extension).[18] Ablation of the sternum completely suppresses this effect. Thoracic spinal stiffness also decreases in cases of severe scoliosis, severe thoracic deformity from lateral flexion, and rotation of the vertebral bodies. These conditions also produce severe respiratory insufficiency.[19]

Furthermore, the mobility of the thoracic region is not uniform throughout its length. The upper segment resembles the cervical vertebrae in respect to the size of the bodies and the discs. The ribs attached to the sternum greatly diminish the range of motion. Flexion and extension become freer in the lower thoracic region where the size of the discs and the vertebral bodies progressively increases. Variations in morphology, however, are common, and congenital malformations, previous infection, trauma, and operative procedures can further distort the normal anatomy. Despite the surgical challenges represented by the thoracic spine and surrounding structures, thoracoscopic vertebrectomies and reconstructions of the thoracic spine are possible.[20]

The nerve root complex is not static. When the spine and the extremities move, the spinal nerves and nerve roots adapt to changes in the position of the spine by stretching and slackening, and the nerves move within the intervertebral foramina.[11,21] The nerve roots, however, are surrounded by cerebrospinal fluid, which may act in conjunction with the dura and arachnoid membranes to protect the nerve roots mechanically.[14]

The first step in the management of various diseases of the spinal cord is to identify the precise anatomical location of the pathology. The cornerstone of achieving excel-lent outcomes after spinal surgery is an astute and accurate clinical assessment of the exact anatomical location of the pathology causing the dysfunction.

Compression of the nerve roots and spinal cord is mainly caused by disc herniations, fractured bone fragments, neoplasms, and congenital spinal abnormalities. Compression may deform the nerve fibers, mainly at the edges of the compressed nerve segment.[22] The ultrastructural appearance of such deformation was first described by Ochoa et al., who found that the nodes of Ranvier were displaced toward the uncompressed parts of the nerve at both the proximal and distal edges of the compressed nerve segment.[11] The nodal displacement was followed by segmental demyelination of the compressed portion of the nerve. Nerve conduction was blocked at this site.[22,23] These and other studies indicate that compression mainly affects large diameter myelinated fibers.[12,13] The nature of a nerve root lesion associated with a herniated nucleus pulposus that compressed the root is probably mixed. Some nerve fibers likely show local demyelination and some fibers likely undergo Wallerian degeneration.[8] Successful surgical outcomes in most of these cases involve removal of the offending compressive pathology.

The instability that follows spinal trauma is a common source of neurological dysfunction and is usually managed by surgical stabilization or bracing to restore function and prevent further deterioration. Rosenthal et al. have described anterior decompression and stabilization in the management of metastatic tumors of the thoracic spine using microsurgical endoscopic techniques.[24] Management of spinal instability from degenerative, neoplastic, or congenital diseases requires a thorough knowledge of anatomy of the spine.

Knowledge of the detailed anatomy of the neurovascular complex of the spinal cord is helpful in diagnosing and treating ischemic complications of the spinal cord. The axonal transport systems and energy-demanding mechanisms that fuel the spinal cord can be blocked by local ischemia and compression.[25] Interference with the axonal transport systems can lead to changes in the normal structure and function of distal nerve fibers as well as in synaptic transmission at neuromuscular junctions. The effects of compression on axonal transport in peripheral nerves have been investigated by Rydevik et al.[25]

Nerve fibers react to trauma with demyelination or axonal degeneration, which leads to changes in nerve function. The impairment of intraneural microcirculation and the formation of intraneural edema are also important factors underlying functional deterioration. In cases of chronic compression, intra- and extraneural fibrosis can develop, leading to further tissue irritation and the establishment of a chronic inflammatory process. Loss of nerve function, manifested as muscle weakness or sensory deficits, can occur. The nerve tissue can also become hyperexcitable. These two conditions can be present simultaneously. In other words, the conduction velocity of nerve fibers at the site of injury may be decreased while the injured segment is still hypersensitive to further mechanical stimulation.[8]

CONCLUSION

A successful clinical evaluation based on a clear understanding of anatomy allows clinicians to identify the anatomic locus of spinal pathology that is causing the dysfunction. Having ascertained this information, clinicians can then plan a specific program of treatment that optimizes the chance of attaining a positive patient outcome. Instrumentation of the thoracic spine continues to grow at a rapid pace. With the advent of neuroendoscopy, thoracic spinal surgery can be even less traumatic for patients. If surgeons are to practice these techniques successfully, they need to master the anatomy of the thoracic spine.

REFERENCES

1. Louis R: *Surgery of the Spine*. Berlin: Springer-Verlag; 1983:26–34.
2. Williams PL, Warwick R, Dyson M, et al: *Gray's Anatomy*, 37th ed. New York: Churchill Livingstone; 1989:319–322, 496–497.
3. Louis R: Topographic relationships of the vertebral column, spinal cord. *Anatomica Clinica* 1978; 1:3–12, 141–145.
4. Maiman DJ, Pintar FA: Anatomy and clinical biomechanics of the thoracic spine. *Clin Neurosurg* 1992; 38:296–324.
5. Scoles PV, Linton AE, Latimer B, et al: Vertebral body and posterior element morphology: The normal spine in middle life. *Spine* 1988; 13(10):1082–1086.
6. Berry JL, Moran JM, Berg WS, et al: A morphometric study of human lumbar and selected thoracic vertebrae. *Spine* 1987; 12(4):362–367.
7. Bailey AS, Stanescu S, Yeasting RA, et al: Anatomic relationships of the cervicothoracic junction. *Spine* 1995; 20(13):1431–1439.
8. Rydevik B, Brown MD, Lundborg G: Pathoanatomy and pathophysiology of nerve root compression. *Spine* 1984; 9(1):7–15.
9. Mixter WJ, Barr JB: Rupture of intervertebral disc with involvement of the spinal canal. *N Engl J Med* 1934; 211:210–215.
10. Epstein JA, Epstein BS, Lavine LS, et al: Lumbar nerve root compression at the intervertebral foramina caused by arthritis of the posterior facets. *J Neurosurg* 1973; 39(3):362–369.
11. Ochoa J, Fowler TJ, Gilliatt RW: Anatomical changes in peripheral nerves compressed by a pneumatic tourniquet. *J Anat* 1972; 113(3):433–455.
12. Seddon H: *Surgical Disorders of the Peripheral Nerves*. Edinburgh: Churchill Livingstone; 1972:32–56.
13. Sunderland S: *Nerves and Nerve Injuries*, 2nd ed. Edinburgh: Churchill Livingstone; 1978.
14. Bailey P, Casamajor L: Osteo-arthritis of the spine as a cause of compression of the spinal cord and its roots, with reports of five cases. *Nerv Ment Dis* 1911; 38:588–609.
15. Golub BS, Silverman B: Transforaminal ligaments of the lumbar spine. *J Bone Joint Surg Am* 1969; 51(5):947–956.
16. Rausching W: Normal and pathologic anatomy of the lumbar root canals. *Spine* 1987; 12(10):1008–1019.
17. Nowicki BH, Haughton VM: Ligaments of the lumbar neural foramina: A sectional anatomic study. *Clin Anat* 1992; 5:126–135.
18. Panjabi MM, Krag MH, Dimnet JC, et al: Thoracic spine centers of rotation in the sagittal plane. *J Orthop Res* 1984; 1(4):387–394.
19. Breig A, Marions O: Biomechanics of the lumbosacral nerve roots. *Acta Radiol (Stockh)* 1963; 1:1141–1160.
20. Dickman CA, Rosenthal D, Karahalios DG, et al: Thoracic vertebrectomy and reconstruction using a microsurgical thoracoscopic approach. *Neurosurgery* 1996; 38(2):279–293.
21. Goddard MD, Reede JD: Movements induced by straight leg raising in the lumbo-sacral roots, nerves and plexus and intra-pelvic section of the sciatic nerve. *J Neurol Neurosurg Psychiatry* 1965; 28:12–18.
22. Fowler TJ, Danta G, Gilliatt RW: Recovery of nerve conduction after a pneumatic tourniquet: Observations on the hind-limb of the baboon. *J Neurol Neurosurg Psychiatry* 1972; 35(5):638–647.
23. Ochs S, Worth RM: Axoplasmic transport in normal and pathological systems. In Waxman S, ed: *Physiology and Pathobiology of Axons*. New York: Raven; 1978:48–61.
24. Rosenthal D, Marquardt G, Lorenz R, et al: Anterior decompression and stabilization using a microsurgical endoscopic technique for metastatic tumors of the thoracic spine. *J Neurosurg* 1996; 84(4):565–572.
25. Rydevik B, Mclean WG, Sjostrand J, et al: Blockage of axonal transport induced by acute, graded compression of the rabbit vagus nerve. *J Neurol Neurosurg Psychiatry* 1980; 43(8):690–698.

CHAPTER **8**

Anesthetic Considerations for Thoracoscopic Spine Surgery

Volker Lischke, M.D., Paul Kessler, M.D., Klaus Westphal, M.D., and Gerhard Matheis, M.D.

Video-assisted thoracoscopic surgery has been used extensively by cardiothoracic surgeons to treat a variety of diseases of the thoracic cavity. The minimal incisional approach using the microsurgical endoscopic technique has been associated with substantial clinical benefits when compared with the standard thoracotomy. The progress achieved in thoracic surgery has been applied to treat abnormalities affecting the anterior thoracic spine. However, new techniques, such as the microsurgical approach to the thoracic spine, confront the anesthetist with new problems, such as an extremely lengthy period of single-lung ventilation. We therefore describe our anesthetic methods and experience with the first group of patients who underwent the new microsurgical endoscopic technique in our hospital.

PREOPERATIVE EVALUATION AND PREPARATION

In addition to routine assessment for major surgery, the preoperative evaluation of patients for microsurgical thoracoscopic neurosurgery should focus on the extent and severity of pulmonary disease and cardiovascular involvement. Most patients with protruding thoracic discs have healthy respiratory and cardiovascular systems. Patients with metastatic tumors of the thoracic spine, however, are often at high risk because their pulmonary or cardiac function is compromised. They may also have coagulation disorders.

In a typical physical examination, patients are evaluated for cyanosis, respiratory rate and pattern, and breath sounds. When thoracoscopy is contemplated, cardiovascular and pulmonary function should also be evaluated. Arterial blood gases should be analyzed, and laboratory studies, electrocardiography, and chest radiography should be performed.

On the day before surgery, hemoglobin, hematocrit, platelets, serum chemistries (Na^+, K^+, Ca^{++}), and coagulation parameters [prothrombin time (PT), partial thromboplastin time (PTT)] should be evaluated. An appropriate amount of "packed red cells" (RBC) should be cross typed.

Beginning at 10:00 P.M. the day before surgery, our patients receive nothing by mouth. They are usually premedicated with diazepam (10 mg by mouth) the evening before surgery and receive midazolam (7.5 mg by mouth) 1 hour before the induction of anesthesia.

PREPARATION FOR ANESTHESIA AND INTRAOPERATIVE MONITORING

Upon arrival in the operating room, all patients undergo continuous electrocardiographic monitoring for heart rate. Pulse oximetry (PO_2), noninvasive blood pressure, and rectal temperature are also monitored.

Before induction of anesthesia, at least one large-bore intravenous line is placed in a forearm vein. For continuous beat-to-beat measurement of arterial blood pressure, an indwelling arterial line (20-gauge Teflon catheter) is placed in the nondominant hand under local anesthesia after adequate collateral circulation has been determined by Allen's test. During both double-lung and single-lung ventilation with the patient in the lateral decubitus position, the arterial line is also used for serial analysis of arterial blood gases.

In addition to the measurement of arterial blood gases, the normal ventilation during double-lung and single-lung ventilation should be confirmed using continuous capnography. The end-tidal CO_2 concentration represents alveolar CO_2, which approximates arterial CO_2 concentration. Normally, there is only a small arterial-to-alveolar CO_2 gradient, depending on the alveolar dead space. The capnogram may be very helpful in diagnosing an airway obstruction, incomplete relaxation, and malpositioning of the double-lumen tube. To detect a malpositioned double-lumen tube, a capnograph is coupled to each port of the double-lumen endotracheal tube. A decrease in end-tidal CO_2 from one lumen of the double-lumen tube suggests that the tube has been malpositioned. Its position should be verified by fiberoptic bronchoscopy. CO_2 is 20 times more diffusible than oxygen, and arterial CO_2 concentration is more dependent on ventilation than the arterial concentration of O_2. Therefore, systemic hypercarbia during single-lung ventilation is a smaller problem than systemic hypoxemia.

The maintenance of neuromuscular blockade is monitored with train-of-four stimulation.

After the induction of anesthesia, one or two additional large-bore intravenous lines are placed for rapid intraoperative volume substitution with colloids, RBCs, or fresh frozen plasma if necessary.

When we first performed thoracoscopic spinal procedures, a pulmonary artery catheter was placed in every patient via the right internal jugular vein for continuous intraoperative hemodynamic monitoring during single-lung ventilation. The pulmonary artery catheter allowed measurement of left-sided cardiac filling pressures, determination of cardiac output by thermodilution, and calculation of derived hemodynamic and respiratory parameters (e.g., systemic and pulmonary vascular resistance and intrapulmonary shunt). Using cross-table radiography, we positioned the pulmonary artery catheter in the west zone 3 of the dependent lung. Currently, we use a central venous catheter rather than a pulmonary artery catheter in most cases.

A double-lumen central venous catheter is inserted via the right jugular vein. Central venous pressure is measured continuously as an indicator of right arterial and right ventricular pressure and to monitor blood volume and venous tone. If it is impossible to insert the pulmonary artery catheter or the central venous catheter via the right internal jugular vein, we puncture the subclavian vein of the nondependent thoracic side (i.e., the side of the operation). If a pneumothorax develops, it can be treated by placing a chest tube intraoperatively. The position of the central venous catheters is verified using in-line electrocardiography or cross-table radiography.

In all patients, a Foley catheter is placed in the bladder to monitor renal function intraoperatively. To verify correct single-lung ventilation, arterial blood gases are analyzed every 30 minutes. Hemoglobin, hematocrit, platelets, serum chemistries (Na^+, K^+, Ca^{++}), and coagulation parameters (PT and PTT) are analyzed hourly.

INTUBATION AND MAINTENANCE OF ANESTHESIA

For intravenous induction of anesthesia, we use an opioid and a hypnotic agent and facilitate intubation with a muscle relaxant.

In the past, we used fentanyl or sufentanil as an opioid for induction and maintenance of anesthesia. With sufentanil, most patients could be primarily extubated because respiratory depression at the end of anesthesia was minimal. In contrast, most patients treated with fentanyl had to be ventilated after surgery and required intensive care. In association with this minimally invasive technique, the new opioid remifentanil may be superior to other opioids because it avoids postoperative respiratory depression. Thiopental as well as etomidate, midazolam, or propofol in normal dosage can be used equally as hypnotic agents for induction of anesthesia, depending more on the maintenance of anesthesia than on the patient's profile. Especially in the beginning of our experience with microsurgical endoscopic techniques and because of potentially long durations of single-lung ventilation, we hesitated to use inhaled anesthetics because of depression of hypoxic pulmonary vasoconstriction by these agents. We therefore primarily used a total-intravenous-anesthetic technique (TIVA) with propofol and sufentanil or fentanyl for most patients using oxygen in air for ventilation.

As our experience with thoracoscopic spinal procedures increased, we started to use a combination (COM) of intravenous-anesthetic techniques using propofol in conjunction with lower concentrations of isoflurane (<1 minimal alveolar concentration) in oxygen and air. We found no significant difference in the oxygenation index (the actual arterial PaO_2 from arterial blood gases divided by inspiratory FiO_2) or other hemodynamic parameters (measured or calculated from pulmonary artery catheter) in patients anesthetized with TIVA or COM. Consequently, we consecutively anesthetized a group of patients primarily with the volatile anesthetic isoflurane, ventilated with oxygen in air, and measured the oxygenation index as well as pulmonary artery catheter-derived parameters. There were no significant differences in the oxygenation index or other hemodynamic parameters between this group and the groups anesthetized with TIVA or COM. We discovered that even when single-lung ventilation lasted as long as 11 hours (695 minutes), patients could be safely anesthetized with TIVA as well as with COM or isoflurane. The suitability of newer volatile anesthetics for these procedures remains to be investigated.

To facilitate intubation with the double-lumen tube, we previously used succinylcholine followed by additional doses of atracurium or continuous infusion of atracurium monitored with train-of-four stimulation. Later, we also used atracurium or vecuronium as a primary agent to facilitate intubation and to maintain neuromuscular blockade during the whole procedure.

Lung Deflation

Single-lung ventilation is essential for performing thoracoscopic spinal surgery. Single-lung ventilation can be accomplished using either a double-lumen endobronchial tube or a bronchial blocker. A double-lumen endotracheal tube, however, is preferred.

Bronchial blockers are placed with the help of a fiberoptic bronchoscope and directed to the nonventilated lung. Inflation of the cuff at the distal end of the blocker stops ventilation of the ipsilateral lung. The lumen of the blocker permits suctioning of the airway distal to the catheter tip. Depending on the clinical situation, oxygen can be insufflated through the catheter lumen. This technique is useful in achieving selective ventilation in smaller patients (i.e., pediatric patients), for whom a normal double-lumen tube may be too large. However, because the blocker balloon requires a high distending pressure, it easily slips out of the bronchus into the trachea, thus obstructing ventilation. This life-threatening situation can occur after changes in body position or surgical manipulations. Consequently, we do not routinely use bronchial blockers.

We prefer disposable double-lumen endotracheal tubes, mostly the Robert Shaw left-sided type. This tube has the advantages of a large diameter, D-shaped lumen that makes suctioning easy. It also offers low resistance to gas flow. A fixed curvature facilitates proper positioning and reduces the possibility of kinking. We *always* prefer left-sided tubes independent of the thoracic side of operation because they prevent occlusion of the right upper lobe.

After the cuff of the double-lumen endotracheal tube has been checked for leakage, the stylet is lubricated and the tube is inserted with the distal concave curvature facing anteriorly. After the tip of the tube is inserted past the vocal cords, the stylet is removed and the tube is rotated 90° to the left side. It is important to remove the stylet before rotating and advancing the tube to prevent bronchial lacerations. The endotracheal tube is advanced into the left main stem bronchus until a moderate resistance to further passage is encountered. This resistance indicates that the tip of the tube has been firmly seated in the main stem bronchus. After the tube is positioned correctly, the tracheal cuff should be inflated and the thorax auscultated for equal ventilation of both lungs. If the sound of the right lung is not equal to the left side, the tube was probably inserted too far down the left main stem bronchus, causing the right main stem bronchus to be occluded by the cuff. In this case, the tube must be withdrawn gently after the tracheal cuff is deflated.

After the position of the endotracheal tube has been verified, the patient is ventilated through the left main stem lumen while the right lumen is disconnected. The bronchial cuff is slowly inflated to prevent an air leak from the lumen around the bronchial cuff into the trachea. To ensure that the left-sided bronchial cuff does not obstruct the contralateral hemithorax, both lungs are ventilated through both lumens of the tube while both cuffs are inflated. Each side is selectively clamped and auscultated for the absence of breath sounds on the ipsilateral side while the contralateral side is ventilated. It should have a clear breath sound and a normal capnographic curve. Normally, with a peak inspiratory airway pressure around 20 cm H_2O during double-lung ventilation, the peak airway pressure should not exceed 40 cm H_2O during single-lung ventilation with the same tidal volume.

After the position of the double-lumen endotracheal tube has been checked clinically, we also always verify the position of the tube with fiber-optic bronchoscopy using a 3.6-mm diameter bronchoscope. With a left-sided double-lumen tube, the bronchoscope is first introduced into the trachea, the carina is visualized, and the bronchial cuff is checked for herniation into the trachea. This part is easily identified during bronchoscopy because it is blue. Next, the bronchoscope is inserted into the bronchial lumen of the tube and the left upper lobe orifice is identified.

The position of the double-lumen tube needs to be verified after each change in the patient's position to ensure correct ventilation, especially after patients are positioned in the stable lateral decubitus position. Therefore, the fiber-optic bronchoscope *must* be available during the entire operation.

VENTILATION

Double-lung ventilation and single-lung ventilation are performed with a Cicero® anesthesia machine (Draeger, Lübeck, Germany), which allows manual as well as controlled or synchronized intermittent mandatory ventilation. During double-lung ventilation in the lateral decubitus position, a larger fraction of the tidal volume goes to the nondependent lung, which has reduced perfusion. A smaller fraction of the tidal volume reaches the dependent lung, which receives better perfusion. This significant ventilation-perfusion mismatch increases by a reduction in the functional residual capacity during anesthesia.

Typically, we use a tidal volume of 10 to 12 ml/kg with an inspiratory oxygen concentration of 50% in air to prevent atelectasis in the dependent lung as well as to reduce the transpulmonary shunt significantly. The respiratory rate is adjusted to maintain end-tidal CO_2 between 35 and 38 mm Hg. Approximately 30 minutes into double-lung ventilation in a lateral decubitus position, we always analyze arterial blood gases and correct the controlled ventilation with regard to the analyzed values. With this regimen, in our department, a median oxygenation index of 410.75 (range: 166.85–861.82) was calculated in 82 patients anesthetized in the lateral decubitus position for microsurgical thoracoscopic spinal surgery.

During single-lung ventilation in a lateral decubitus position, the dependent lung is also ventilated with a tidal volume of 10 to 20 ml/kg. If peak inspiratory airway pressure exceeds 30 mm H_2O, we typically decrease tidal volume while increasing the respiratory rate to a frequency of 14 to 16 cycles/minutes.

Single-lung ventilation creates an *obligatory* right-to-left-transpulmonary shunt through the nonventilated, nondependent lung, where the ventilation-perfusion ratio is zero. However, because of the hypoxic pulmonary vasoconstriction in the nondependent lung, the total shunt during single-lung ventilation in the lateral decubitus position is approximately 30%. Because of general anesthesia, paralysis, intraabdominal pressure, compression by the weight of mediastinal structures, and the patient's position on the operating table, the functional residual capacity is reduced. Due to the risk of absorption atelectasis, the accumulation of secretions, and the formation of transudate in the dependent lung, ventilation of this lung is further impaired. Therefore, a low ventilation-perfusion ratio results in a large alveolar-to-arterial O_2 gradient.

As expected, the oxygenation index always significantly decreased during the initiation of single-lung ventilation to a minimum approximately 60 minutes after the onset of single-lung ventilation in a lateral decubitus position. This decrease may reflect absorption atelectasis in connection with a high oxygen concentration. However, as the duration of single-lung ventilation increased, the oxygenation index continuously and significantly increased to a maximum approximately 300 minutes after the onset of single-lung ventilation. This increase in the oxygenation index during the later phase of single-lung ventilation was independent of the kind of anesthesia (TIVA, COM, or isoflurane) used—there were no significant differences between groups. Consequently, we were unable to verify the previously described depression of hypoxic pulmonary vasoconstriction by volatile anesthetics.

At the end of the thoracoscopic spinal procedure, double-lung ventilation is reestablished and the previously collapsed lung is completely reexpanded by manual ventilation with elevated peak inspiratory pressures and increased inspiratory flow. After double-lung ventilation is reestablished, the oxygenation index typically is expected to increase markedly after 30 minutes. Peak inspiratory airway pressure *always* increases during single-lung ventilation. This elevated peak inspiratory airway pressure decreases after double-lung ventilation has been reestablished, returning to its normal level (i.e., its level before single-lung ventilation was instituted).

Although its use is reported in the literature, we never had to apply continuous positive airway pressure on the nondependent lung. A continuous positive airway pressure of 5 to 10 cm H_2O by insufflation of oxygen under positive pressure induced by a pressure relief valve keeps the nondependent lung quiet and prevents it from collapsing completely. Therefore, continuous positive airway pressure on the nondependent lung seems to be superior to a positive expiratory pressure on the dependent lung.

Volume Therapy During Operation

To maintain hemodynamic stability and renal function intraoperatively as well as to substitute pre- and intraoperative volume deficiency, we infuse 6 to 8 ml/kg/hour of crystalloids, primarily Ringer's lactate solution. In cases of mild hemodynamic instability from moderate bleeding, we substitute the volume deficiency with 500 to 1000 ml of the colloid hetastarch.

Increased blood loss, with hemoglobin levels significantly below 10 mg/ml, requires an intraoperative transfusion of RBCs. If a significant intraoperative transfusion of RBCs is needed, we also substitute fresh frozen plasma. Platelets are given when blood platelet counts are below 60,000–70,000 platelets/mm^3. With this regimen, we obtain adequate diuresis. Inadequate urine production is treated with volume replacement and with dopamine (3 μg/kg/minute) to increase renal perfusion.

POSTOPERATIVE CARE

At the end of the operation, the surgeon inspects the mediastinal contents and evaluates the lungs for air leaks. One or two chest tubes are placed through thoracoscopic portals and positioned using direct visualization with the thoracoscope. If necessary, the chest tubes are connected to 20 cm H_2O of suction. Chest tubes are left in place for full-lung expansion, which is verified by chest radiographs. The tubes can also be used to drain fluid from the chest.

Depending on the operative procedure and their hemodynamic and respiratory status, patients are usually extubated primarily and transferred to the recovery room while a nurse supervised by the anesthesiologist on call monitors heart rate, PO_2, and noninvasive blood pressure. Patients are transferred to a neurosurgical ward under stable hemodynamic and respiratory conditions after a few hours.

If the patient's status, especially respiratory status, is critical or unstable, the double-lumen tube is removed, and the patient is reintubated using normal endotracheal tubes for further double-lung ventilation. When reintubation is necessary, most patients are transferred to the neurosurgical intensive care unit. Provided that no further complications arise, patients are discharged from the hospital or transferred to an aftercare hospital within a week.

Problems

Most patients who have surgery for herniated thoracic discs are healthy (ASA-class I–II). In this group of patients, the microsurgical endoscopic approach to the thoracic spine is as challenging for the anesthesiologist as other thoracic surgery procedures. Thoracoscopic spinal surgery typically requires several hours of single-lung ventilation, which is longer than the duration of single-lung ventilation for thoracic procedures. In our opinion, patients with respiratory insufficiency or multisystem organ failure should be excluded from this procedure. Individuals with severe cardiac disease, anemia, or coagulopathies are at much greater risk for severe intraoperative bleeding, hemodynamic instability, and death. If an intraoperative complication were to occur, the surgeon and anesthesiologist should always be prepared to convert to a conventional thoracotomy.

CONCLUSION

The minimal incisional approach using microsurgical endoscopic technique provides a viable alternative to thoracotomy for thoracic spine procedures. Because of its technical complexity and sophisticated demands for providing intraoperative single-lung ventilation for several hours, thoracoscopy demands a maximum effort from the anesthesiologist.

CHAPTER **9**

Anesthetic Management and Intraoperative Monitoring

Paul W. Detwiler, M.S., M.D., Randall W. Porter, M.D., Michael Lemole, M.D., and Steven Shedd, M.D.

R ecent advances in thoracoscopic instruments and minimally invasive thoracoscopy have facilitated approaches to the anterior spinal column and spinal cord.[1–5] For the most part, anesthetic considerations are the same as those associated with a thoracotomy. The patient's cardiopulmonary history and examination should be emphasized and the neurosurgical preoperative evaluation conducted as it would be for any other neurosurgical procedure. Intraoperative management, although not complicated, usually requires single-lung ventilation with a double-lumen endotracheal tube. Spinal cord function is routinely monitored by recording somatosensory evoked potentials (SSEPs) or motor evoked potentials (MEPs), an emerging technology that permits neurophysiological assessment of the anterior spinal cord. Postoperative care focuses on the patient's cardiac and respiratory function, and the need for intensive care unit (ICU) monitoring is determined by the patient's medical history, intraoperative course, and degree of surgical manipulation.

PREOPERATIVE EVALUATION

Patients who undergo thoracoscopic surgery range from uncomplicated young patients with a herniated disc to elderly patients with multiple medical problems. Spinal pathology ranges from a simple herniated disc to neoplastic destruction of the spinal column and spinal cord compression. The anesthesiologist should perform a routine history and physical examination, focusing on any cardiac or pulmonary history.[6] A chest radiograph is routinely ordered in patients older than 40 years. Pulmonary function and arterial blood gases must be evaluated in patients with chronic obstructive pulmonary disease and morbid obesity. Patients with significant pulmonary or cardiac disease are referred

for appropriate consultation before they proceed to surgery.[7] Preoperative laboratory studies include a complete blood cell count, evaluation of electrolytes, liver function enzymes, renal function, coagulation parameters, urinary analysis, and electrocardiography (if over age 40). Banked blood is reserved if significant intraoperative blood loss is anticipated. Active smokers are encouraged to abstain from tobacco before and after the operative procedure to enhance bone fusion.

INTRAOPERATIVE MANAGEMENT

Before the patient is transferred to the operating room, the neurosurgical team performs a detailed neurological examination. Surface electrodes for intraoperative monitoring are placed and the patient is brought to the operating theater. Although local anesthesia is effective for minor procedures such as biopsies of the pleura, most neurosurgical procedures require general endotracheal anesthesia.[1] In adults, the use of a double-lumen endotracheal tube permits single-lung ventilation on the nonoperative side.[8] Whether to approach the spine from the patient's left or right side is determined by the location of the pathology. Single-lung ventilation of the dependent lung is performed on the "down-side lung" with collapse of the lung on the side of exposure. The distal endotracheal tube and balloon cuff (Fig. 9–1) are placed in the proximal left main stem bronchus. A second proximal cuff is inflated in the trachea. The endotracheal tube can be placed under fiber-optic guidance or direct visualization using a bronchoscope. Both lungs are auscultated to ensure bilateral ventilation. The tube is then secured to prevent its migration while the patient is rotated into the lateral decubitus position. After the patient is repositioned, the placement of the endotracheal tube is again verified with bronchoscopy. When its

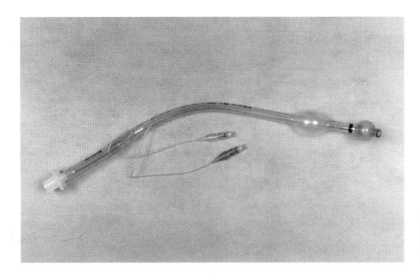

Figure 9–1. Double-lumen endotracheal tube permits single-lung ventilation. The proximal balloon is inflated in the trachea; the distal balloon is inflated in the main stem bronchus of the ventilated lung.

bronchus is obstructed, the nonventilated lung slowly collapses. During the initial part of the thoracoscopic procedure, the surgeon uses a fan retractor to retract the collapsed lung away from the surface of the spine. As the procedure progresses, the fan is removed and the lung remains collapsed, using gravity to keep it off the surface of the spine.

In pediatric patients, several options are available for single-lung ventilation, including a double-lumen endotracheal tube or a single-lumen endotracheal tube with an obstructive device (bronchial blocker) in the bronchus of the nonventilated lung.[9,10]

Normal ventilator parameters for a patient with no significant cardiorespiratory history would be a tidal volume of approximately 10 to 15 ml/kg and an inspired oxygen content of 100%. Respiratory rate is titrated to obtain an end-tidal pCO_2 between 35 and 40 mm Hg. If the oxygen saturation drops during the operative procedure, auscultation over the inflated lung should be performed to verify proper placement of the endotracheal tube. If one is unsure of the tube placement, bronchoscopy is a useful adjunct.[11,12] Blood oxygen saturation can be increased by intermittently reexpanding the nonventilated lung and/or by adding 5 to 10 mm Hg of continuous positive airway pressure to the lung on the operative side. When pediatric patients are ventilated with a single-lumen endotracheal tube, the tube can be repositioned in the trachea and the noninflated lung ventilated until the cardiorespiratory system is stabilized. To minimize the occurrence of postoperative atelectasis, the deflated lung is reinflated intraoperatively 5 to 10 minutes each hour of operating time.

INTRAOPERATIVE MONITORING

Cardiopulmonary Parameters

Placement of an arterial catheter facilitates real-time monitoring of arterial blood pressure and permits rapid determination of blood pH, pCO_2, PO_2, and oxygen saturation.[13] A pulse oximeter probe attached to a finger,

toe, or ear lobe permits continuous monitoring of oxygen saturation.[14] The latter is especially useful if the extremities are vasoconstricted. This modality correlates well with oxygen saturation determined by arterial blood gas assessment. The continuous measurement of end-tidal CO_2 ensures proper ventilation and should be correlated with arterial blood gases.[15]

Central venous pressure is a gross estimation of volume status in healthy patients. If significant cardiac or respiratory disease is present or significant blood loss is anticipated or encountered, a Swan-Ganz catheter is placed before or during the operative procedure. Single-lung ventilation can lead to unique changes in pulmonary arterial pressures. With significant atelectasis in the nonventilated lung, the resistance to blood flow is greatly increased and pulmonary blood flow is shunted preferentially to the ventilated lung (right-to-left shunt) in most scenarios. This situation can lead to erroneous hemodynamic calculations because use of the Swan-Ganz catheter is based on a thermodilution technique that assumes uniform pulmonary capillary resistance.[16]

Somatosensory Evoked Potentials

The use of SSEPs has been accepted widely among spinal surgeons.[17–28] The sensitivity and specificity of SSEP monitoring appear to be high.[17–28] However, new postoperative neurological deficits, especially paraparesis and paraplegia, have also been associated with normal intraoperative SSEPs.[18,20–22] Peripheral nerves are stimulated with subdermal or cutaneous electrodes; the resultant evoked potentials over the sensory cortex are monitored with scalp electrodes. Stimulation on one side of the body is coupled with passive monitoring on the contralateral scalp. The pathway of this response has been localized to the posterior columns and therefore is believed to be most sensitive at detecting injury to the posterior part of the spinal cord.

Typically, scalp electrodes are placed on both sides of the head before anesthesia is initiated. After general endotracheal anesthesia has been initiated, dermal needle electrodes are placed on both legs for stimulation of the common peroneal and posterior tibial nerves. Initially, the common peroneal nerve is stimulated at 12 mA and the posterior tibial nerve at 16 to 20 mA. In both cases, the stimulus is gradually increased to 1.5 times the motor threshold. The placement of a cutaneous lumbar electrode proximal to the surgical level permits troubleshooting during a procedure. The repetition rate of the stimulus is 4.7 Hz and its duration is 2 to 3 msec. The recording or sampling window is approximately 100 msec. Five hundred to 2000 responses are recorded and averaged. The number of responses required is based on the reproducibility of the recorded evoked potential.

Anesthesia is initiated and a baseline response is recorded before the patient is rolled from the prone to the lateral decubitus position. Once the patient is positioned, but before the surgical site is prepared, a second set of SSEPs is recorded. The surgical team is alerted if a significant change occurs. Any significant changes in amplitude or latency during a procedure should be evaluated to prevent irreversible neurological compromise to the spinal cord. Examples of potentially injurious maneuvers include placing a patient with a stenotic canal in a position that increases the degree of spinal cord compression, spinal cord impingement during bone removal, and changes in the geometry of the spinal canal during instrumentation.

A decrease in SSEP amplitude greater than 50% or an increase in latency greater than 10% is highly suggestive of neurological injury to the spinal cord. Factors known to produce changes in the SSEPs, not attributable to neurological compromise, include changes in anesthetic technique, electrode malfunction, a change in the patient's body temperature, hypotension, and hypoxemia. A decrease in the patient's body temperature can increase the latency of the SSEP. Two techniques can rule out a malfunction of the electrode. After the stimulating electrode has been activated, the stimulated muscle should twitch. The competency of the recording electrode also can be assessed by checking its impedance.

Motor Evoked Potentials

MEPs enable the ventral spinal cord to be monitored.[18,29–33] Experimental studies indicate that the evoked responses are conducted by the corticospinal tract. The Food and Drug Administration has not yet approved this technique for clinical use, but it has been employed successfully, either alone or in combination with SSEPs, at clinical institutions in the United States.[18,22,30,31,33] In addition to providing a useful intraoperative monitoring technique, a correlation between pre- and postoperative motor function and motor evoked potentials has been demonstrated.[22] The technique is more sensitive to the effects of anesthesia than SSEPs.

Once the patient has been anesthetized, electrodes are placed in major muscle groups of the extremities to record the compound action potentials that occur after transcranial stimulation of the cortical motor strip, spinal epidural stimulation, or direct stimulation of the spinal cord at the level of surgery. Both the amplitude and latency of the MEPs are evaluated.[23] Most work has indicated that a significant change in amplitude is indicative of neurological injury.[18,29–33] In contrast to SSEPs, changes in the latency of the MEPs are inconsistently associated with injury, which can occur even when the latency is stable.

Theoretically, a combination of SSEPs, which monitor the dorsal spinal cord, and MEPs, which monitor the ventral spinal cord, would be the most sensitive method for determining potential spinal cord injury, given the present status of technology. The use of SSEPs is well established, but the utility of MEPs has yet to be defined. For instance, transcranial stimulation, either by electrodes or a magnetic field, has yielded inconsistent results.

POSTOPERATIVE CARE

After surgery, the patient is observed in the postanesthesia recovery room for about 2 hours. A postoperative chest radiograph is obtained to verify full inflation of the lungs and to rule out residual pneumothorax; a small thoracostomy tube is usually left behind in the operative site to drain any fluid or blood collecting in the chest. Occasionally, these tubes can be removed in the recovery room; however, they are usually left in place 24 hours after surgery. Blood gases are assessed and compared to their intraoperative and preoperative values. Aggressive pulmonary care, which may include bronchodialators, deep suctioning, and deep coughing, is initiated if the patient has a significant respiratory history. If the patient is transferred to a critical care unit, intravascular volume status can be monitored using central venous pressure or pulmonary capillary wedge pressure and urine output. The hematocrit should be followed daily for the first 48 hours after surgery or more frequently if intraoperative blood loss is significant.

The decision to place the patient in an ICU, stepdown unit, or general care ward is made collaboratively by the anesthesiologist and operative team and is based on the patient's medical history, intraoperative course, and expected level of postoperative pain. Obesity, preexistent pulmonary disease, and lengthy procedures are associated with postoperative pulmonary insufficiency. Postoperative pain is treated aggressively to prevent atelectasis, pneumonia, and discomfort. Pulmonary secretions are aggressively suctioned and patients are mobilized as soon as possible.[1] Thoracostomy tubes, if left in place, are typically removed the day after surgery. Stockings and compression boots are applied to prevent deep venous thrombosis.

CONCLUSION

With the increasing interest in and demand for minimally invasive surgery, thoracic endoscopic approaches are being performed with increasing frequency. Anesthetic technique for such endoscopic procedures requires a thorough preoperative cardiopulmonary evaluation. Single-lung ventilation allows the lung on the operative side to be collapsed and retracted. Changes in cardiopulmonary parameters, including a right-to-left shunt of pulmonary blood flow, necessitate modification of the anesthetic technique to maintain proper ventilation and oxygenation. Intraoperatively, evoked sensory and motor potentials can be monitored to assess the integrity of spinal cord function.

REFERENCES

1. Mulder DS: Pain management principles and anesthesia techniques for thoracoscopy. *Ann Thorac Surg* 1993; 56:630–632.

2. Sugarbaker DJ: Thoracoscopy in the management of anterior mediastinal masses. *Ann Thorac Surg* 1993; 56:653–656.

3. Graeber GM, Jones DR: The role of thoracoscopy in thoracic trauma. *Ann Thorac Surg* 1993; 56:646–648.

4. Daniel TM: Diagnostic thoracoscopy for pleural disease. *Ann Thorac Surg* 1993; 56:639–640.

5. Hazelrigg SR, Nunchuck SK, Landreneau RJ, et al: Cost analysis for thoracoscopy: Thoracoscopic wedge resection. *Ann Thorac Surg* 1993; 56:633–635.

6. Roizen MF: Preoperative evaluation. in Miller RD, ed: *Anesthesia*, 4th ed. New York: Churchill Livingstone; 1994:827–882.

7. Gal TJ: Pulmonary function testing. in Miller RD, ed: *Anesthesia*, 4th ed. New York: Churchill Livingstone; 1994:883–901.

8. Horswell JL: Anesthetic techniques for thoracoscopy. *Ann Thorac Surg* 1993; 56:624–629.

9. MacGillivray RG: Evaluation of a new tracheal tube with a movable bronchus blocker. *Anaesthesia* 1988; 43:687–689.

10. Inoue H, Shohtsu A, Ogawa J, et al: New device for one-lung anesthesia: Endotracheal tube with movable blocker [letter]. *J Thorac Cardiovasc Surg* 1982; 83(6):940–941.

11. Benumof JL, Partridge BL, Salvatierra C, et al: Margin of safety in positioning modern double-lumen endotracheal tubes. *Anesthesiology* 1987; 67:729–738.

12. Brodsky JB, Shulman MS, Mark JBD: Malposition of left-sided double-lumen endobronchial tubes. *Anesthesiology* 1985; 62:667–669.

13. O'Rourke MF, Yaginuma T: Wave reflections and the arterial pulse. *Arch Intern Med* 1984; 144:366–371.

14. Tremper KK, Barker SJ: Pulse oximetry. *Anesthesiology* 1989; 70:98–108.

15. Murray IP, Modell JH: Early detection of endotracheal tube accidents by monitoring carbon dioxide concentration in respiratory gas. *Anesthesiology* 1983; 59:344–346.

16. Pearl RG, Rosenthal MH, Nielson L, et al: Effect of injectate volume and temperature on thermodilution cardiac output determination. *Anesthesiology* 1986; 64:798–801.

17. Jones SJ, Edgar MA, Ransford AO, et al: A system for the electrophysiological monitoring of the spinal cord during operations for scoliosis. *J Bone Joint Surg Br* 1983; 65(2):134–139.

18. Owen JH, Jenny AB, Naito M, et al: Effects of spinal cord lesioning on somatosensory and neurogenic-motor evoked potentials. *Spine* 1989; 14(7):673–682.

19. Loder RT, Thomson GJ, LaMont RL: Spinal cord monitoring in patients with nonidiopathic spinal deformities using somatosensory evoked potentials. *Spine* 1991; 16(12):1359–1364.

20. Lesser RP, Raudzens P, Lüders H, et al: Postoperative neurological deficits may occur despite unchanged intraoperative somatosensory evoked potentials. *Ann Neurol* 1986; 19:22–25.

21. Machida M, Weinstein SL, Yamada T, et al: Dissociation of muscle action potentials and spinal somatosensory evoked potentials after ischemic damage of spinal cord. *Spine* 1988; 13(10):1119–1124.

22. Owen JH, Laschinger J, Bridwell K, et al: Sensitivity and specificity of somatosensory and neurogenic-motor evoked potentials in animals and humans. *Spine* 1988; 13(10):1111–1118.

23. Stechison MT: Neurophysiological monitoring in spinal surgery. In Menezes AH, Sonntag VKH, eds: *Principles of Spinal Surgery*. New York: McGraw-Hill; 1996:315–333.

24. Ryan TP, Britt RH: Spinal and cortical somatosensory evoked potential monitoring during corrective spinal surgery with 108 patients. *Spine* 1986; 11(4):352–361.

25. Brinker MR, Willis JK, Cook SD, et al: Neurologic testing with somatosensory evoked potentials in idiopathic scoliosis. *Spine* 1992; 17(3):277–279.

26. Perlik SJ, VanEgeren R, Fisher MA: Somatosensory evoked potential surgical monitoring. Observations during combined isoflurane-nitrous oxide anesthesia. *Spine* 1992; 17(3):273–276.

27. Kalkman CJ, tenBrink SA, Been HD, et al: Variability of somatosensory cortical evoked potentials during spinal surgery. Effects of anesthetic technique and high-pass digital filtering. *Spine* 1991; 16(8):924–929.

28. Lubicky JP, Spadaro JA, Yuan HA, et al: Variability of somatosensory cortical evoked potential monitoring during spinal surgery. *Spine* 1989; 14(8):790–798.

29. Levy WJ, McCaffrey M, York DH, et al: Motor evoked potentials from transcranial stimulation of the motor cortex in cats. *Neurosurgery* 1984; 15(2):214–227.

30. Levy WJ, York DH, McCaffrey M, et al: Motor evoked potentials from transcranial stimulation of the motor cortex in humans. *Neurosurgery* 1984; 15(3):287–302.

31. Calancie B, Klose KJ, Baier S, et al: Isoflurane-induced attenuation of motor evoked potentials caused by electrical motor cortex stimulation during surgery. *J Neurosurg* 1991; 74:897–904.

32. Jellinek D, Platt M, Jewkes D, et al: Effects of nitrous oxide on motor evoked potentials recorded from skeletal muscle in patients under total anesthesia with intravenously administered propofol. *Neurosurgery* 1991; 29(4):558–562.

33. Edmonds HL, Jr., Paloheimo MPJ, Backman MH, et al: Transcranial magnetic motor evoked potentials (tcMMEP) for functional monitoring of motor pathways during scoliosis surgery. *Spine* 1989; 14(7):683–686.

CHAPTER *10*

Perioperative Management for Thoracoscopic Spine Surgery

Noel I. Perin, M.D., Curtis A. Dickman, M.D., Stephen M. Papadopoulos, M.D., and Daniel J. Rosenthal, M.D.

Before thoracoscopic surgery is considered, patients should be evaluated for severe pulmonary disease, which would prohibit the surgery. Thoracoscopic spinal surgery is also contraindicated when selective intubation cannot be achieved (e.g., tracheal stenosis, age younger than 5 years), when a pulmonary disease or a parenchymal process within the lung prohibits single-lung ventilation, when dense pleural adhesions would prevent exposure for endoscopic access, or when a medical contraindication is present (Table 10–1).

PREOPERATIVE ASSESSMENT

Preoperatively, patients should be screened to assess their activity level and exercise tolerance, pulmonary signs and symptoms, and their history of smoking, prior chest surgery or injury, toxic exposure (e.g., silicon, asbestos), tuberculosis, and chronic or acute pulmonary diseases, especially pneumonia, empyema, lung trauma, and rib fractures. Diagnostic studies should include anteroposterior and lateral radiographs of the thoracic spine, posteroanterior and lateral chest radiographs, and any other pertinent imaging studies of the spine [i.e., magnetic resonance (MR) imaging, myelography, or computed tomography (CT)]. The number of ribs should be counted *carefully* on the chest radiograph to rule out an anomalous number. The chest and spine radiographs, MR images, or CT scans also can provide helpful cues for localizing pathology (e.g., osteophytes) during surgery.

If potential pulmonary contraindications exist, arterial blood gases spirometry and consultation with a pulmonologist should be obtained.

Preoperatively, the patient's pulmonary function and medical conditions are optimized by adjusting medications as needed or by adding new treatments. If reactive airway disease is present, the patient may need perioperative aerosolized bronchodilator inhalation therapy and oral or intravenous (IV) theophylline. The serum levels of theophylline and cardiac drugs (e.g., digoxin) and complete serum chemistries, blood counts, and clotting parameters should also be assessed.

The patient should shower the morning of the surgery, washing with antibacterial soap. An antibiotic for prophylaxis is administered on call to the operating room. If the patient has myelopathy, methylprednisolone can be administered prophylactically according to the doses used for spinal cord injury (i.e., 30 mg/kg IV bolus followed by 5.4/mg/kg/hr IV over 23 hours). Antiembolism stockings and pneumatic compression stockings are applied before surgery to prevent venous stasis and the development of deep venous thrombosis.

POSTOPERATIVE MANAGEMENT

When chest tubes are used, pleuritic pain causes moderate postoperative discomfort and splinting of deep respirations. The pleuritic pain is usually referred to the apex of the chest and the scapula. This pleuritic pain and postoperative incisional pain are managed by parenteral narcotics, a patient-controlled analgesia pump, oral narcotics, lumbar epidural narcotics, or a transdermal narcotic patch. After general thoracoscopy, thoracic surgeons often deliver postoperative local anesthetic solutions to the pleural surfaces. If, however, the dura has been exposed, intrapleural local anesthetic solutions should be *avoided* after spinal thoracoscopy. A spinal anesthetic block might occur that could cause sudden respiratory arrest.

Usually, endotracheal tubes are removed postoperatively in the operating or recovery room. If patients have atelectasis or copious bronchial secretions, they may be kept

TABLE 10–1   Contraindications to Spinal Thoracoscopy

I. Inability to Perform Selective Intubation
    Age less than 5 years (trachea and bronchi too small)
    Tracheobronchial stenosis
    Prior tracheostomy
    Tracheobronchial neoplasm
    Tracheobronchial scar tissue
    Congenital tracheobronchial stenosis or aplasia

II. Pulmonary Pathology Preventing Single-Lung Ventilation
    Parenchymal consolidation processes
        Pulmonary edema
        Acute respiratory distress syndrome
        Pneumonia
        Acute congestive heart failure
        Primary or metastatic lung neoplasms
    Diffuse pulmonary processes affecting ventilation
        Chronic obstructive pulmonary disease
        Emphysema
        Severe reactive airway disease/asthma
        Interstitial pulmonary fibrosis or pneumonitis
        Pulmonary hypertension
    Miscellaneous processes causing acute or chronic respiratory
        insufficiency
    Miscellaneous processes prohibiting single-lung ventilation
        Contralateral bronchopleural fistula
        Contralateral pulmonary artery aplasia
        Contralateral pneumothorax
        Contralateral lobectomy or pneumonectomy
        Contralateral lung aplasia
        Congenitally anomalous tracheobronchial tree
        Paralytic hemidiaphragm (contralateral)
        Contralateral pleural effusion or empyema

III. Lung Adhesions (Relative Contraindications)
    Prior ipsilateral thoracotomy
    Prior ipsilateral thoracoscopy
    Sclerotherapy (ipsilateral)
    Prior empyema (ipsilateral)
    Prior hemothorax (ipsilateral)

IV. Spinal Contraindications (Relative Contraindications)
    Intradural extension of the pathology
    Pathology also affecting the posterior spine or contralateral side
    Prior CSF leak from surgical site
    Prior spine surgery at surgical site (scar tissue)
    Highly vascular tumor (e.g., renal cell carcinoma, hemangioma,
        aneurysmal bone cyst, hypernephroma)
    Vascular anomalies (AVM of bone, hemangioma laterally ectatic
        aorta or azygos veins)

V. Medical Contraindications
    Bleeding diatheses
        Hemophilia, congenital diathesis, etc.
        Iatrogenic (heparin, Coumadin®, etc.)
        Thrombocytopenia
        Disseminated intravascular coagulopathy
    Cardiac disease
        Recent myocardial infarction
        Severe cardiac arrhythmias
        Acute or chronic uncontrolled cardiac failure
        Pericardial effusion
    Pulmonary or pleural disease (see sections I and II)
    Miscellaneous
        Inability to tolerate general anesthesia
        Limited life expectancy
        Severe dementia

AVM = arteriovenous malformation; CSF = cerebrospinal fluid.

intubated and ventilated mechanically to promote positive pressure reexpansion of the lung and to access lung secretions for suctioning. Atelectasis can be *minimized* by reinflating the lung intraoperatively 5 to 10 minutes for every hour of surgical time. Postoperatively, breathing treatments with positive pressure inhalation (incentive spirometry and intermittent positive pressure breathing treatments) are used. If atelectasis persists after surgery, mucolytic agents and bronchoscopy may be needed to clear inspissated secretions from the bronchi.

Chest radiographs are obtained in the recovery room and subsequently as needed. If the lung remains fully expanded and drainage from the chest tube is minimal, additional chest films can be obtained just before and after the chest tubes are removed.

The chest tubes remain in place until the fluid output diminishes to less than 100 ml/day. The output can be reduced by obtaining meticulous hemostasis at the surgical site, especially of the epidural veins. The chest tubes are usually placed to suction −20 cm of H_2O pressure until the output diminishes. Then they are placed to water seal and checked for air leaks. If there are no problems, the chest tubes can be removed. If the dura was opened intraopera-

tively, the chest tubes are placed to gravity drainage (water seal) rather than to suction to prevent the formation of a subarachnoid pleural fistula. In such cases, the dura is closed, and a lumbar drain or lumboperitoneal shunt should be used to divert the flow of cerebrospinal fluid (CSF) and to reduce the intraspinal hydrostatic pressure until the dura seals.

Postoperative spinal radiographs should be obtained, in addition to the intraoperative radiographs or fluoroscopy, to assess spinal alignment and to confirm the localization of surgery. If the spinal cord was decompressed, the adequacy of the decompression at the surgical site should be evaluated on postoperative MR imaging or CT. CT is used if the pathology was calcified or bony.

If the thoracoscopic procedure was brief and the patient experienced little blood loss or other intraoperative difficulties, he or she may be placed in an intermediate care or general care ward after surgery. If the procedure was prolonged or the patient requires special nursing care, he or she should be placed in an intensive care unit.

Patients often can be mobilized within 24 hours of surgery. A spinal brace such as a thoracolumbosacral orthosis or Jewett hyperextension brace can be used if indicated by the spinal procedure.

AVOIDANCE AND MANAGEMENT OF COMPLICATIONS

There are many potential complications of thoracoscopic spinal surgery—both intrathoracic (Table 10–2) and neurological (Table 10–3)—just as there are for any anterior transthoracic approach. Although thoracoscopy and thoracotomy share the same potential risks, the incidence of complications associated with each procedure varies.[1–19]

Compared to thoracoscopy, thoracotomy is associated with higher incidences of chest wall and incisional pain syndromes (postthoracotomy pain), intercostal neuralgia, shoulder girdle and scapular dysfunction, atelectasis, pneumonia, pulmonary dysfunction, and acute postoperative pain.[1–6,8–11,19] Because of these complicating factors, hospital stays and recovery times are also longer after thoracotomy.[1–6]

When attempting to perform an endoscopic spinal procedure, the surgeon should not necessarily consider the procedure a failure if an open thoracotomy is required to accomplish the surgical dissection. Lung adhesions, severely distorted spinal anatomy, brisk epidural bleeding, a dural tear with an accompanying CSF leak, or an inability to expose or visualize the lesion satisfactorily are excel-

lent reasons for using thoracotomy as the alternative for access. The surgeon should employ the method of access that achieves the surgical goals and is the safest for the patient. The method should also be within the individual surgeon's experience, skill level, and expertise. Preoperatively, patients should be informed that a thoracotomy could be needed so that they are prepared for it, should the occasion arise.

Emergency conversion to a thoracotomy may be needed to treat vascular (aorta or azygos vein), visceral, or cardiac injuries. The surgeon and scrub nurse should always be prepared to perform a thoracotomy immediately. Chest retractors and open thoracotomy instruments are kept *open* on the sterile back table. A sponge stick that can fit through a portal is also prepared before the operation begins in case it is needed for the gentle tamponade of a bleeding vessel until the chest can be opened.

Surgeons can anticipate and prevent most complications. To do so, however, requires comprehensive knowledge of the thoracic, mediastinal, and spinal anatomy; the factors unique to the patient's pathology; practice and skill in handling endoscopic dissection tools (e.g., stability, precision, triangulation); and experience with strategies to approach, retract, and dissect structures safely endoscopically. Remember that experience with open surgery does not adequately prepare the surgeon to perform thoracoscopy! Even if the surgeon has done *hundreds* of thoracotomies for spine pathology, special, dedicated, and intensive practice and training are required to learn the new psychomotor skills needed for performing thoracoscopy safely. The specific strategies to prevent or treat complications related to each type of spinal procedure are discussed throughout the text; only the major principles are reemphasized below.

Injury to the lung is avoided by minimizing or avoiding retraction of the lung, using gravity to facilitate retraction (rotating the patient anteriorly), observing all repositioning

TABLE 10–2 Potential Pulmonary, Pleural, and Intrathoracic Complications of Thoracoscopy or Thoracotomy

Acute respiratory distress syndrome
Atelectasis
Air leak (secondary lung laceration)
Air embolism
Bronchopleural fistula
Cerebrospinal fluid leak (subarachnoid-pleural fistula)
Chylothorax (thoracic duct injury)
Hemothorax
Hiccoughs
Hypercarbia
Hypoxemia
Hemoptysis
Pneumonia
Pleural effusion
Pneumothorax
Pulmonary contusion
Paralytic hemidiaphragm (phrenic nerve injury)
Pulmonary edema
Respiratory failure
Empyema
Subcutaneous emphysema
Tumor dissemination from spine (pleural spread or chest wall seeding)
Infection dissemination (empyema, osteomyelitis, wound infection)
Acute hemorrhage/major vascular injury
Diaphragm penetration with visceral injury (liver or splenic injury)
Cardiac arrhythmias
Myocardial infarction
Cardiac arrest
Cardiac laceration
Hypotension
Decreased venous return
Esophageal injury

TABLE 10–3 Potential Spinal and Neurological Complications of Thoracoscopy or Thoracotomy

Cerebrospinal fluid leak
Dural tear
Excessive epidural bleeding
Graft migration
Hardware loosening
Horner's syndrome (stellate ganglion)
Inadequate decompression
Inadvertent sympathectomy
Intercostal neuralgia
Misidentified level
Nerve root avulsion
Nonunion
Persistent myelopathy
Persistent radicular pain
Recurrent laryngeal nerve, vagus nerve, or phrenic nerve injury
Retained disc herniation
Spinal cord injury
Spinal deformity
Spinal instability

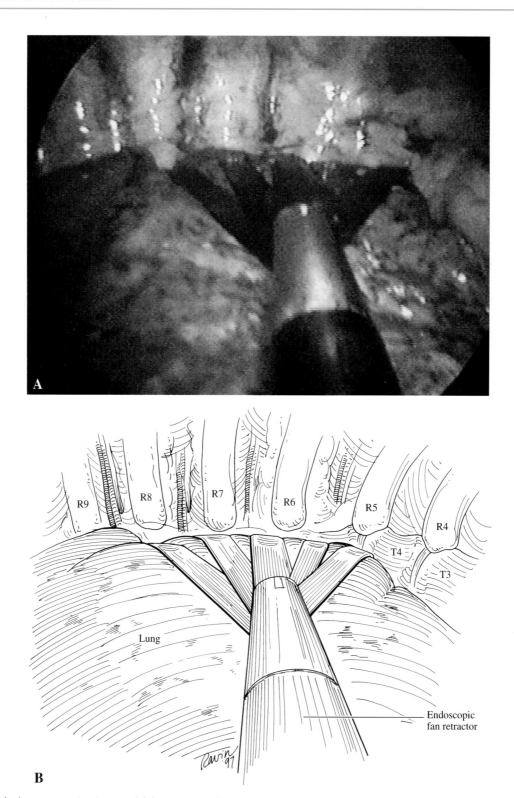

Figure 10–1. **(A)** Thoracoscopic view and **(B)** corresponding illustration showing an endoscopic retractor being used to gently retract the lung from the surface of the spine. The retractor must be used carefully to avoid injuring the lung. The retractor should be positioned, opened, and closed while it is directly visualized with the endoscope.

maneuvers of the fan retractor, and carefully detaching any adhesions under direct observation (Fig. 10–1). If an air leak from the lung occurs, it can be sealed with an endoscopic lung stapler. The lung surface should be inspected with the endoscope before and during reinflation to assess for injury.

Atelectasis and bronchial mucous plugging are minimized with humidified ventilation, intraoperative aerosols, frequent bronchial suctioning through the endotracheal tube, and intraoperative bronchoscopy, if needed. Postoperative atelectasis can be minimized by intraoperatively reinflating the lung 5 to 10 minutes for each hour of surgical time and using postoperative intermittent positive pressure breathing treatment and incentive spirometry. Removing the chest tube as soon as output decreases reduces the patient's pleuritic pain, facilitating deeper respirations.

Persistent pneumothorax may indicate an air leak from the lung, malpositioning of the chest tube, or an inadequate seal at the entry site of the chest tube. If the pneumothorax is from an air leak and does not respond to continued suction, reoperation to staple the lung or to administer sclerotherapy may be required.

Hemothorax may occur from removing the chest tube too soon before the output ceases, from injuring an intercostal vessel during removal of a portal or a chest tube, from inadequate ligation of a segmental vessel on the surface of the spine, or from persistent epidural venous bleeding. If a large hemothorax occurs after the chest tube is removed, it can be evacuated surgically using thoracoscopy to remove the clot and to control the source of the hemorrhage.

Meticulous epidural hemostasis should be achieved with bipolar cauterization and precise application of small pieces of hemostatic material (Fig. 10–2). We prefer compressed fibrillar collagen (sheets of compressed avitene) to cover the epidural vessels after the thorax has been irrigated. The fibrillar material sticks to the surface of the vessels and is less likely to be washed away as easily as a single piece of gelatin foam. The portal incisions should be inspected with the endoscope internally after the portals are removed to rule out bleeding from the incision. The segmental vessels should be isolated and individually doubly ligated with hemoclips for secure hemostasis.

Chylothorax, a rare complication, can occur from injury to the thoracic duct or to lymphatics within the chest. It appears as milky fluid draining into the chest tube and requires reoperation. Before the thoracic duct is repaired, the flow of chylomicrons can be promoted by administering

olive oil to the patient by nasogastric tube for several hours before surgery. This technique helps identify the source of the chyle leak intraoperatively. The thoracic duct can be ligated with hemoclips; smaller lymphatic vessels can be oversewn with surgical pledgets. If the leak persists despite reoperation, the patient is treated with total parenteral nutrition and complete bowel rest for several months.

A simple pleural effusion can be treated with percutaneous thoracentesis. If, however, a CSF-pleural fistula occurs, it can be difficult to stop: The normal negative intrathoracic pressure creates a gradient that promotes a persistent CSF leak. The best approach, therefore, is to prevent a CSF leak. Dural tears should be sutured with watertight closures, even if it means converting to thoracotomy.

The dura can be closed with sutures or dural clips [20] and sealed with fibrin glue and a fascial patch. If the dura was opened intraoperatively, a lumbar drain or lumboperitoneal shunt is used to reduce intraspinal pressure and to divert the flow of CSF. The chest tube should *not* be placed to suction; this would create a gradient for CSF to flow into the chest. Instead, the chest tube is placed to water seal for gravity-dependent drainage of any fluid from within the thorax.

To avoid cardiac arrhythmias, monopolar cauterization is avoided near the heart, and the shafts of many of the tools used with cauterization are insulated to prevent conducting the current.

Visceral, soft tissue, and spinal injuries are prevented by using stable, controlled, precise, two-handed anchoring and dissection techniques whenever heavy or sharp tools are needed.

Neurological complications (i.e., spinal cord and/or nerve root injury) are prevented by several strategies. The intercostal nerves are preserved by subperiosteally separating them from the undersurfaces of any ribs that need to be removed. For decompression of the spinal cord, the pedicle

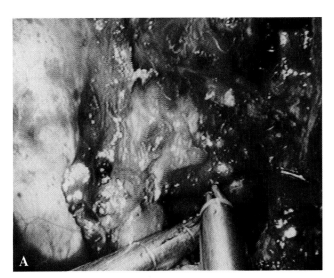
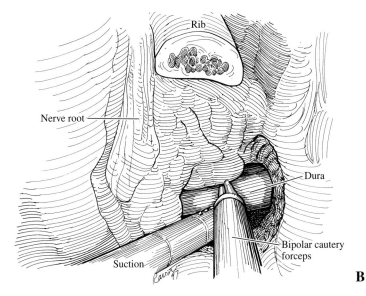

Figure 10–2. **(A)** Thoracoscopic view and **(B)** corresponding illustration showing an insulated endoscopic bipolar cautery forceps being used to obtain hemostasis of the epidural veins. The bipolar cautery is performed identical to the techniques in open surgery.

is removed *first* so that the dura can be visualized clearly before the decompression is actually performed. Furthermore, a cavity in the vertebral body must be made sufficiently large so that tools can be inserted and the pathology delivered away from the spinal canal. Tools should *never* be inserted into the compromised epidural space.

Intercostal neuralgia can be minimized by using flexible rather than rigid portals, by locally blocking the intercostal nerve at a portal site with 1% marcaine with epinephrine, and by inserting the portal adjacent to the superior rib surface to avoid the neurovascular bundle.

Horner's syndrome is prevented by preserving the stellate ganglion, which is located adjacent to the head of the first rib.

Mislocalization of a level may be avoided by using preoperative radiographs and imaging studies for preliminary confirmation of the level of the pathology, employing intraoperative fluoroscopy or radiography, and by counting the ribs directly endoscopically to identify the level of the pathology (Fig. 10–3).

Incomplete spinal cord decompression can be avoided by providing an adequate cavity in the vertebrae so that the entire ventral surface of the dura can be visualized. The

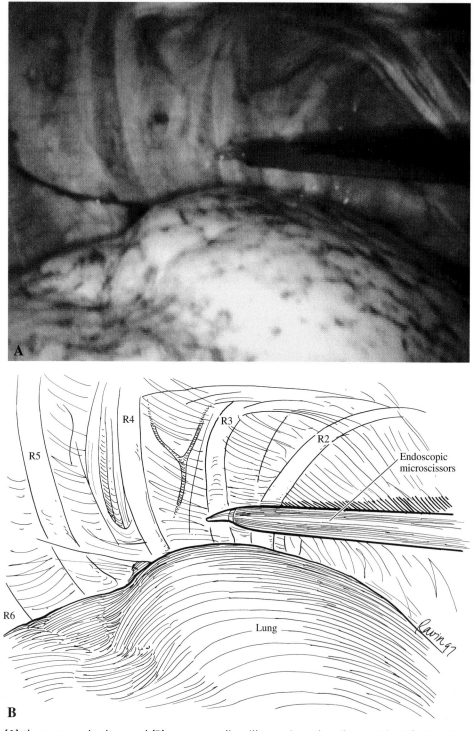

Figure 10–3. In this **(A)** thoracoscopic view and **(B)** corresponding illustration, the ribs are identified, palpated, and counted internally to help localize the spinal segments. The second rib is usually the first visible rib structure in the apex of the hemithorax. The first rib is usually not visible. The internal localization of the spinal level is confirmed fluoroscopically.

depth of the dissection in the spine can be judged using calibrated markings on the tools and intraoperative radiographs. Postoperative spinal radiographs, CT, or MR imaging is suggested to evaluate whether a decompression is complete.

Visceral injury to the liver or spleen by penetrating through the diaphragm or to the lung can be avoided by inserting all portals under direct endoscopic vision, especially if they are placed below the seventh intercostal space. The surgeon inserts a finger through the first portal incision and feels for lung adhesions (and lung deflation) before the first trocar and portal are inserted. The first portal is the only insertion site that is not visualized internally with the endoscope. Similarly, portals should not be placed in the first and second intercostal spaces to avoid injuring the subclavian vessels.

CONCLUSIONS

The principles for perioperative management of patients undergoing thoracoscopic spinal surgery are straightforward. Complications can be prevented and treated effectively using a variety of simple management strategies.

REFERENCES

1. Regan JJ, Mack MJ, Picetti GD, III, et al: A comparison of video-assisted thoracoscopic surgery (VATS) with open thoracotomy in thoracic spinal surgery. *Today's Therapeutic Trends* 1994; 11:203–218.
2. Landreneau RJ, Hazelrigg SR, Mack MJ, et al: Postoperative pain-related morbidity: Video-assisted thoracic surgery versus thoracotomy. *Ann Thorac Surg* 1993; 56:1285–1289.
3. Hazelrigg SR, Landreneau RJ, Boley TM, et al: The effect of muscle-sparing versus standard posterolateral thoracotomy on pulmonary function, muscle strength, and postoperative pain. *J Thorac Cardiovasc Surg* 1991; 101:394–401.
4. Ferson PF, Landreneau RJ, Dowling RD, et al: Comparison of open *versus* thoracoscopic lung biopsy for diffuse infiltrative pulmonary disease. *J Thorac Cardiovasc Surg* 1993; 106:194–199.
5. Dickman CA, Rosenthal D, Karahalios DG, et al: Thoracic vertebrectomy and reconstruction using a microsurgical thoracoscopic approach. *Neurosurgery* 1996; 38:279–293.
6. Dickman CA, Karahalios DG: Thoracoscopic spinal surgery. *Clin Neurosurg* 1996; 43:392–422.
7. Rosenthal D, Dickman CA, Lorenz R, et al: Thoracic disc herniation: Early results after surgical treatment using microsurgical endoscopy. *J Neurosurg* 1996; 84(2):334A.
8. Kaiser LR, Bavaria JE: Complications of thoracoscopy. *Ann Thorac Surg* 1993; 56:796–798.
9. McAfee PC, Regan JR, Zdeblick T, et al: The incidence of complications in endoscopic anterior thoracolumbar spinal reconstructive surgery. A prospective multicenter study comprising the first 100 consecutive cases. *Spine* 1995; 20(14):1624–1632.
10. Faciszewski T, Winter RB, Lonstein JE, et al: The surgical and medical perioperative complications of anterior spinal fusion surgery in the thoracic and lumbar spine in adults. A review of 1223 procedures. *Spine* 1995; 20(14):1592–1599.
11. Dajczman E, Gordon A, Kreisman H, et al: Long-term postthoracotomy pain. *Chest* 1991; 99:270–274.
12. Landreneau RJ, Mack MJ, Hazelrigg SR, et al: Video-assisted thoracic surgery: Basic technical concepts and intercostal approach strategies. *Ann Thorac Surg* 1992; 54:800–807.
13. Landreneau RJ, Hazelrigg SR, Ferson PF, et al: Thoracoscopic resection of 85 pulmonary lesions. *Ann Thorac Surg* 1992; 54:415–420.
14. Allen MS, Deschamps C, Jones DM, et al: Video-assisted thoracic surgical procedures: The Mayo experience. *Mayo Clin Proc* 1996; 71:351–359.
15. Lewis RJ, Caccavale RJ, Sisler GE: Special report: Video-endoscopic thoracic surgery. *N Engl J Med* 1991; 88(7):473–475.
16. Kaiser LR: Video-assisted thoracic surgery. Current state of the art. *Ann Surg* 1994; 220(6):720–734.
17. Coltharp WH, Arnolc JH, Alford WC, Jr., et al: Videothoracoscopy: Improved technique and expanded indications. *Ann Thorac Surg* 1992; 53:776–779.
18. Mack MJ, Aronoff RJ, Acuff TE, et al: Present role of thoracoscopy in the diagnosis and treatment of diseases of the chest. *Ann Thorac Surg* 1992; 54:403–409.
19. Naunheim KS, Barnett MG, Crandall DG, et al: Anterior exposure of the thoracic spine. *Ann Thorac Surg* 1994; 57:1436–1439.
20. Kirsch WM, Zhu YH, Gaskill D, et al: Tissue reconstruction with nonpenetrating arcuate-legged clips. Potential endoscopic applications. *J Reprod Med* 1992; 37(7):581–586.

CHAPTER *11*

Operating Room Setup and Patient Positioning

Daniel J. Rosenthal, M.D., and Curtis A. Dickman, M.D.

*U*sing local anesthesia, Jacobeus was able to perform diagnostic thoracoscopic procedures at a patient's bedside in the early 1900s.[1] Modern thoracoscopy, however, is performed in an operating room with the patient under general anesthesia. The complexity of thoracoscopy has increased significantly, and a wide variety of different surgical procedures can now be performed.

OPERATING ROOM SETUP

The largest available operating room should be used for thoracoscopic procedures, which require extensive equipment and a large number of personnel. In addition to the patient, at least nine people are typically present in the operating room, including the spine surgeon, the surgical assistant, a thoracic surgeon, the scrub nurse, two circulating nurses, a clinical neurophysiology monitoring technician, an x-ray technician, a videographer–medical photographer, the anesthesiologist, plus any observers.

Ideally, two circulating nurses should be available at the beginning of surgery to prepare and connect the endoscopes, suctions, electrocautery devices, and drills; to open the tools; to prepare pressurized, warmed irrigation solution; to calibrate the endoscopes; and so on. Later, during surgery, usually one circulating nurse is needed.

A variety of different options can be used to position the equipment and personnel in the operating suite (Fig. 11–1). The scrub nurse can stand next to the surgeon or across the operating table from the surgeon next to a Mayo stand. Several large sterile back tables are needed to hold the extensive amount of dissection equipment used in thoracoscopic spinal surgery. Space is also necessary for the video monitors, the C-arm and fluoroscopic monitors, instrument tables and Mayo stands, personnel, and other equipment.

In case of an intraoperative emergency, tools for converting to open thoracotomy are always open in the sterile field. A sterile sponge stick is also prepared for insertion through a portal should a rapidly bleeding vessel need to be tamponaded.

Ideally, two or more video monitors should be used. The primary monitor is placed across the operating table from the surgeons toward the cranial end of the table. Other monitors are positioned for the scrub nurse and the operative team to view the procedure. The surgeons should be looking in the direction in which the surgery is performed (Fig. 11–1).

A complete *backup endoscopic system* should be available in case the operating endoscopic system fails or becomes contaminated. A backup system includes additional sterilized telescopes, a video camera, light cables, an additional monitor, a light source, extra light bulbs, and a signal processor.

The scrub nurse and circulating nurses coordinate the routing of the wires, cables, and tubes from the operating table in an organized fashion. Suction tubing, drill cables, the endoscope camera wires, fiber-optic light cables, irrigation tubing, and monopolar and bipolar cautery cables can easily become entangled in the operating field. The resulting "spaghetti" makes it difficult to pass tools between the surgeon and scrub nurse.

We minimize the tangling of lines and cables by using an extra Mayo stand placed near the patient's head (Fig. 11–1E). This stand holds the bone drills, cables for the endoscopes, and bipolar cautery tools. The cables for these tools are routed to the head of the operating table. The scrub nurse stores the suction, irrigation, and monopolar cautery device on the caudally positioned Mayo stand and routes the cables to the foot of the table. The cables can be routed along the surfaces of the drape by securing the cables

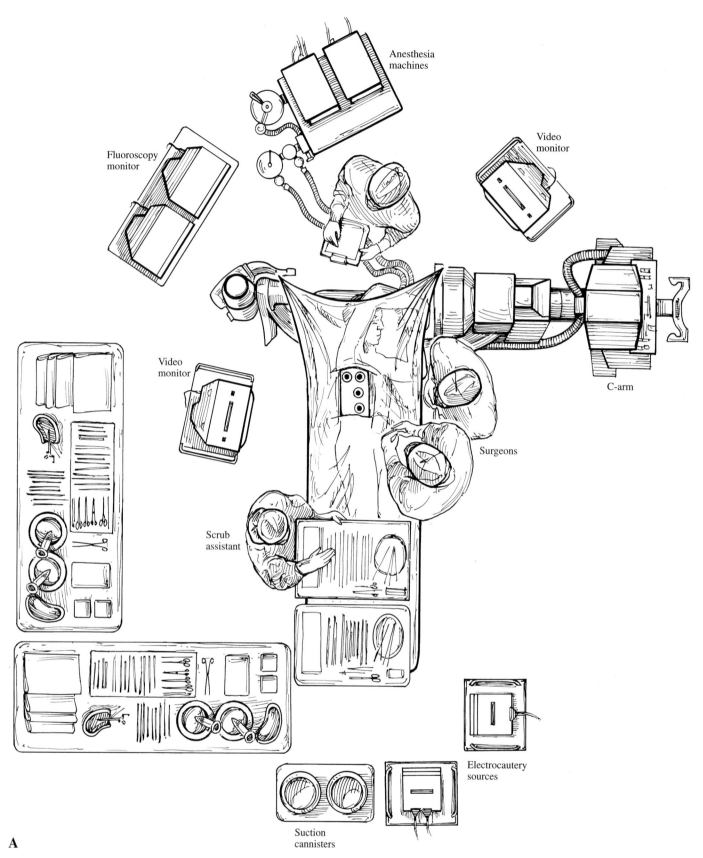

A

Figure 11–1. Options for setting up the operating room for thoracoscopic spinal surgery. The anesthesiologist and related equipment are positioned at the head of the table. Both the surgeon and assistant are best positioned on the same side, facing the anterior surface of the patient's chest. Video monitors are positioned directly across from the surgeon and assistants so they can observe the surgical procedure. The position of the C-arm, scrub assistant, sterile tables, video monitors, fluoroscopy monitors, and other equipment can vary depending on the location of the pathology in an individual case. The fluoroscopic C-arm can be draped in the sterile field and positioned (**A** and **B**) cephalad or (**C** and **D**) caudal to the patient. The C-arm is moved into position when it is used to visualize the anatomy.

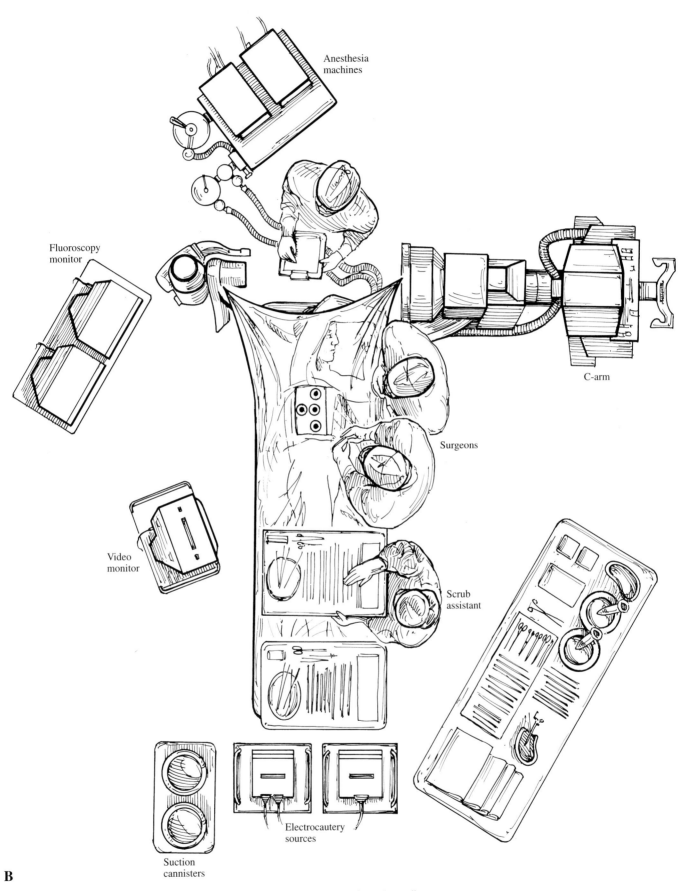

Anesthesia
machines

Fluoroscopy
monitor

C-arm

Surgeons

Video
monitor

Scrub
assistant

Electrocautery
sources

Suction
cannisters

B

Figure 11–1. *(continued)*

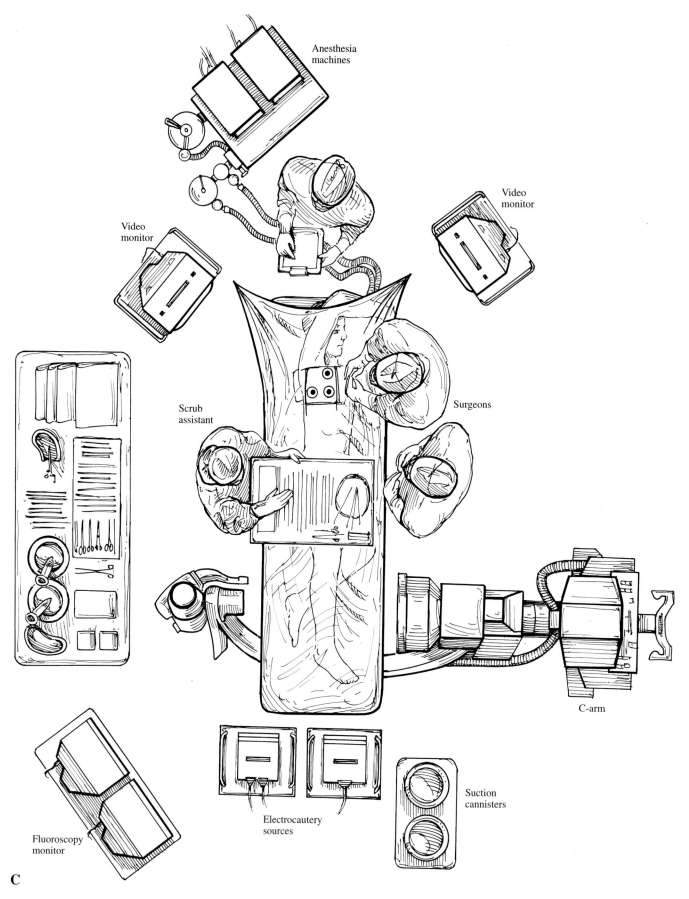

Anesthesia
machines

Video
monitor

Video
monitor

Scrub
assistant

Surgeons

C-arm

Fluoroscopy
monitor

Electrocautery
sources

Suction
cannisters

C

Figure 11–1.   *(continued)*

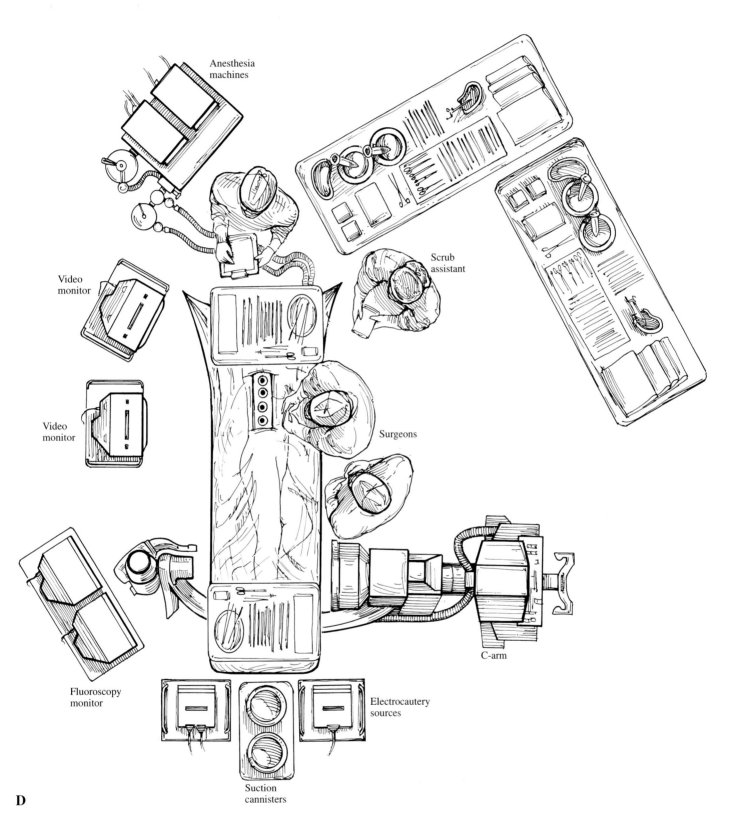

Anesthesia
machines

Scrub
assistant

Video
monitor

Video
monitor

Surgeons

C-arm

Fluoroscopy
monitor

Electrocautery
sources

Suction
cannisters

D

Figure 11–1. *(continued)*

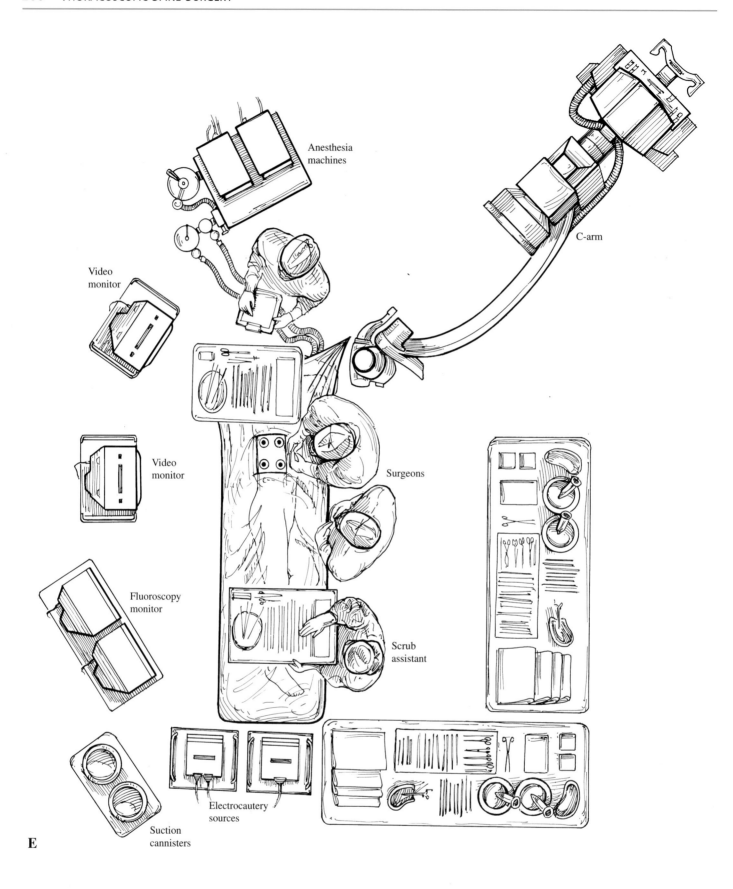

Figure 11–1. *(continued)* **(E)** The C-arm also may be positioned out of the field and brought in when needed.

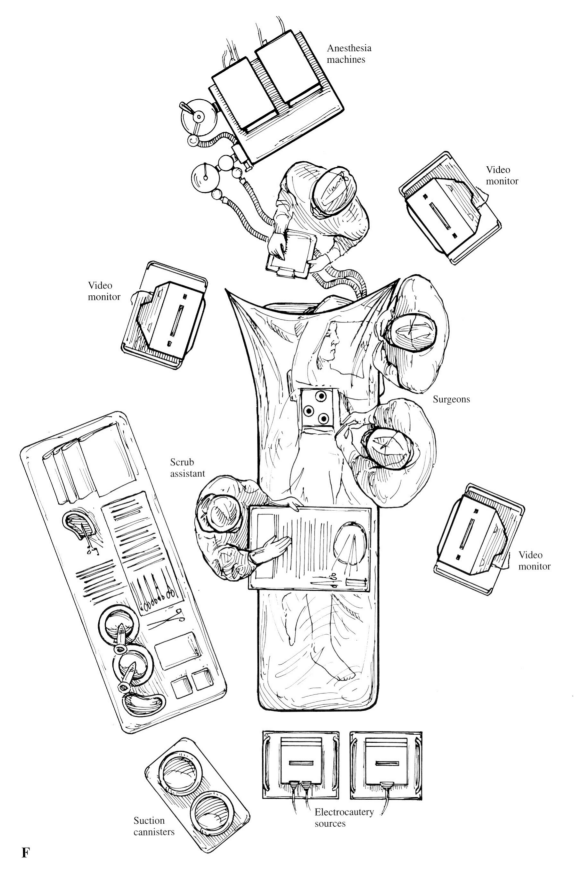

Anesthesia
machines

Video
monitor

Video
monitor

Surgeons

Scrub
assistant

Video
monitor

Suction
cannisters

Electrocautery
sources

F

Figure 11–1.   *(continued)*   **(F)** For a sympathectomy, no C-arm is needed. Without it, there is more room for the surgical team and equipment.

with Allis clamps within creased horizontal pockets created in the drapes.

Warmed irrigation solution must be supplied continuously throughout the operation. The solution must be warm to prevent the lens of the endoscope from becoming fogged during irrigation. The irrigation stream must be forceful to be effective. Irrigation can be administered using pressurized tubing and a pressurized IV bag connected to a suction and irrigation tool. Irrigation can also be delivered manually through a 50-ml syringe and a long IV catheter (i.e., Swan-Ganz catheter introducer or central venous pressure introducer).

Several surgical tools require foot pedals, including pneumatic drills, bipolar and monopolar cautery devices, and the C-arm. The surgeon should control the positioning and use of the pedals for both the drills and cautery. The fluoroscopic pedal can be controlled by an assistant. It can be challenging to maintain unobstructed access to the four foot pedals during the surgery.

Before surgery, the surgeon should select the spine and soft-tissue dissection tools that he or she anticipates using and review them with the scrub nurse. The scrub nurse should be familiar with the needed tools and keep them accessible on the Mayo stands.

After all the surgical equipment is set up and all the tools are opened and organized, the endoscopes are activated and assembled. The lens of the endoscope is prewarmed to body temperature by soaking it in warmed irrigation solution. The lens is dried and a lens defogging solution (FRED) is applied to it. The camera and light cables are attached to the endoscope. The light source, signal processor, and monitors are turned on and connected to the endoscope. The color processing and color images on the monitor are balanced and prepared. The relative color intensity is prepared by "white balancing" the image. The surgeon assesses the orientation of the endoscopic image before inserting the endoscope into the patient's body.

During the thoracoscopic portion of the procedure, the overhead operating room lights are turned off. The sterile surgical lamps are dimmed, but kept as spotlights for the scrub nurse and the anesthesiologist. The darkened room improves the quality of the images on the monitor. The images appear more brilliant and intense, and there is less reflection on the screen. The darkness also minimizes distractions for the surgeon caused by movement within the operating room. The surgeon's attention is directed to the video monitor rather than downward at the operating field.

PATIENT POSITIONING

Initially, the patient is placed supine on the operating table while the anesthesiologist inserts the double-lumen endotracheal tube, an arterial line, and a central venous catheter. The circulating nurse inserts a Foley catheter and applies sequential pneumatic compression stockings to the legs to prevent deep venous thrombosis. During this time, the neurophysiological monitoring technician applies leads to monitor somatosensory evoked potentials (SSEPs), motor evoked potentials, or both. A radiolucent operating table is used so that anteroposterior (AP) and lateral fluoroscopy can be obtained intraoperatively.

The anesthesiologist must keep a flexible fiber-optic bronchoscope available in the operating room to insert the double-lumen endotracheal tube and to reposition the endotracheal tube and suction secretions from the tube if needed intraoperatively. The anesthesiologist is usually positioned at the head of the operating table (Fig. 11–1), and the monitoring equipment, anesthetic equipment, ventilator, and bronchoscope should be accessible. The patient's intravenous (IV) arterial line and Foley catheter are routed to the anesthesiologist at the head of the table.

After these preliminary preparations, the patient is turned and placed in a lateral decubitus position on the operating table with the operative side up. After the patient has been repositioned, the anesthesiologist should reassess the position of the double-lumen endotracheal tube, which can migrate when the patient is turned. The side for access to the spine is positioned up; the ventilated side of the thorax is positioned dependently. The latter is often referred to as the *down-side* lung.

Once the patient is in the lateral decubitus position, a foam axillary roll is used to pad the dependent axilla. The dependent leg is flexed, and the patient's knees and bony prominences are padded with pillows and foam padding (Fig. 11–2). The hips are securely taped to the operating table so that the table can be safely tilted anteriorly during surgery. Tilting is often used intraoperatively to allow the atelectatic lung to fall away from the surface of the spine. Gravity thereby increases the surgical exposure after a passive pneumothorax and atelectasis have been achieved (Fig. 11–3). Using gravity to retract the lung reduces the need to retract it mechanically.

The patient's dependent arm is usually placed on a padded arm board; the upper arm is elevated on a pillow or secured to a sling or an ether screen (Fig. 11–2). The upper arm is abducted to move the scapula dorsally to provide greater exposure to the chest wall (Fig. 11–4). If the middle or lower thoracic spinal levels are to be accessed surgically, elevating the arm on a pillow provides sufficient exposure. If upper thoracic spinal (T1 to T5) exposure is needed, the arm is abducted and taped to an ether screen to provide surgical access to the axillae for placement of the portals in the upper intercostal spaces (Fig. 11–4A–C). After the patient is positioned, the abdomen and legs are covered with a warming blanket to prevent hypothermia.

A C-arm is then positioned to provide a clear AP view of the patient's thoracic spine. Fluoroscopy is used to count the ribs to identify the level(s) of the patient's pathology (Figs. 11–4 and 11–5). The seventh rib leads to the T6–T7 disc space, the eighth rib leads to the T7–T8 disc space, and

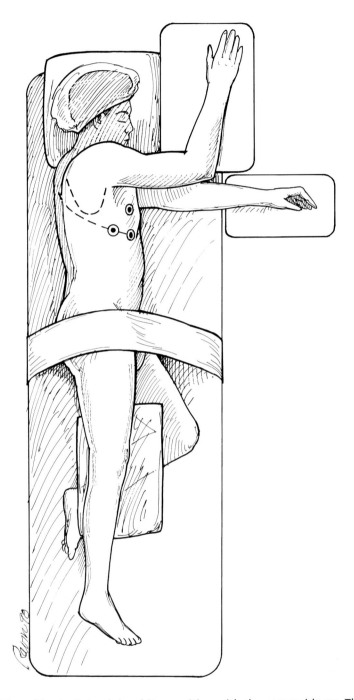

Figure 11–2.   The patient is positioned in the lateral decubitus position with the access side up. The axillae and all bony prominences are padded. An axillary roll is used to protect the dependent axillae, chest wall, brachial plexus, and scapula. The patient is taped securely to the operating table to permit intraoperative rotation. The positions of the pathology, portals, scapula, and a potential thoracotomy incision are marked on the chest wall. The upper arm is elevated to move the scapula dorsally and cephalad, away from the lateral chest wall. A unilateral pneumothorax is provided by blocking the endotracheal tube unilaterally. The nonventilated lung becomes atelectatic, providing exposure to the spine.

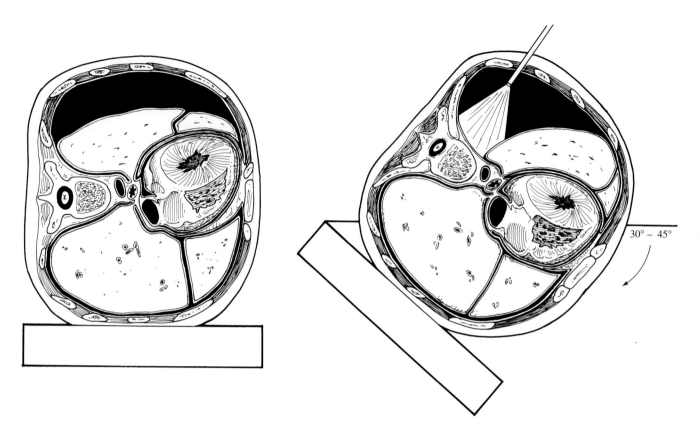

Figure 11–3. Rotating the patient anteriorly 30 to 45° allows gravity to retract the atelectatic lung. This technique reduces or eliminates the need for mechanical lung retraction. The patient's body should be securely taped to the operating table with wide cloth tape to permit the table to be rotated this extensively.

so on. When the level of pathology has been identified radiographically, the overlying skin is marked with indelible ink to help identify the level of pathology intraoperatively and plan the position of the portals. The positions of the portals, the scapula, and the potential thoracotomy incision also are marked on the patient's chest wall (Fig. 11–5).

If possible, one or two portals should be positioned along the line of the potential thoracotomy incision. This placement minimizes the number of additional incisions needed on the chest if the procedure must be converted to an open thoracotomy. If the patient requires endoscopic internal fixation with a screw plate, the portals should be positioned coaxial to the intended trajectory of the bolts and screws into the spine. AP and lateral fluoroscopy are used to plan the portal sites.

The patient's entire chest, axilla, proximal arm, back, and abdomen are sterilely scrubbed with a standard surgical cleansing solution. If an autograft harvest is anticipated, the skin over the iliac crest is also prepared (Fig. 11–6). Sterile towels and drapes are applied to maintain wide access to the chest. Wide exposure is needed in case the procedure must be converted to an open thoracotomy. The C-arm unit is also draped sterilely and positioned for intraoperative use.

The surgeon and the surgical assistant stand anterior to the patient, facing the patient's anterior thorax (Figs. 11–1 and 11–7). This position easily allows the surgeons to recognize the spinal anatomy and to dissect the spine. If the assistant stands posterior to the patient facing the surgeon, his or her dissection and movements will be mirror images of those on the monitor because the visual orientation is reversed from that of the surgeon's endoscopic orientation. This configuration can confuse an assistant and hinder his or her intraoperative movements.

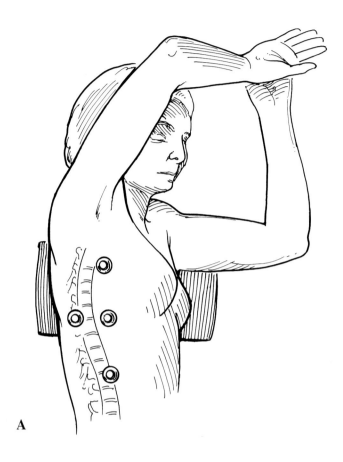

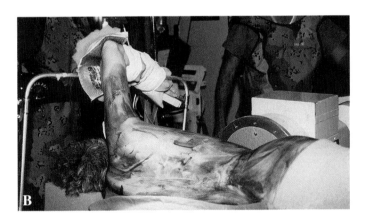

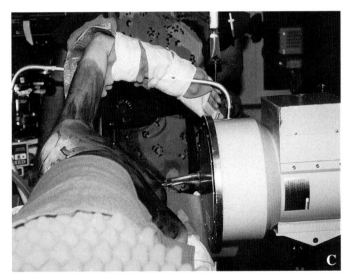

Figure 11–4. **(A)** Exposure to the upper thoracic spine requires abducting the patient's arm to provide exposure to the axillae and upper intercostal spaces. A foam roll is used to pad the dependent axillae and chest wall. The portals are spread apart on the surface of the chest, centered around the target level of the pathology. **(B)** Posterior and **(C)** inferior intraoperative views showing the patient's arm secured to an ether screen in a padded cradle for access to the upper thoracic spine. A C-arm is used to identify the level of the pathology and to plan the incisions for the portals. [B used with permission from Barrow Neurological Institute.]

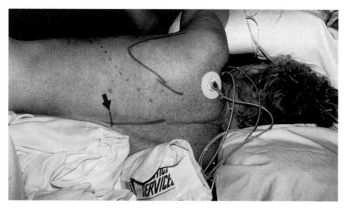

Figure 11–5. Anteroposterior fluoroscopy is used for accurate identification of the level of pathology. The twelfth ribs are identified and the cephalad ribs and vertebrae are counted sequentially. The skin over the level of the pathology is marked to aid in identification intraoperatively (*arrow*). A potential thoracotomy incision, the portal incisions, and the position of the scapula also are marked on the chest wall. The C-arm is sterilely draped and used intraoperatively to judge the level and extent of the spinal dissection. [Used with permission from Barrow Neurological Institute.]

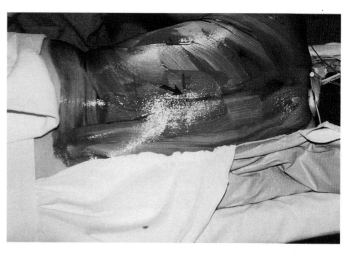

Figure 11–6. Before a thoracoscopic corpectomy, fusion, and fixation with a screw plate are performed, the level of the pathology is marked on the skin with a surgical pen (*arrow*). In this case, the sterile surgical preparation of the skin was very wide and included the iliac crest; the entire back, chest, and abdomen; the shoulder; and the arm.

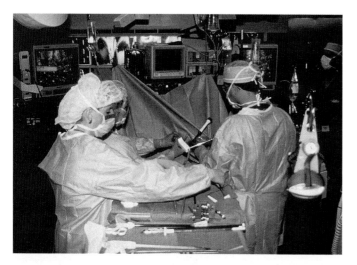

Figure 11–7. The surgeon and assistant stand anteriorly facing the patient's chest, observing an identical endoscopic image on the video monitors. The primary surgical video monitor screen is positioned across the operating table from the surgeon (*left*). The scrub nurse stands across the operating table from the surgeon. Two Mayo stands are used to hold the endoscopic dissection tools.

CONCLUSIONS

Unique positioning and preparatory strategies facilitate thoracoscopic spinal surgery and require an extensive amount of equipment and personnel. Several simple strategies, including the use of large operating rooms, extra backup equipment, and several circulating nurses, can streamline the preparation for surgery.

REFERENCES

1. Jacobeus HC: The pratical importance of thoracoscopy in surgery of the chest. *Surg Gynecol Obstet* 1921; 34:493–500.

RECOMMENDED READINGS

1. Dickman CA, Rosenthal D, Karahalios DG, et al: Thoracic vertebrectomy and reconstruction using a microsurgical thoracoscopic approach. *Neurosurgery* 1996; 38(2):279–293.
2. Rosenthal D, Rosenthal R, de Simone A: Removal of a protruded thoracic disc using microsurgical endoscopy. A new technique. *Spine* 1994; 19:1087–1091.
3. Kaiser LR: Video-assisted thoracic surgery. Current state of the art. *Ann Surg* 1994; 220:720–734.
4. Landreneau RJ, Mack MJ, Hazelrigg SR, et al: Video-assisted thoracic surgery: Basic technical concepts and intercostal approach strategies. *Ann Thorac Surg* 1992; 54:800–807.
5. Coltharp WH, Arnold JH, Alford WC, Jr., et al: Videothoracoscopy: Improved technique and expanded indications. *Ann Thorac Surg* 1992; 53:776–779.
6. Mack MJ, Aronoff RJ, Acuff TE, et al: Present role of thoracoscopy in the diagnosis and treatment of diseases of the chest. *Ann Thorac Surg* 1992; 54:403–409.
7. Dickman CA, Mican CA: Multilevel anterior thoracic discectomies and anterior interbody fusion using a microsurgical thoracoscopic approach. *J Neurosurg* 1996; 84:104–109.
8. Dickman CA, Mican C: Thoracoscopic approaches for the treatment of anterior thoracic spinal pathology. *BNI Quarterly* 1996; 12(1):4–19.

CHAPTER **12**

Thoracoscopic Access Strategies: Portal Placement Techniques and Portal Selection

Curtis A. Dickman, M.D. and Daniel J. Rosenthal, M.D.

The selection and positioning of the endoscopic portals are crucial portions of a thoracoscopic procedure and require forethought and careful planning. If the portals are malpositioned, the surgeon will struggle throughout the operation. If the portals are positioned appropriately, the operation is much easier to perform.

PRINCIPLES OF PORTAL POSITIONING

Several general principles are used to guide positioning of the portals. The portals should be spread far enough apart over the surface of the chest so that the surgeon's hands are placed neither too close together nor too close to the endoscope. If the portals are clustered together too closely, the surgeon's surface movements for manipulating the tools will be restricted. Consequently, he or she will "sword fight" or "fence" with the tools in an attempt to perform the dissection.

Because the surgeon stands anteriorly facing toward the patient's chest during spinal thoracoscopy, the working portals for the insertion of tools, retractors, and suction devices are best positioned anterolaterally in the zone between the anterior and middle axillary lines (i.e., in the working zone, Fig. 12–1). The portal for the endoscope is best positioned posterolaterally between the middle and posterior axillary lines within the "viewing zone" for the spine. Separating the entry site of the endoscope from the area where the surgeon's hands are actively working facilitates unencumbered, unrestricted dissection. The anterolaterally positioned working portals allow the surgeon's hands and arms to rest in a natural, comfortable position during the dissection.

When the thoracoscope is inserted into the thoracic cavity and a 0°-angled endoscope is used, the portal must be positioned directly over the spinal segment where the pathology is located (Fig. 12–2). If a 30°-angled endoscope is used, the portal position may be offset above or below the level of the pathology and the endoscope is angled obliquely to provide a direct view of the spine. Using the 30°-angled endoscope brings the end of the endoscope camera away from the working portals, allowing the surgeon's hands more room to work on the surface of the chest (Fig. 12–2).

The orientation and field of view of the 30°-angled endoscope can change if the telescope lens is inadvertently rotated intraoperatively. Such movement is counterproductive because the field of view is rotated away from the surgical target (Fig. 12–3). The surgeon should verify the desired orientation of the 30°-angled endoscope before inserting it into the chest and, if needed, remove the endoscope to reorient the lens properly.

The positions of the working portals are triangulated. Ideally, they should be spaced evenly rostral and caudal to the surgical target. During the dissection, the surgeon can then stand comfortably, with his or her hands at approximately equal medial trajectories (Fig. 12–4). This portal configuration has been referred to as a baseball diamond with the surgeon positioned at home plate, the target pathology at second base, and the working portals at first and third base, respectively. If the working portals are both offset above or below the target, the surgeon must twist his or her body and hold the arms in an awkward position to use the endoscopic tools (Fig. 12–4). If the working portals are positioned too posteriorly, the surgeon must elevate his or her arms in an awkward position, which is unstable and susceptible to fatigue (Fig. 12–5A). A natural, comfortable arm position for the surgeon is facilitated by placing working portals anterolaterally and rotating the patient anteriorly 30 to 40° (Fig. 12–5B).

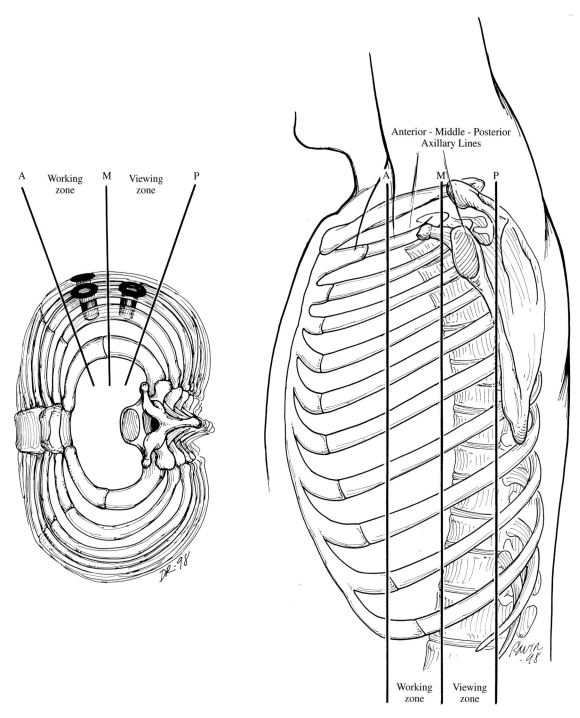

Figure 12–1. The posterior axillary line is superficial to the thoracic vertebrae in a coronal plane over the spinal canal. The space between the middle and posterior axillary lines, the *viewing* zone, provides the best region to insert the endoscope for spinal thoracoscopy. The space between the anterior and middle axillary lines, the *working* zone, provides the best region to insert portals for tools to perform dissections of the spine. This configuration brings the surgeon's hands anteriorly away from the endoscope, allowing more space to maneuver.

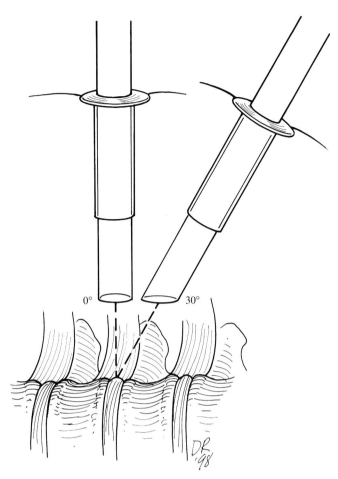

Figure 12–2. A 0°-angled endoscope has a field of view directly ahead of the tip of the telescope. It must be placed directly over its surgical target to provide a direct view of the pathology. A 30°-angled endoscope can offer a clear view of the surgery from an oblique trajectory, which moves the camera and endoscope away from the surgeon's hands on the surface of the chest. The 30°-angled telescope provides more room for the surgeon's hand on the surface of the chest because the endoscope is positioned farther from the working portals.

If a fan retractor is needed to move or hold the lung away from the spine manually, the retractor can be placed between the anterior and middle axillary lines offset rostral or caudal to the working portals. The retractor is inserted obliquely so it can retract the lung but not interfere with the surgeon's hand movements (Fig. 12–6). Once the lung is gently moved away from the spine, the patient can often be rotated anteriorly to allow gravity to keep the lung away from the spine.

PORTAL SELECTION

Flexible portals are used for thoracoscopy rather than rigid portals that can contuse or compress the intercostal nerves and cause intercostal neuralgia postoperatively. The portals are protective, plastic tissue sheaths that maintain the space into the chest through the intercostal spaces. Portals are needed at the site where the endoscope is inserted to keep blood and debris off the endoscope. Portals are also useful at the working sites where tools are inserted and removed from the channel repetitively. For sites where a single tool is inserted and held in position (i.e., the site for a fan retractor or suction device), a portal is probably unnecessary. The tool can be inserted directly through a small incision, through the intercostal space, and into the chest.

The diameter of the flexible thoracoscopic portal must be able to accommodate the size of the tools or objects that will pass through the portal. An 11-mm or a 15-mm portal is adequate for most purposes during thoracoscopy: they fit the endoscope and most tools. A 7-mm portal can be used for a suction-irrigation tool. A 20-mm diameter portal is needed if bone grafts or screw plates will be placed (end-on) through the portal (Fig. 12–7). Large diameter objects (i.e., 16–25 mm) can also be passed by dilating the soft tissues with a speculum (Fig. 12–8) or by extending the intercostal incision to 1 to 2 inches (i.e., a mini-utility thoracotomy). The 7- and 11-mm portals have a round cross section. The 15- and 20-mm portals have an oval cross section so that they can fit into the intercostal space without compressing the intercostal nerve.

TECHNIQUES OF PORTAL INSERTION

Before a portal is inserted, the skin, muscle, and intercostal nerve at the sites are blocked with a local anesthetic by the local infiltration of 1% Marcaine® with epinephrine solution. The anesthetic reduces the incidence of intercostal neuralgia at the portal sites.

For insertion of the first portal, the skin and subcutaneous tissue are incised (10 to 15 mm) parallel to the superior surface of the rib to avoid the neurovascular bundle. A hemostat is passed through the intercostal muscles directly adjacent to the superior surface of the rib. The blunt

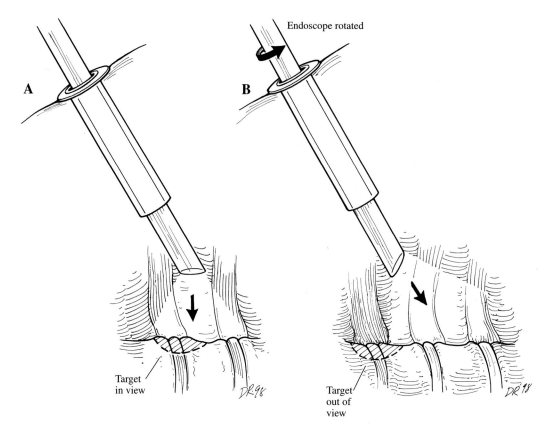

Figure 12–3. **(A)** The lens of the 30°-angled endoscope can be rotated to view the anatomy from a new perspective. This off-axis telescope can be positioned to look around corners of the dissection site. **(B)** If the 30°-angled endoscope is inadvertently rotated, the target can move out of the field of view.

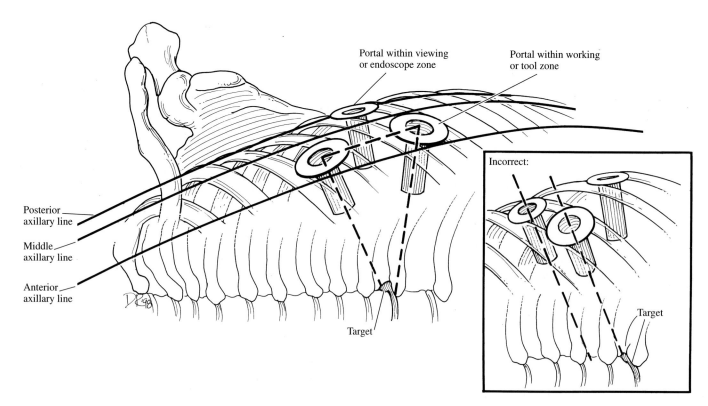

Figure 12–4. The working portals are ideally positioned equidistant rostral and caudal to the surgical target so that the surgeon's hands rest in a comfortable position during the dissection. (*Inset*) If both portals are above or below the spinal target, the surgeon's arm position can become awkward and uncomfortable.

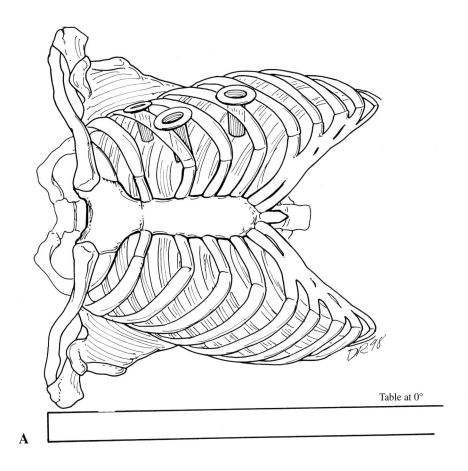

Table at 0°

A

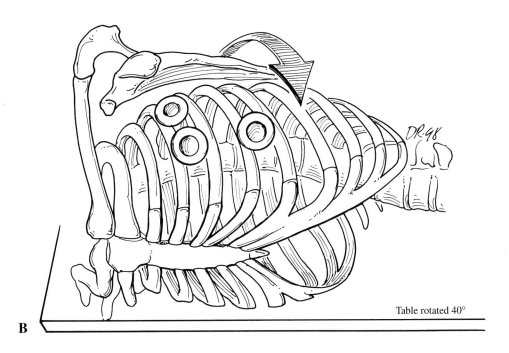

Table rotated 40°

B

Figure 12–5. **(A)** Positioning the working portals too posteriorly forces surgeons to elevate their arms in an awkward, unstable, fatiguing position. **(B)** The surgeon's arms rest in a comfortable position when the working portals are placed near the anterior axillary line, and the patient is rotated anteriorly 30 to 40°.

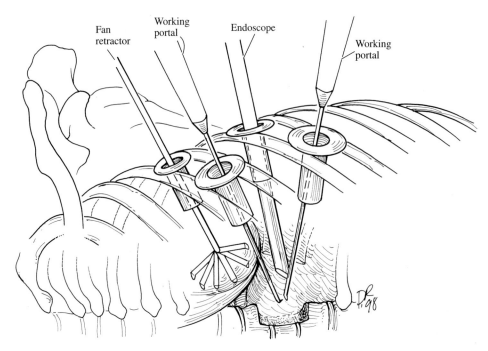

Figure 12–6. The endoscope is positioned between the middle and posterior axillary lines to provide an anterolateral perspective of the thoracic spine. The working portals and retractors are placed more anteriorly. When a lung retractor is needed, its portal should be positioned so that its handle does not interfere with the surgeon's hand movements on the chest surface.

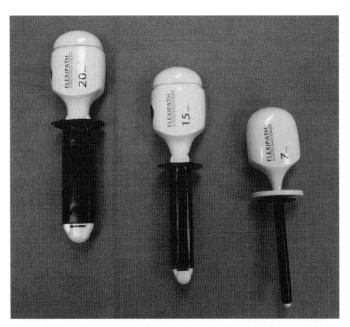

Figure 12–7. Flexipath™ (Ethicon Endosurgery, Cincinnati, OH) flexible thoracoscopic portals are available in diameters of 20, 15, and 7 mm.

tips of the closed hemostat penetrate through the parietal pleura into the thoracic cavity. The tips of the hemostat are opened and widely spread apart to dissect the intercostal muscles from the upper edge of the rib to create a space for the trocar and portal (Fig. 12–9). The surgeon then inserts a gloved finger through the incision into the chest and feels for lung adhesions that would preclude inserting a portal at that site. The method for preparing the portal insertion site is similar to the method for inserting a chest tube, except that an oblique tunneled incision is unnecessary. The portal

penetrates through the intercostal space directly beneath the skin incision (Fig. 12–10).

A rigid trocar is inserted into the flexible portal to guide the portal through the chest wall. After the surgeon excludes the presence of local pleural adhesions, the first portal and the trocar are inserted through the intercostal space into the chest (Figs. 12–9 and 12–10). The rigid trocar is removed from the portal, leaving the flexible tissue sheath within the chest wall (Fig. 12–10B). The length of the soft flexible portal can be customized to fit the individual patient. If needed, the tip of the portal can be shortened with scissors. The proximal end of the flexible portal has a cuff that can be stapled or sutured to the skin to keep the portal anchored in a stable position during the procedure (Fig. 12–11).

After the first portal is inserted, the endoscope is inserted into the chest, the extent of atelectasis is assessed, and the contents of the thoracic cavity are inspected systematically. All additional portals are inserted under direct visualization using techniques identical to those employed for the first portal. Direct endoscopic visualization is needed to prevent penetration of the diaphragm and visceral injury. Particularly when portals are inserted below T7, the surgeon must exercise caution to avoid penetrating the diaphragm. Far anterior portal placement should be avoided to prevent injury to the internal mammary artery and the mediastinal structures. The first and second intercostal spaces should be avoided to prevent injury to the subclavian artery and vein.

When present, focal pleural adhesions may be detached by sharp dissection with scissors or blunt dissection (digital separation or cotton-tipped dissectors) to mobilize the lung (Fig. 12–12). Dense, diffuse pleural adhesions (i.e., pleural

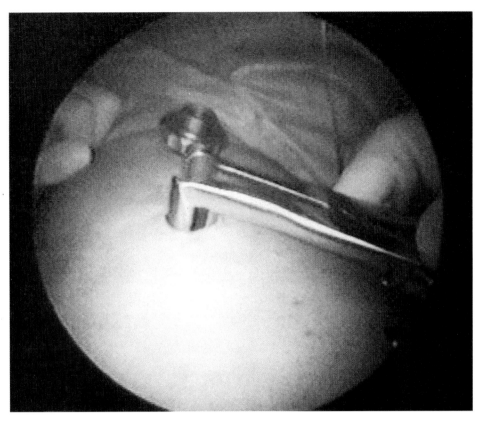

Figure 12–8. Photograph of a speculum for dilating soft tissue incisions. This tool was designed as an extractor for gallbladders full of gallstones, but it may be used to dilate thoracoscopic portal incisions for the insertion or removal of objects that are larger than the incision (i.e., bone grafts, screws, plate).

fusion, pleural symphysis) usually cannot be detached endoscopically. Such adhesions preclude endoscopic access and require conversion to a thoracotomy. If adequate atelectasis was not achieved initially or if the lung was partially ventilated, the anesthesiologist should reposition the double-lumen endotracheal tube using a fiber-optic bronchoscope. As the lung is deflated, dense atelectasis is achieved. The lung may be moved gently away from the surface of the spine with a tool or retractor. Rotating the operating table 30 to 40° anteriorly reduces or eliminates the need to retract the lung. If an endoscopic fan retractor is needed for mechanical retraction of the lung, it should be opened, repositioned, and closed under direct endoscopic visualization to avoid lacerating the lung.

PORTAL CONFIGURATIONS

The configuration of the portals can vary depending on the surgeon's preferences, the patient's body habitus, the type of pathology, the type of spinal procedure performed, and the location of the spinal pathology (Figs. 12–13 to 12–20). Most simple spinal procedures (i.e., sympathectomy, discectomy, biopsies) can be performed with three portals (Figs. 12–13 to 12–15). Four portals (sometimes more) may be needed for more complex procedures (i.e., corpectomy, tumor resection, multilevel anterior release, screw plate fix-

ation) or when a lung or diaphragm retractor is needed (Figs. 12–16 to 12–22).

Portals for Upper Thoracic Access

T1 to T5 are accessed by inserting portals close to the inferior edge of the axillae. The arm is abducted and secured to an ether screen to provide access to the axillae and to rotate the scapula posteriorly away from the portal insertion sites. The axillary space is *never* entered so that the brachial plexus and axillary vessels are not injured. Likewise, neither the first nor second intercostal space is entered so that the subclavian vessels can be avoided. Working portals are inserted in the third and fifth intercostal spaces. The portal for the endoscope is inserted more posteriorly in the fourth or fifth intercostal space, anterior to the edge of the latissimus dorsi muscle (Fig. 12–13).

Portals for Middle Thoracic Access

T5 to T10 are the easiest levels to expose because they are centrally located in the thoracic cavity, and the diaphragm seldom must be retracted to expose the spine. The portal configurations are individually customized for the patient's surgical procedure. Three or four portals are used for most procedures; occasionally, another portal may be needed. A T-shaped portal configuration is used with a 0°-angled telescope. An L-shaped portal configu-

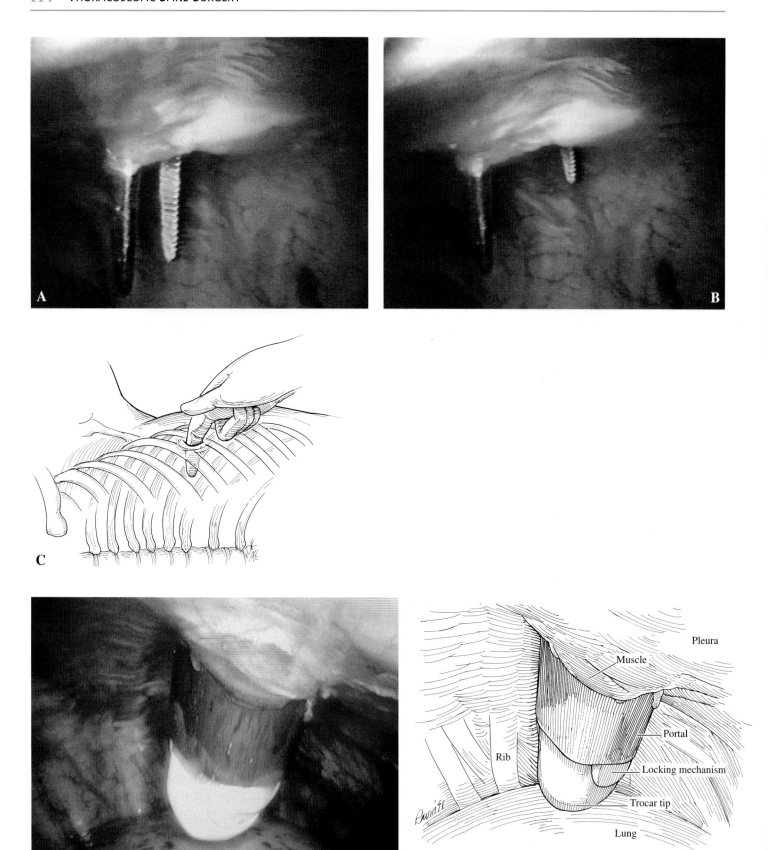

Figure 12–9. Technique for insertion of flexible portals. A small incision is made parallel to the superior surface of the rib over the intercostal space. **(A)** A closed hemostat penetrates through the intercostal muscles over the superior surface of the rib. **(B)** The hemostat is spread to dissect the muscles apart. **(C)** Before the first portal for the endoscope is inserted, the surgeon inserts a gloved finger to feel for lung adhesions and to ensure that the lung is deflated to prevent its injury. **(D)** Intraoperative photograph and **(E)** corresponding illustration showing the insertion of the portal and trocar.

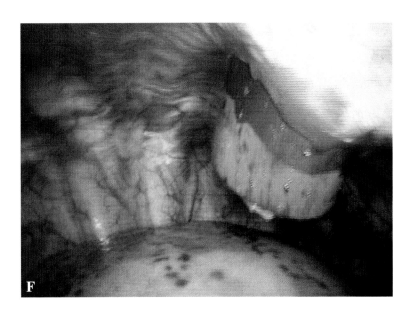

Figure 12–9. *(continued)* **(F)** The trocar is removed, leaving the portal in place.

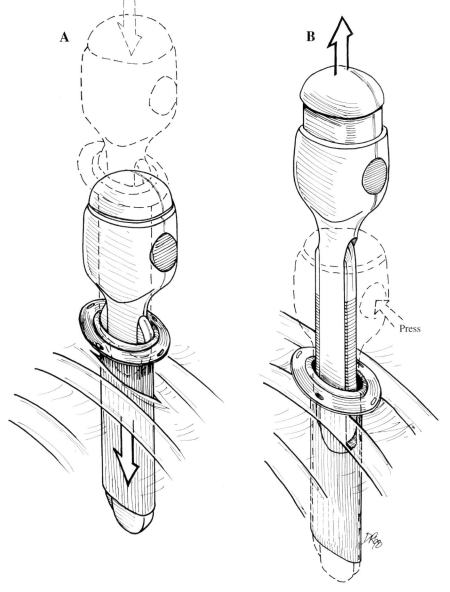

Figure 12–10. **(A)** The flexible portal and trocar are inserted into the incision in the intercostal space. **(B)** The trocar is removed, leaving the portal in place. The portals are sutured or stapled to the skin to anchor them into position.

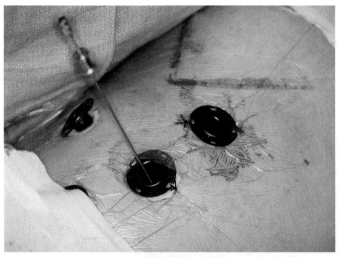

Figure 12–11. Flexible portals are anchored to the skin with staples or sutures. A long needle can be inserted through one of the portals into a disc space so that the spinal level can be localized radiographically. [With permission of Barrow Neurological Institute.]

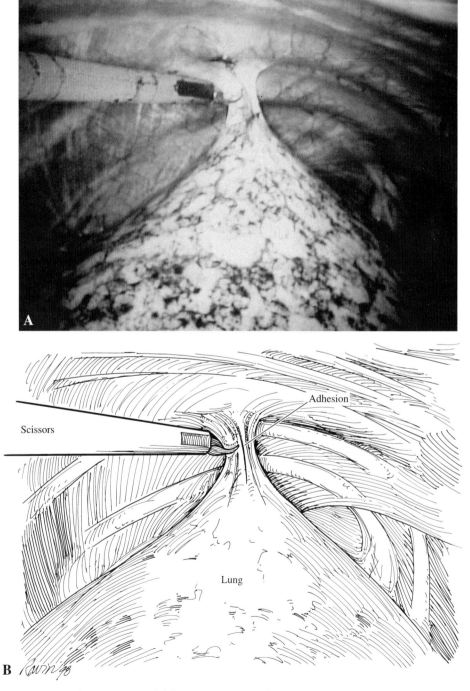

Figure 12–12. **(A)** Intraoperative photograph and **(B)** corresponding illustration showing local pleural adhesions being detached with endoscopic scissors. The adhesions are cut close to the surface of the parietal pleura to avoid lacerating the lung.

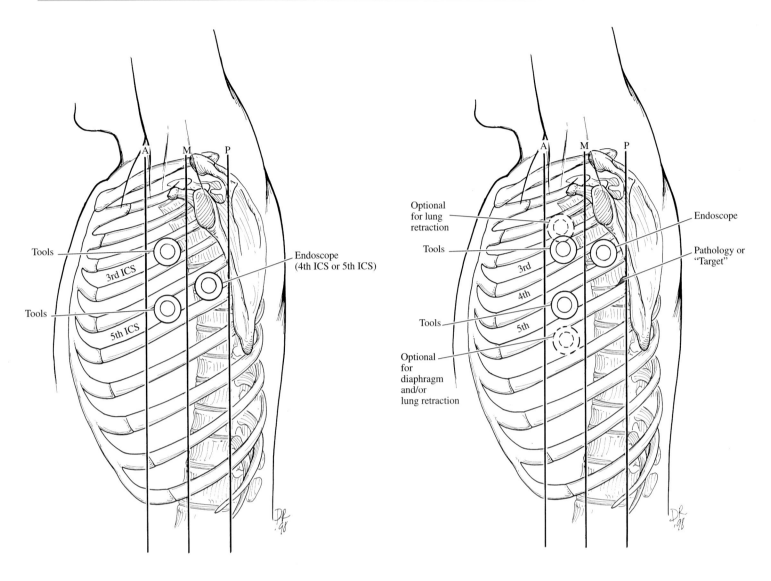

Figure 12–13. Illustration of portal placements for approaching the upper thoracic spine. This configuration is useful for sympathectomy or lesions affecting the T1 to T4 vertebrae. The working portals are positioned in the third and fifth intercostal spaces (ICS). The second ICS should not be used to avoid injuring the subclavian vessels. The viewing portal for insertion of the endoscope is positioned posterior to the working portals.

Figure 12–14. Three portals are usually used for thoracoscopic microdiscectomy. The portals are triangulated above and below the spinal target level. An additional portal may be needed in the working zone, rostral or caudal to the working portals, to insert a retractor for the lung or the diaphragm.

ration is used with a 30°-angled telescope (Figs. 12–13 to 12–17). Positioning the portals linearly or in an L shape is often used for anterior release of scoliosis or kyphosis (Fig. 12–19). A trapezoidal portal configuration is required for screw plates so that the portal positions are coaxial with the trajectories needed to insert the screws into the vertebral bodies (Figs. 12–20 to 12–22).

Portals for Lower Thoracic Access

T9 to L1 are adjacent to the diaphragm, which usually must be gently retracted caudally to expose the spine within the costophrenic recess (Fig. 12–18). A reverse Trendelenburg position, with the head of the table elevated, permits gravity to retract the liver, spleen, and contents of the peritoneal cavity caudally to reduce the amount of diaphragm retraction needed. For exposure of the T12 and L1 vertebral bodies, the pulmonary ligament is detached. The pleura is mobilized so that the caudal retropleural space can be entered. The crus of the diaphragm is incised and the diaphragm is retracted caudally. This strategy allows the surgeon to expose T12 and L1 transthoracically without inserting separate portals in the retroperitoneal space. If needed for reconstruction and dissection, additional retroperitoneal portals can be used for access. Typically, L-shaped or T-shaped portal configurations are employed for these purposes.

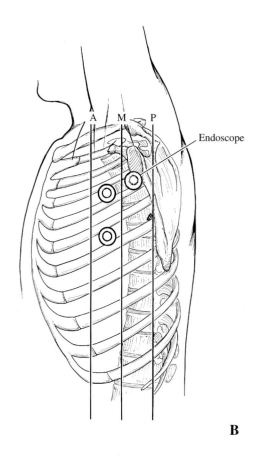

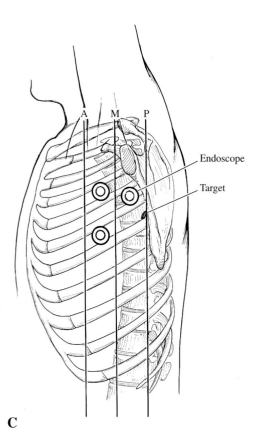

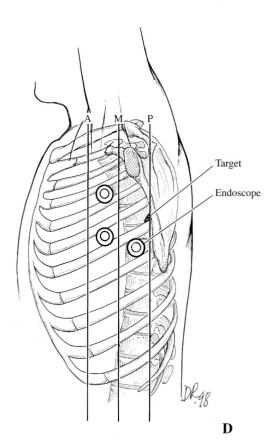

Figure 12–15.   When three portals are needed, various positions and shapes can be used to configure the working portals and the viewing portal for a thoracoscopic microdiscectomy. **(A)** The working portals are spaced equidistant rostral and caudal to the target. When a 0°-angled endoscope is used, it must be positioned directly over the target. **(B, C, and D)** To move the endoscope away from the working portals, the endoscope portals are offset when the 30°-angled endoscope is used.

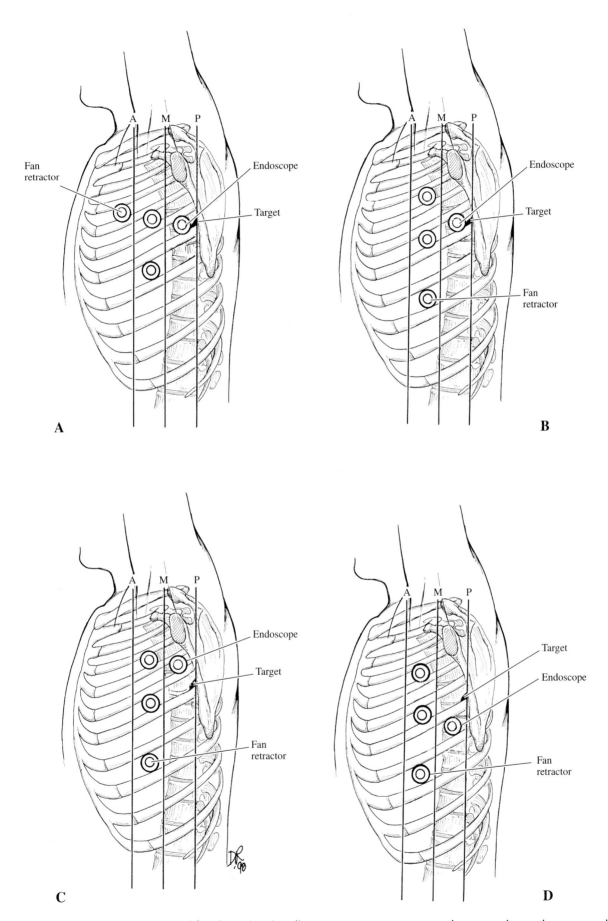

Figure 12–16. When four portals are used for thoracic microdiscectomy, corpectomy, or other procedures, the surgeon has more options to vary the positions of the portals. Retractors are inserted through offset portals so that access to the working portals is unobstructed. Typically, T- or L-shaped portal configurations are used. 0°-angled endoscope with fan retractor positioned **(A)** anterior and **(B)** caudal to working portals. 30°-angled endoscope positioned **(C)** rostral and **(D)** caudal to target.

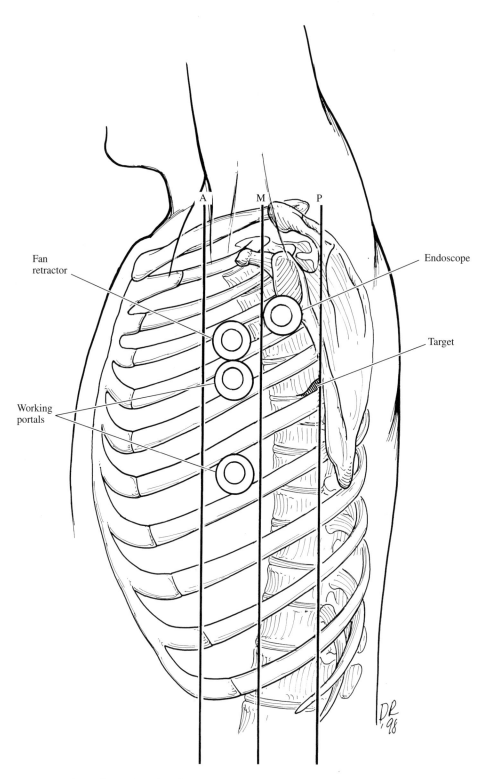

Figure 12–17. A common portal configuration for thoracoscopic microdiscectomy positions a 30°-angled endoscope obliquely to the target, bringing the endoscope's camera farther away from the surface of the chest over the working portals. The working portals are positioned near the anterior axillary line, spaced equidistantly above and below the pathology.

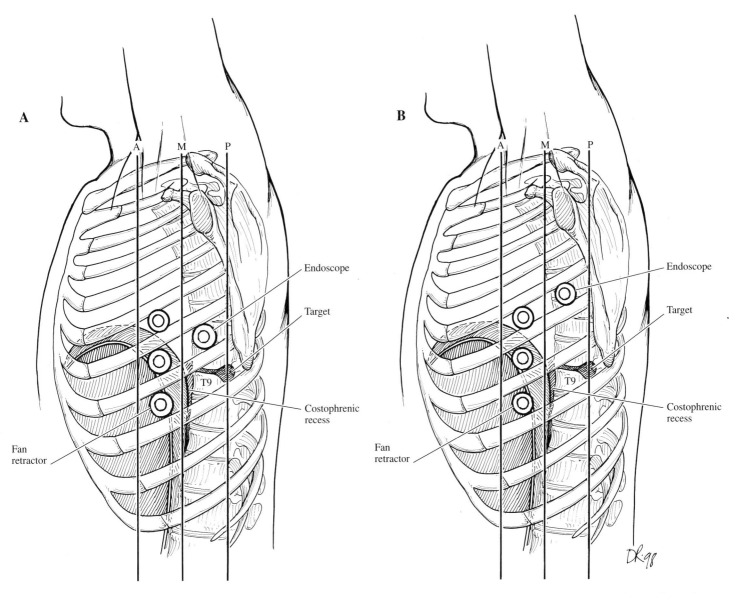

Figure 12–18.   Portal configurations to access the lower thoracic spine and thoracolumbar junction. A portal is devoted to a fan retractor to retract the diaphragm caudal to the costophrenic recess to expose the spine. A reverse Trendelenburg position can be used to allow gravity to aid in the retraction of the viscera and diaphragm caudally.

CLOSURE OF PORTAL SITES

After the spinal dissection and hemostasis have been completed, the thorax has been irrigated and cleared of debris, and the lung surface inspected, the portals are removed from the chest wall. The endoscope is kept inside the thorax so that the portal incisions can be examined internally. A bleeding portal incision can be controlled internally using thoracoscopy or externally by inserting a speculum into the incision to identify the bleeding vessel and using bipolar cauterization to seal it. After most thoracoscopic procedures, chest tubes typically are inserted into the chest through the existing portal incisions and secured with heavy-gauge silk purse-string sutures. The surgeon may wish to make a separate skin stab incision to create an oblique subcutaneous tunnel through which the chest tube can be inserted into the portal site. The skin over the portal site can then be sutured directly to obtain an airtight closure. For postoperative analgesia, the subcutaneous tissues adjacent to the portal incisions are anesthetized with a 1% Marcaine® injection just before the incisions are closed. The portal incisions are then closed with separate subcutaneous and subcuticular layers of interrupted absorbable sutures to provide an airtight tissue closure.

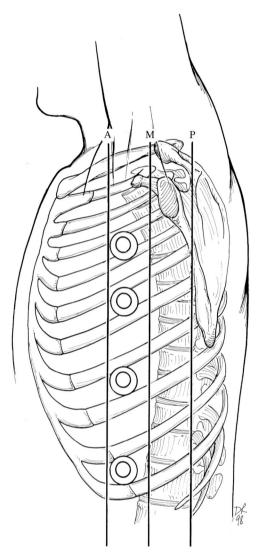

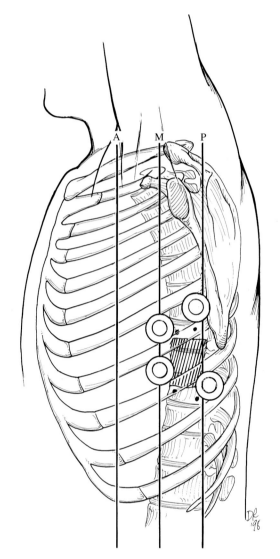

Figure 12–19.   For an anterior release of an extensive multilevel scoliotic deformity, the convex surface of the spine is approached using portals positioned linearly. Most of the portals are positioned near the anterior or middle axillary lines. This configuration allows the surgeon to view and expose the anterior longitudinal ligament and the disc spaces over multiple levels of the spine.

Figure 12–20.   When a screw plate is needed for internal fixation, the portals must be positioned coaxial to the intended trajectory of the screws and bolts. The positions of the portals are evaluated fluoroscopically.

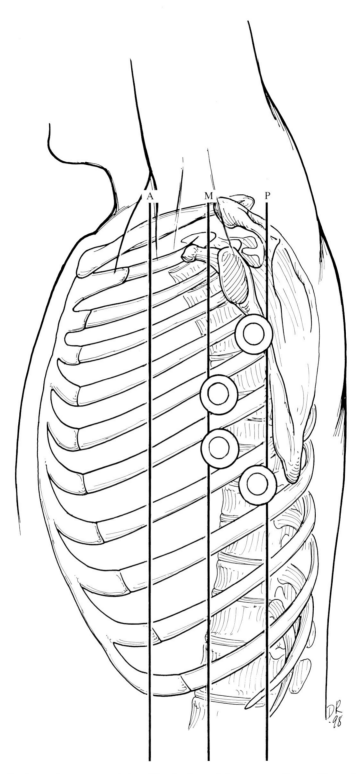

Figure 12–21.   Portal positions for inserting screw plates. The bolt portals are usually positioned near or behind the posterior axillary line. The screw holes are positioned more anteriorly yet posterior to the midaxillary line.

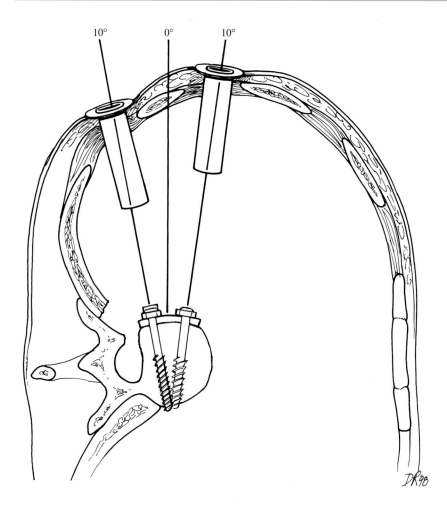

10°   0°   10°

Figure 12–22. An axial cross section of the thorax demonstrates the portal positions required for a screw plate. The bolt is positioned more posteriorly, angled 10° away from the spinal column. The screw is positioned anterior to the bolt, converging 20° toward the bolt.

CONCLUSIONS

Selection and positioning of the portals are crucial steps that can facilitate intraoperative access and dissection. The tech- niques for inserting thoracoscopic portals into the chest are relatively simple, and various strategies can be individual- ized to fit a patient's pathology, the level of the spine, and the particular operative procedure being used. If the portals are malpositioned, however, surgery will be hindered.

RECOMMENDED READINGS

1. Dickman CA, Rosenthal D, Karahalios DG, et al: Thoracic verte- brectomy and reconstruction using a microsocurgical thoracoscopic approach. *Neurosurgery* 1996; 38(2):279–293.
2. Horowitz MB, Moossy JJ, Julian T, et al: Thoracic discectomy using video assisted thoracoscopy. *Spine* 1994; 19:1082–1086.
3. Rosenthal D, Rosenthal R, de Simone A: Removal of a protruded thoracic disc using microsurgical endoscopy. A new technique. *Spine* 1994; 19:1087–1091.
4. Regan JJ, Mack MJ, Picetti GD, III: A technical report on video- assisted thoracoscopy in thoracic spinal surgery. *Spine* 1995; 20:831–837.
5. Kaiser LR: Video-assisted thoracic surgery. Current state of the art. *Ann Surg* 1994; 220:720–734.
6. Landreneau RJ, Mack MJ, Hazelrigg SR, et al: Video-assisted tho- racic surgery: Basic technical concepts and intercostal approach strategies. *Ann Thorac Surg* 1992; 54:800–807.
7. Coltharp WH, Arnold JH, Alford WC, Jr., et al: Videothoracoscopy: Improved technique and expanded indications. *Ann Thorac Surg* 1992; 53:776–779.
8. Mack MJ, Aronoff RJ, Acuff TE, et al: Present role of thoracoscopy in the diagnosis and treatment of diseases of the chest. *Ann Thorac Surg* 1992; 54:403–409.
9. Dickman CA, Mican CA: Multilevel anterior thoracic discectomies and anterior interbody fusion using a microsurgical thoracoscopic approach. *J Neurosurg* 1996; 84:104–109.
10. Robertson DP, Simpson RK, Rose JE, et al: Video-assisted endoscopic thoracic ganglionectomy. *J Neurosurg* 1993; 79: 238–304.
11. Kao M-C, Tsai J-C, Lai D-M, et al: Autonomic activites in hyper- hidrosis patients before, during, and after endoscopic laser sympa- thectomy. *Neurosurgery* 1994; 34:262–268.
12. Dickman CA, Mican C: Thoracoscopic approaches for the treat- ment of anterior thoracic spinal pathology. *BNI Quarterly* 1996; 12(1):4–19.

CHAPTER 13

Spinal Exposure and Pleural Dissection Techniques

Curtis A. Dickman, M.D. and Daniel J. Rosenthal, M.D.

The most important initial step in facilitating thoracoscopic spinal surgery is proper positioning of the portals. Malpositioned portals hinder the surgeon's movements, interfering with the procedure. Portal designs and the techniques for inserting portals are discussed in Chapter 12. Once the portals are inserted, they serve as "windows" into the thorax for viewing the surgery and performing the dissection with surgical tools.

GENERAL CONSIDERATIONS FOR SPINAL EXPOSURE

Thoracoscopic spinal surgery requires a thorough familiarity with the anatomy of the thoracic spine, spinal cord, thorax, and mediastinum.[1,2] The decision to approach the spine from the left or right side depends on several factors, including the location, lateralization, and extent of the pathology. The position of the great vessels is also important to consider and can be evaluated on preoperative computed tomography or magnetic resonance imaging. A right-sided approach is most commonly used for midline lesions because more spinal surface area tends to be available behind the azygos vein than behind the aorta. If a lesion is lateralized to the left, a left-sided approach is more appropriate. If a lesion is located below T9, a left-sided approach is also preferred because at this level the diaphragm rides higher on the right side. In general, an exposure from T1–T2 to the T12–L1 interspace is possible via the thoracoscopic approach.

SURGICAL ANATOMY OF THE THORACIC SPINE

Several anatomical relationships are reemphasized because of their relevance to the surgical approaches. The 12 thoracic vertebrae have cylindrical, slightly oval vertebral bodies. The size of the thoracic vertebrae increases progressively from the first to the twelfth thoracic level. The height of each vertebral body is slightly shorter than its anteroposterior diameter and width. The thoracic disc spaces are relatively narrow, reflecting the limited motion that occurs across the thoracic motion segments.

Surface contours are important clues for determining anatomical relationships intraoperatively. Between each disc space, the middle surface of the thoracic vertebral bodies is slightly concave. The segmental arteries and veins course over the middle of the vertebral bodies. The disc spaces and end plates form a convex surface.

The pedicles connect the vertebral bodies with the remainder of the posterior arch (i.e., transverse processes, pars interarticularis, facets, laminae, and spinous processes, Fig. 13–1). The pedicles, dense oval cylinders of bone with a cancellous center, are adjacent to the upper third of the vertebral body. Understanding the relationship of the pedicle to the disc space, vertebral body, and spinal canal is critical for intraoperative anatomical orientation. The pedicles of two adjacent vertebrae form the boundaries of the neural foramen through which the nerve roots traverse. The pedicle therefore surrounds the lateral aspect of the dura over the spinal cord. The nerve roots within the neural foramen are surrounded by foraminal ligaments, a large amount of epidural fat, a rich epidural venous plexus, and radiculomedullary veins and arteries.[1,2] Therefore, the dura is best exposed by removing the thoracic pedicles rather than by dissecting through tissue within the neural foramen. The upper surface of the pedicles is contiguous with the superior surface of the vertebral end plates. Consequently, tracing the upper surface of the pedicle anteriorly leads the surgeon into the disc space. To obtain adequate exposure of the spinal canal for neural decompression, a portion of the

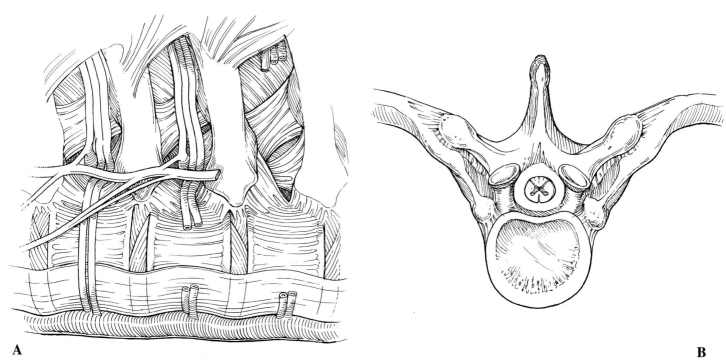

Figure 13–1. **(A)** Illustration of the thoracic vertebral anatomy. The ribs attach to the vertebrae via the costotransverse and costovertebral ligaments. The head of the ribs articulates with the base of the pedicle and the vertebral body just below the disc or at the disc space. The segmental vessels cross over the middle of the concave surface of the vertebral bodies. The sympathetic chain lays over the rib heads. **(B)** Axial view of a thoracic vertebrae showing the relationship of the rib and pedicle to the spinal cord. [With permission from Barrow Neurological Institute.]

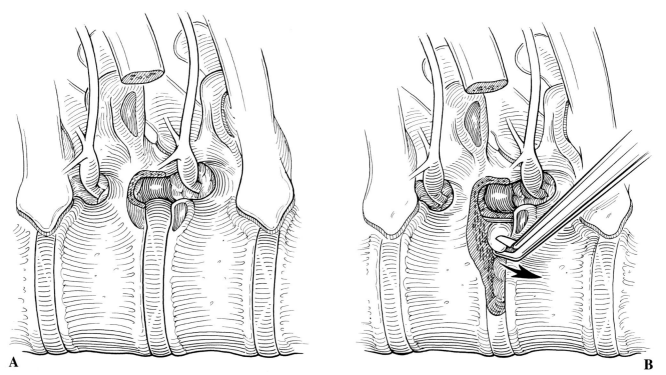

Figure 13–2. Illustration of a thoracoscopic microdiscectomy. **(A)** The superior half of the pedicle caudal to the herniated disc is removed to visualize the dura adjacent to the disc space. **(B)** A cavity is made in the dorsal disc space and the adjacent vertebral bodies to create a working space. Microdissection tools are used to remove the disc material away from the epidural space into the cavity. [With permission from Barrow Neurological Institute.]

pedicle of the caudal vertebrae *must* be removed to visualize the dura (Fig. 13–2).

The rib heads are essential landmarks for localization. The sympathetic ganglia and sympathetic chain are just lat-

eral to the rib heads beneath the parietal pleura. The ribs articulate with the transverse processes and the pedicles by strong ligamentous attachments. The costotransverse and costovertebral ligaments are dense, thick, and relatively

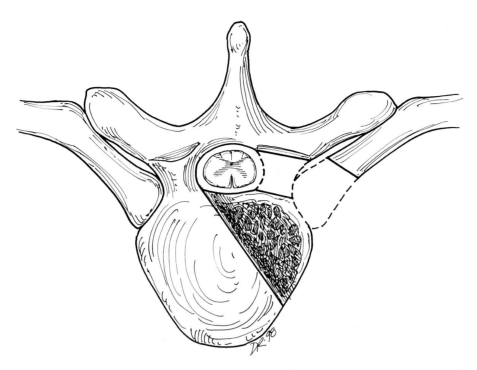

Figure 13–3.   The rib head forms an important triangular space that overlays the transverse process, pedicle, vertebral bodies, and disc space. The proximal rib head must be removed to access the spinal canal; next, the pedicle is removed. If the anterior surface of the spinal cord is to be decompressed, a pyramidal-shaped cavity is made in the vertebral bodies to provide access across the entire spinal canal.

inelastic. The rib forms a triangular space overlying the transverse process, the pedicle, the disc space, and the adjacent vertebral bodies (Fig. 13–3). The rib head, which articulates with the base of the pedicle and the vertebral body just caudal to or at the level of the disc space, serves to orient the surgeon to the relative position of the disc space and the pedicles. The T9 rib leads to the T8–T9 disc space; the T8 rib leads to the T7–T8 disc space, and so on. This relationship holds for most thoracic levels except at the T11 and T12 levels where the ribs articulate with the vertebral bodies caudal to the pedicle and disc spaces. The costovertebral joint is a shallow ball-and-socket type joint. The glistening surfaces of the cartilage in this joint are a helpful anatomical feature for verifying that the rib head has been resected completely.

The key to unlocking the spinal canal and visualizing the nerve roots, dura, and spinal cord is the *costovertebral triangle* between where the rib joins the transverse process and the vertebral body. The proximal 2 to 3 cm of the rib is removed *en bloc* to expose the surface of the pedicle. The pedicle is then removed to unlock the lateral aspect of the thecal sac. Removing the pedicle early in the dissection allows the dura to be visualized clearly so the surgeon can remain oriented to the position of the spinal cord and ensure its protection during the dissection.

Predictable anatomical relationships exist among the intercostal vein, artery, and nerve. The segmental artery and vein course over the middle of the concave surface of the vertebral body. At the neural foramen, the vessels give off radiculomedullary branches and the segmental nerve joins the segmental vessels.[2] As the neurovascular bundle extends laterally, from cephalad to caudal, the vein, artery, and nerve run in the groove on the undersurface of each rib.

SPINAL EXPOSURE AND LUNG MOBILIZATION

The nonventilated lung becomes densely atelectatic within a few minutes after its airflow is blocked. Adhesions that prevent spinal exposure may be present. Filamentous adhesions are easily detached using cautery scissors. However, extensive, dense pleural adhesions (caused by sclerotherapy, pneumonia, empyema, hemothorax, prior thoracotomy, or prior thoracoscopy) rigidly scarring a broad area of the lungs' surface can prohibit endoscopic access. Focal, dense adhesions can be detached surgically (Fig. 13–4), but entry into the pulmonary parenchyma should be avoided so that an air leak from the lung does not occur. Once the lung has been mobilized, it is retracted manually or with gravity by rotating the patient anteriorly. Mechanical retraction of the lung should be performed cautiously to avoid injury to the lung parenchyma (Fig. 13–5). The diaphragm may also need to be retracted to access the lower thoracic disc spaces.

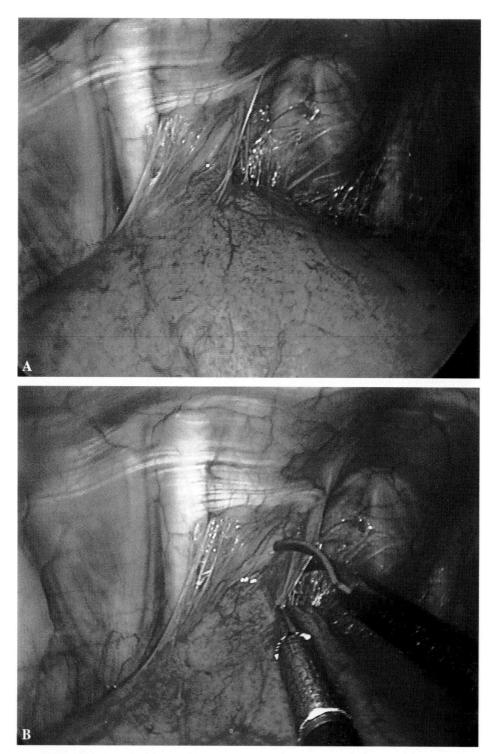

Figure 13–4. **(A)** Intraoperative photograph of pleural adhesions. **(B)** The focal adhesions were sharply detached from the chest wall with scissors to mobilize the lung.

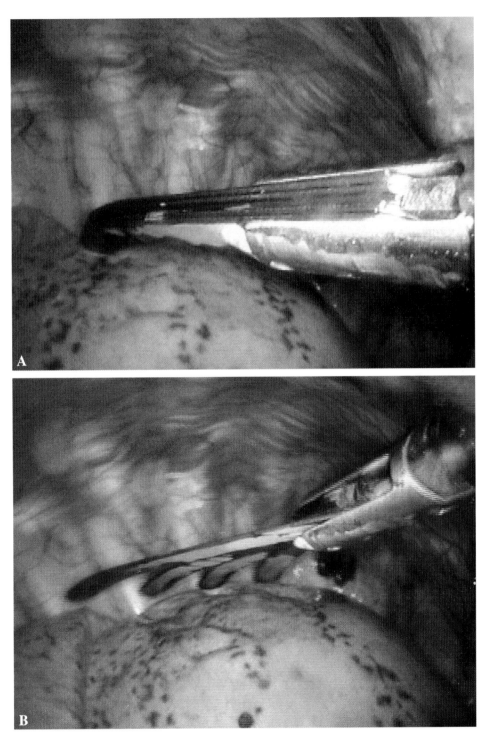

Figure 13–5.   **(A)** A fan retractor is inserted into the chest to mobilize and retract the lung away from the surface of the spine.
(B) The fan retractor is always opened, closed, and repositioned under direct visualization to avoid injuring the lung.

SPINAL LOCALIZATION

Direct visualization and fluoroscopy are used together to verify the correct level of spinal exposure. Misidentification of a disc level can be avoided if the level is carefully localized visually and radiographically.

Identification of the appropriate spinal level can be challenging. Counting the ribs endoscopically from within the thoracic cavity is an excellent way of initially localizing the proper level. Usually, the first visible rib at the apex of the thoracic cavity is the second rib. Each subsequent rib is directly visualized, palpated, and counted (Fig. 13–6). A long, blunt-tipped needle can then be inserted into the disc space and a radiograph obtained. Anteroposterior images are preferable to lateral images to enable reliable rib counting. The twelfth rib is identified first and the adjacent ribs are identified sequentially.

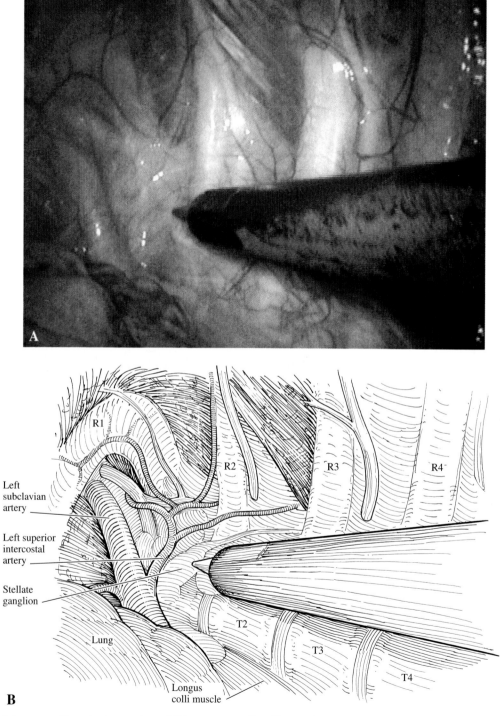

Figure 13–6. **(A)** Intraoperative photograph and **(B)** corresponding illustration showing the second rib being identified in the apex of the left hemithorax. The ribs are counted sequentially and palpated to identify the level of spinal pathology correctly. R = rib.

PLEURAL MOBILIZATION

The incision made in the parietal pleura over the spine depends on the spinal procedure that is being performed (Fig. 13–7). The pleura is incised and the pleural edges are folded away from the region of interest to expose the bone surfaces, blood vessels, and sympathetic chain.

Scissors or monopolar cauterization is used for the initial pleural incision, which is made over the rib head or the disc space to avoid the segmental vessels. The surgeon then grasps the edge of the pleura with an endoscopic Debakey forceps and elevates the pleural edges away from the spine or chest wall. An endoshears (scissors) or a pleural dissector is used to incise the pleura, undermine the edges of the elevated pleura, and mobilize the pleura away from the segmental arteries and veins on the surface of the spine (Fig. 13–8). The pleural flaps are folded away from the operative field.

At the end of the procedure, the parietal pleural incisions can sometimes be closed with sutures (if the patient is

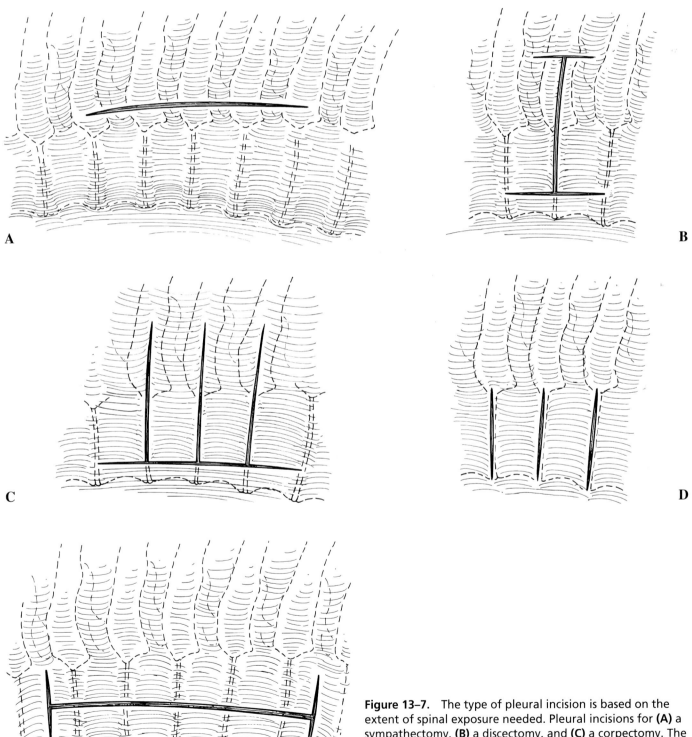

Figure 13–7. The type of pleural incision is based on the extent of spinal exposure needed. Pleural incisions for **(A)** a sympathectomy, **(B)** a discectomy, and **(C)** a corpectomy. The incision for an anterior release can be **(D)** centered over the disc space for a focal lesion or **(E)** span several disc spaces for a larger lesion.

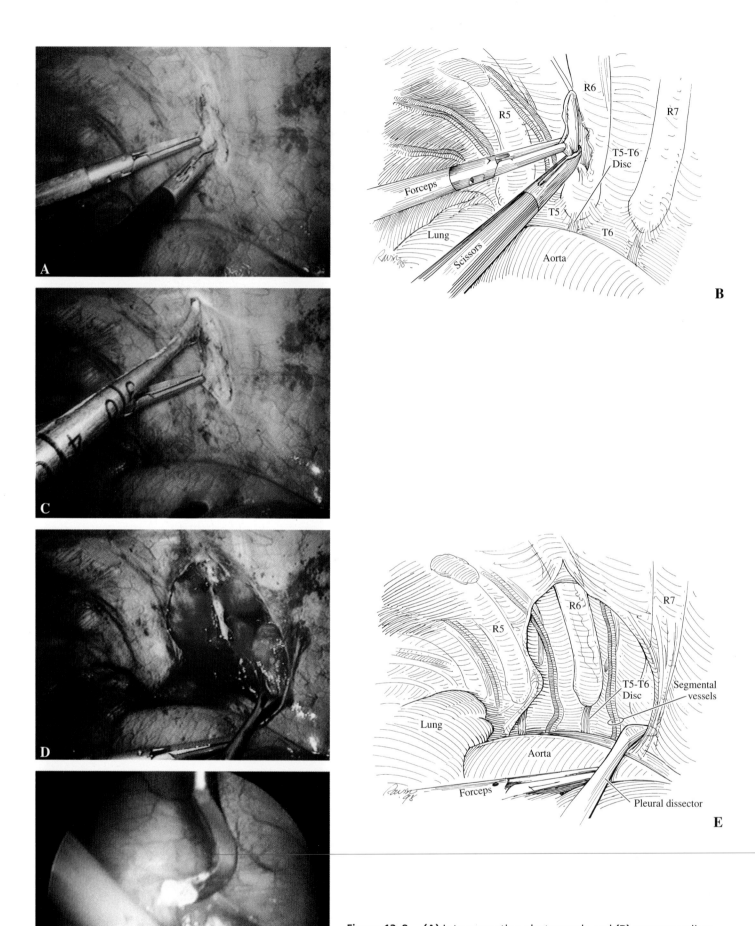

Figure 13–8. **(A)** Intraoperative photograph and **(B)** corresponding illustration showing the pleura being grasped with a forceps and incised with scissors. **(C)** The pleural incision is extended with a pleural dissector. **(D)** Intraoperative photograph and **(E)** corresponding illustration showing the pleural dissector being used to lift the parietal pleura away from the surface of the spine and to incise the pleura. **(F)** Intraoperative photograph of a pleural hook dissector used to mobilize the pleura. R = rib.

young and has thick pleura), which minimize blood oozing from the spinal surface. Most patients, however, have a thin pleura that shrinks after it is mobilized. In such cases, the surgeon is unable to close the pleura.

VASCULAR MOBILIZATION AND LIGATION

The segmental vessels course over the concave recesses in the midportion of the vertebral bodies. The segmental arteries and veins connect directly to the aorta and the azygos or hemiazygos veins with no intervening structures to reduce the intravascular pressure. Laterally, the segmental vessels have branches that perforate the neural foramen and supply the nerve roots and spinal cord. As the vessels course laterally, they are joined by the intercostal nerve. Together, this intercostal neurovascular bundle runs beneath the caudal edge of each rib (Fig. 13–1A).

The segmental vessels should be protected and preserved when possible. Often in spinal procedures, however, they must be mobilized, ligated, or both. The segmental vessels are mobilized by gently grasping and elevating the vessels with a Debakey forceps and undermining them with right-angle forceps. Once the vessel has been isolated, it is ligated with an endoscopic hemoclip (Fig. 13–9). The segmental vessels are most easily isolated along the center of the lateral surface of the vertebral bodies, midway between the great vessels and the neural foramen. Hemoclips are required to provide secure permanent hemostasis for these vessels. The hemoclips should be spaced far enough apart (i.e., 1 cm) to allow the vessels to be transected sharply between the ligatures. The vessels should not be coagulated and divided without permanent ligation.

Along with the intercostal nerve, the segmental intercostal vessels are preserved when the proximal rib is being dissected for exposure of the pedicle and spinal canal. The vessels and nerve are carefully detached from the rib using

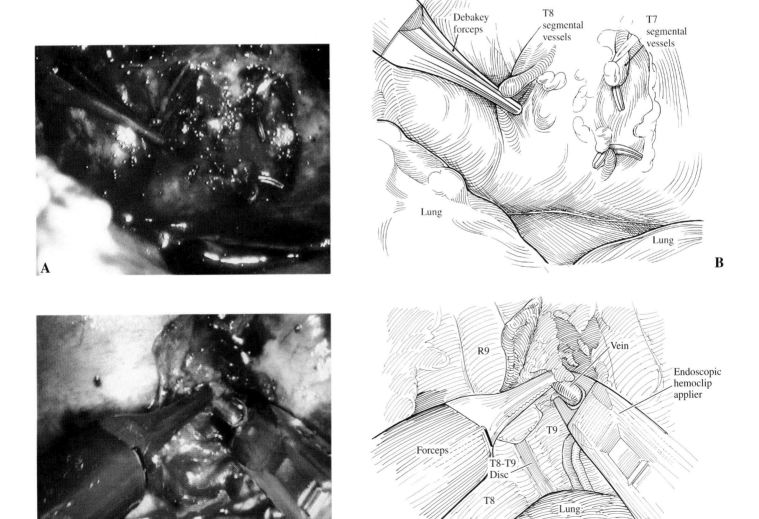

Figure 13–9. **(A)** Intraoperative photograph and **(B)** corresponding illustration showing the segmental vessels being mobilized, isolated, and ligated with hemoclips. The vessels were transected between the clips. [A and B from Dickman CA, Mican C: Multilevel anterior thoracic discectomies. *J Neurosurg* 1996;84:104–109. With permission from the Journal of Neurosurgery.] **(C)** Intraoperative photograph and **(D)** corresponding illustration showing a segmental vein grasped with a forceps. An endoscopic hemoclip is applied with a multiloaded clip applier. R = rib.

subperiosteal dissection with Cobb dissectors, curved curettes, and rib dissectors. If the vessels bleed during mobilization of the neurovascular bundle, the hemorrhage is controlled with *bipolar* cauterization to avoid injury to the intercostal nerve.

Occasionally, the aorta or the azygos vein may need to be mobilized to provide access for the spinal dissection. These vessels can be mobilized by ligating several adjacent sets of segmental vessels and gently retracting the great vessels anteriorly with a sponge stick. Gauze sponges can also be inserted to maintain the space between the mobilized vessels and the surface of the spine. The aorta may need to be mobilized during a left-sided approach for a discectomy, corpectomy, or an anterior release. The azygos vein must be mobilized for an anterior release from a right-sided approach, but rarely for a discectomy or a corpectomy. An anterior release requires more extensive vascular mobilization because the entire ventral surface of the spine is exposed. The anterior longitudinal ligament must be transected at multiple levels to facilitate the releases.[3,4]

When multiple segmental blood vessels are sacrificed (especially on the left at the lower thoracic segments), there is a risk of spinal cord infarction from occlusion of the artery of Adamkiewicz and its collateral vessels. Because of the extensive multisegmental collateral supply of the arterialis radicula magna to the spinal cord, infarction is seldom a concern if only one or two sets of segmental vessels are ligated. The potential for this complication is more of a concern when extensive vascular mobilization is required for an anterior release. The risk can be minimized by temporarily occluding the segmental vessels before their ligation and transection. If the evoked potentials diminish, flow to the vessel should be restored and preserved.

SPINAL CANAL EXPOSURE

Exposing the spinal cord is an important maneuver if the nerve roots and spinal cord need surgical decompression (i.e., for a discectomy, corpectomy, or removing a neural foraminal nerve sheath tumor).[1,2,5–11] The spinal canal does not need to be exposed for a sympathectomy or an anterior release or to biopsy the vertebral body.[3,4,11–13]

The spinal canal *cannot* be easily accessed by traversing the neural foramen, which is covered by ligaments and contains the nerve roots, a rich vascular plexus, and epidural fat. The most *reliable* way to expose the spinal canal is to remove the rib and the pedicle from the lateral surface of the dura (Fig. 13–3).

The proximal 2 cm of the rib and the rib head are removed to expose the pedicle. First, the neurovascular bundle is carefully detached from the undersurface of the rib. The intercostal muscles are detached from the rib using a periosteal elevator and a right-angled rib dissector (Fig. 13–10). The costotransverse ligaments are cut with a right-

angled rib dissector (Fig. 13–11). The costovertebral ligaments are cut with a Cobb periosteal elevator, which is inserted into the costovertebral joint (Fig. 13–12) parallel to the articular surface of the joint. Visualizing the glistening cartilage of the costovertebral joint surface confirms that the rib head has been completely removed.

After the neurovascular bundle, ligaments, and soft tissues have been detached from the rib, the proximal 2 cm of the rib is removed to provide access to the pedicle and spinal canal. The proximal rib can be removed piecemeal (i.e., with a burr, drill, or Kerrison rongeur) or transected sharply (i.e., with a drill, osteotome, rib cutting tool, Kerrison rongeur, or oscillating saw) and removed as a single piece (Fig. 13–13). The bone can be saved for grafting, if desired.

The pedicle is identified after the proximal rib is removed. The lateral surface of the pedicle is exposed with a periosteal elevator. The superior surface of the pedicle is defined with a small curved microsurgical curette. The foraminal ligaments are cut from the superior edge of the pedicle to provide access to the epidural space (Fig. 13–14). Once the upper border of the pedicle is delineated, a Kerrison rongeur is used to remove the pedicle to expose the epidural space (Fig. 13–15). If the pedicle is wide, it may need to be thinned by applying a burr to its lateral surface. The medial half of the pedicle can then be removed with a Kerrison punch.

If the pathology is positioned at the level of the disc space, the cephalad half of the pedicle (of the vertebrae caudal to that disc space) must be removed to provide access to the epidural space. If the compressive pathology is broad based or extends caudally to the disc space, the entire pedicle must be resected (Fig. 13–15).

During resection of the pedicle, the epidural veins can bleed moderately, requiring suction to clear the surgical field. After the pedicle is resected, epidural hemostasis is achieved with bipolar cauterization or with small pieces of hemostatic material precisely delivered to the epidural space with cottonoids ($\frac{1}{2} \times \frac{1}{2}$ inch). These methods are identical to those used for epidural hemostasis in open surgery. If a cottonoid is used, the end of the string should be grasped with a hemostat outside the portal to prevent the loss of the patty within the thorax. Clear identification of the epidural space allows the decompression to be performed under direct visualization.

Removing the rib head and pedicle exposes the *lateral* surface of the dura. To expose the *ventral* surface of the dura, a cavity must be created in the vertebral body using a drill (Fig. 13–16). For a microdiscectomy exposure, this cavity is pyramidal with its base along the posterior margin of the vertebral body adjacent to the disc space. A 1- to 2-cm wide cavity is created to work toward the opposite side of the spinal canal (Fig. 13–16A–D). For adequate exposure of the spinal canal to access large lesions (i.e., large calcified discs or intradural discs), a corpectomy is required. The normal dura must be exposed above and below the compressive lesion. The size of

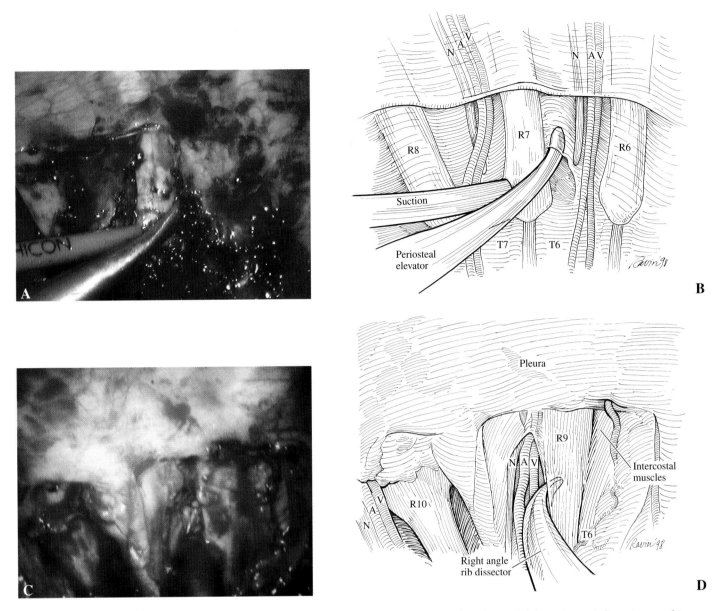

Figure 13–10.   **(A)** Intraoperative photograph and **(B)** corresponding illustration showing a Cobb periosteal dissector used to detach the neurovascular bundle, muscles, and ligaments from the proximal rib. **(C)** Intraoperative photograph and **(D)** corresponding illustration showing a right-angle rib dissector used to detach soft tissue from the lateral aspect of the rib. N = nerve, A = artery, V = vein, and R = rib.

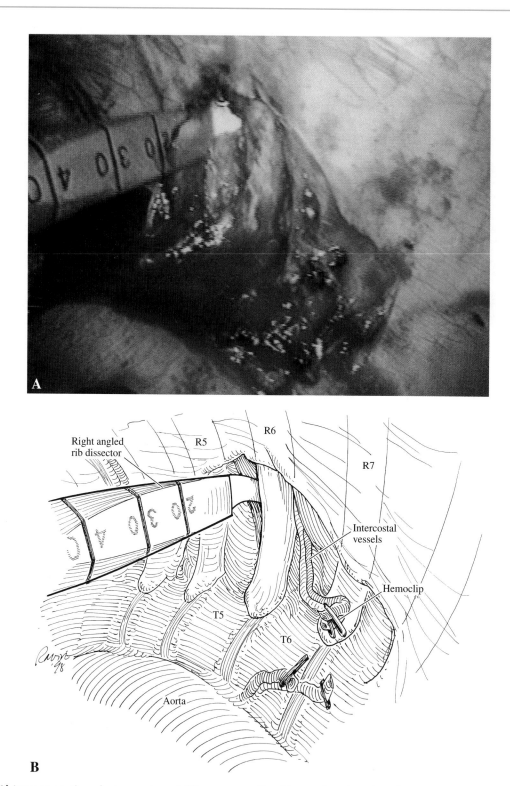

Figure 13–11.   (A) Intraoperative photograph and **(B)** corresponding illustration showing the costotransverse ligaments being cut with a right-angled rib dissector. R = rib.

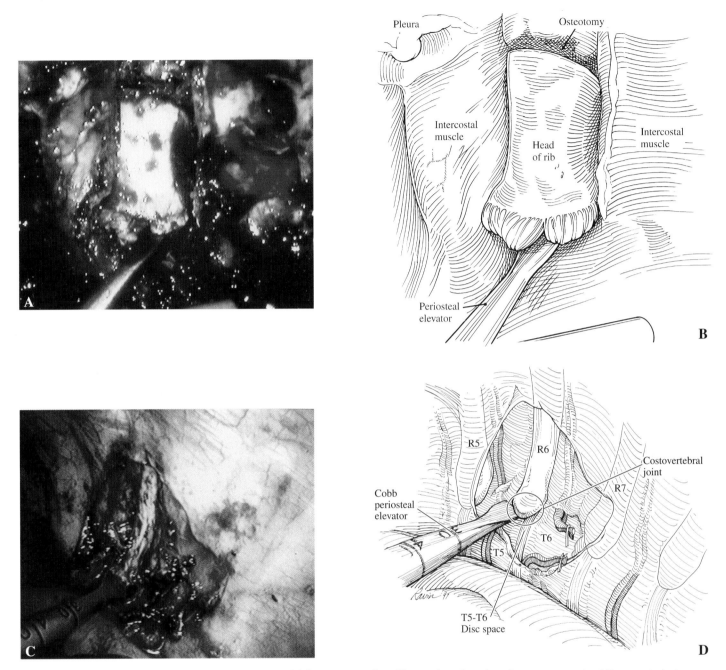

Figure 13–12. **(A)** Intraoperative photograph and **(B)** corresponding illustration showing the costovertebral ligaments being detached with a Cobb periosteal elevator. [A and B from Dickman CA, Mican C: Multilevel anterior thoracic discectomies. *J Neurosurg* 1996;84:104–109. With permission from the Journal of Neurosurgery.] **(C)** Intraoperative photograph and **(D)** corresponding illustration showing the neurovascular bundle detached from the caudal rib margin and the intercostal muscles detached from the rib. A Cobb periosteal elevator is inserted into the costovertebral joint to cut the ligaments and disarticulate the joint.

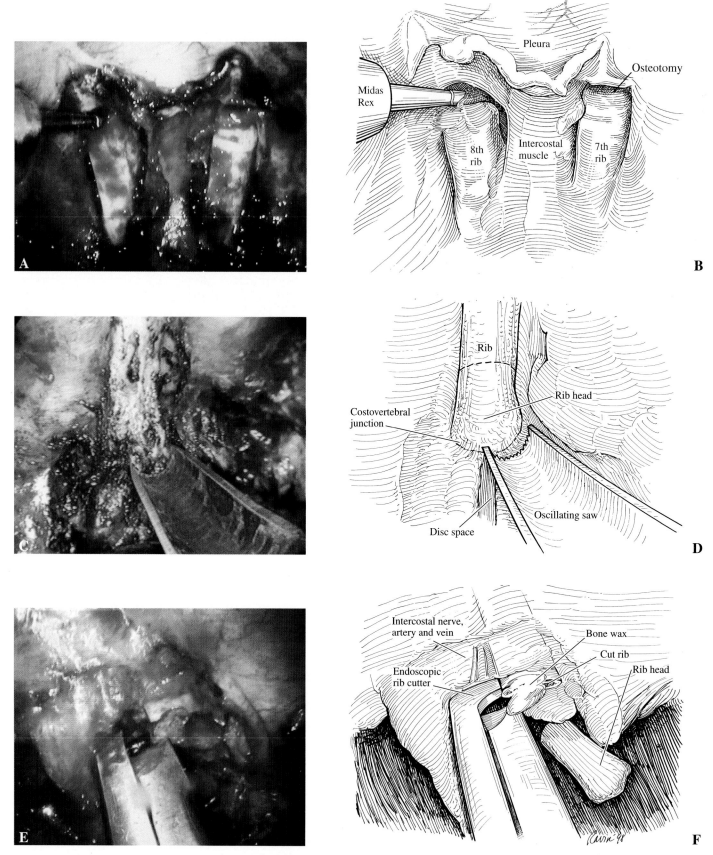

Figure 13–13. Methods of proximal rib resection. **(A)** Intraoperative photograph and **(B)** illustration showing the rib being transected with a drill. [A and B from Dickman CA, Mican C: Multilevel anterior thoracic discectomies. *J Neurosurg* 1996;84:104–109. With permission from the Journal of Neurosurgery.] **(C)** Intraoperative photograph and **(D)** corresponding illustration showing transection with an oscillating saw. **(E)** Intraoperative photograph and **(F)** illustration showing transection with a rib cutting tool. R = rib.

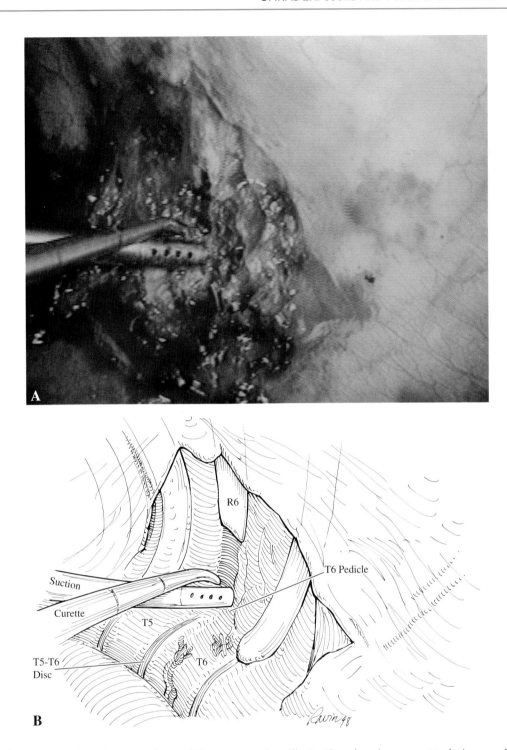

Figure 13–14. **(A)** Intraoperative photograph and **(B)** corresponding illustration showing a curette being used to cut the foraminal ligaments from the superior edge of the pedicle to expose the edge of the pedicle. R = rib.

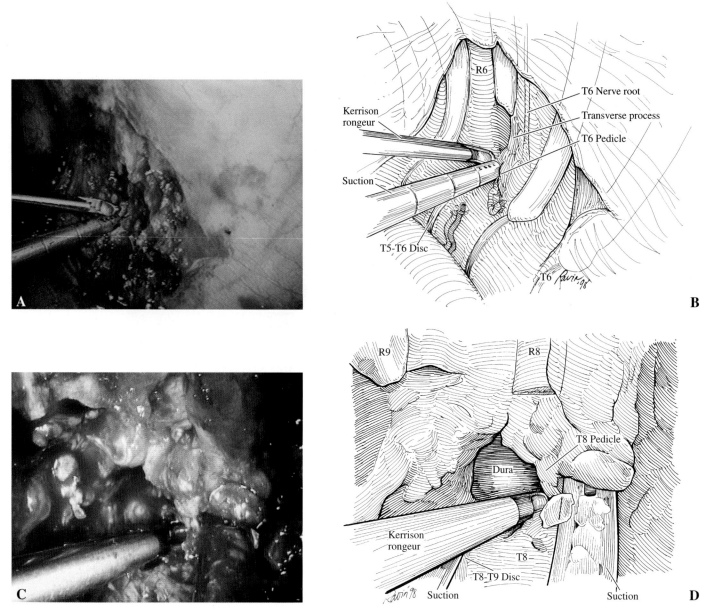

Figure 13–15. **(A)** Intraoperative photograph and **(B)** corresponding illustration showing a Kerrison rongeur being used to remove the cephalad portion of the pedicle to expose the epidural space. **(C)** Intraoperative photograph and **(D)** corresponding illustration showing that when the pathology extends caudal to the disc space, the entire pedicle must be removed to provide adequate visualization of the dura. R = rib.

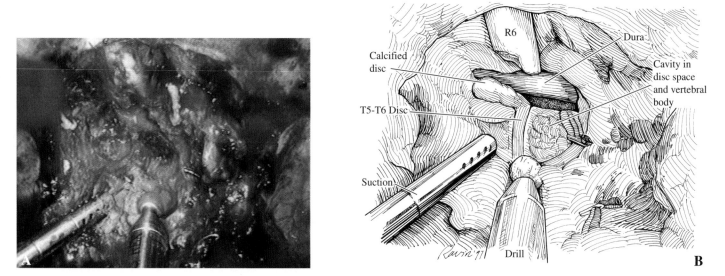

Figure 13–16. **(A)** Intraoperative photograph and **(B)** corresponding illustration showing a cavity drilled into the dorsal disc space and vertebral body to expose the ventral surface of the dura.

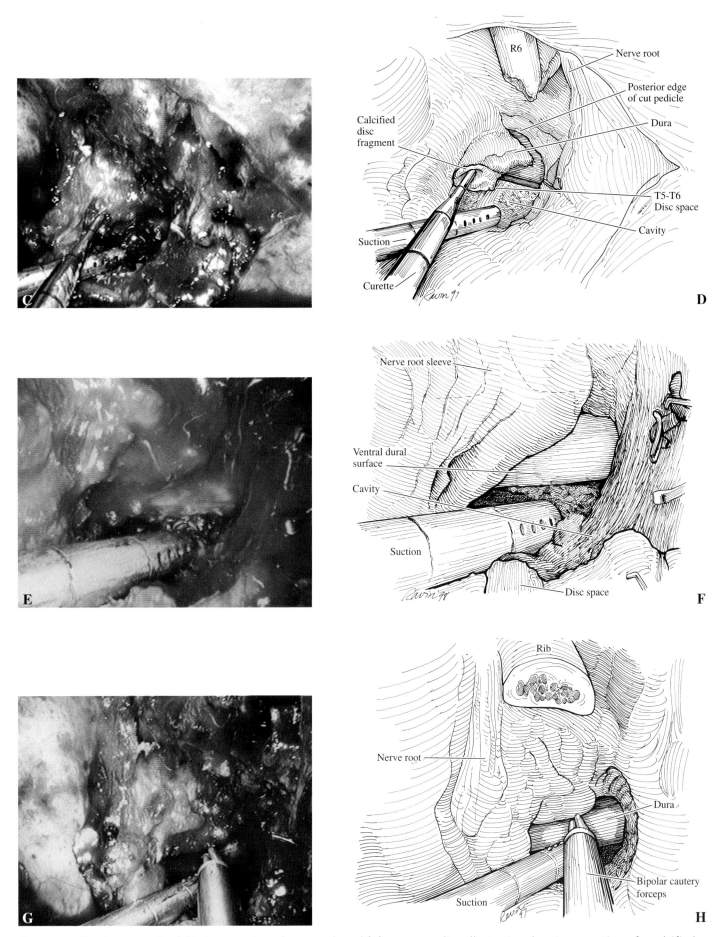

Figure 13–16. *(continued)* **(C)** Intraoperative photograph and **(D)** corresponding illustration showing resection of a calcified herniated thoracic disc with microsurgical curettes. **(E)** Intraoperative photograph and **(F)** corresponding illustration showing the entire ventral surface of the dura after resection of the calcified disc. **(G)** Intraoperative photograph and **(H)** corresponding illustration showing epidural hemostasis being achieved with insulated bipolar cauterization. R = rib.

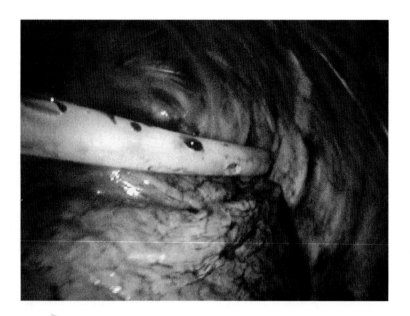

Figure 13–17. The endoscope is used to assess the position of the chest tubes before the lung is reinflated and the incisions are closed.

the working space needed is *directly* proportional to the size of the lesion compressing the spinal cord. Larger lesions require more working space (i.e., a corpectomy) to visualize the entire pathology and to minimize the risk of any tool entering the epidural space.

After the spinal dissection has been completed, the thorax is irrigated and inspected. Any loose bone, disc, or debris is removed from the chest cavity. Epidural hemostasis is best completed using compressed sheets of microfibrillar collagen, which are laid gently over the dural surface. The pleura is closed with suture, if desired. The portals are removed from the chest wall, and the incisions are inspected with the endoscope to determine if the portal sites are bleeding. Chest tubes are inserted through the portal incisions under direct endoscopic vision (Fig. 13–17). An apical chest tube is used to promote reexpansion of the lung. A dependent inferior-posterior chest tube is used to drain fluid from the chest. The chest tubes are secured to the chest with heavy gauge silk purse-string sutures. As the lung is reinflated, it is inspected for air leaks and the position of the chest tubes is inspected endoscopically. The endoscope is then removed, and the remaining portal incisions are closed with subcutaneous and subcuticular sutures. The chest tubes are positioned to −20 cm of suction and usually remain in place until the output is less than 100 ml/day.

REFERENCES

1. Naunheim KS, Barnett MG, Crandall DG, et al: Anterior exposure of the thoracic spine. *Ann Thorac Surg* 1994; 57:1436–1439.
2. Safdari H, Baker RL, II: Microsurgical anatomy and related techniques to an anterolateral transthoracic approach to thoracic disc herniations. *Surg Neurol* 1985; 23:589–593.
3. Dwyer AF, Schafer MF: Anterior approach to scoliosis. Results of treatment in fifty-one cases. *J Bone Joint Surg Br* 1974; 56(2): 218–224.
4. Simmons ED, Jr., Kowalski JM, Simmons EH: The results of surgical treatment for adult scoliosis. *Spine* 1993; 18(6):718–724.
5. Rosenthal D, Marquardt G, Lorenz R, et al: Anterior decompression and stabilization using a microsurgical endoscopic technique for metastatic tumors of the thoracic spine. *J Neurosurg* 1996; 84(4):565–572.
6. Dickman CA, Rosenthal D, Karahalios DG, et al: Thoracic vertebrectomy and reconstruction using a microsurgical thoracoscopic approach. *Neurosurgery* 1996; 38(2):279–293.
7. Horowitz MB, Moossy JJ, Julian T, et al: Thoracic discectomy using video assisted thoracoscopy. *Spine* 1994; 19(9):1082–1086.
8. Rosenthal D, Rosenthal R, de Simone A: Removal of a protruded thoracic disc using microsurgical endoscopy. A new technique. *Spine* 1994; 19(9):1087–1091.
9. Regan JJ, Mack MJ, Picetti GD, III: A technical report on video-assisted thoracoscopy in thoracic spinal surgery. Preliminary description. *Spine* 1995; 20(7):831–837.
10. Rosenthal D, Lorenz R: The use of the microsurgical endoscopic technique for treating affections of the dorsal spine: Indications and early results (abstract). *J Neurosurg* 1995; 82:342A.
11. Dickman CA, Mican C: Thoracoscopic approaches for the treatment of anterior thoracic spinal pathology. *BNI Quarterly* 1996; 12(1):4–19.
12. Krasna MJ, Mack MJ: Sympathectomy, in Krasna MJ, Mack MJ, eds: *Atlas of Thoracoscopic Surgery*. St. Louis: Quality Medical; 1994:139.
13. Robertson DP, Simpson RK, Rose JE, et al: Video-assisted endoscopic thoracic ganglionectomy. *J Neurosurg* 1993; 79(2): 238–240.

14

Thoracoscopic Sympathectomy

Stephen M. Papadopoulos, M.D. and Curtis A. Dickman, M.D.

Thoracic sympathectomy may be used to surgically treat palmar hyperhidrosis, axillary hyperhidrosis, reflex sympathetic dystrophy affecting the upper extremities, or ischemic syndromes of the hands such as Raynaud's disease. The surgical procedure for these problems involves removing the second, third, and fourth sympathetic ganglia with the sympathetic chain. The open surgical approaches used for thoracic sympathectomy include the extrapleural or subpleural posterior approach, the transaxillary approach, the supraclavicular approach, or the anterior thoracotomy approach.[1-3] Thoracoscopy, however, is the most efficient, least traumatic surgical method for the direct surgical access of the upper sympathetic chain to visualize and remove the upper sympathetic ganglia.[1,4-9]

SURGICAL INDICATIONS

Palmar hyperhidrosis can be disabling, interfering with a patient's personal and social functions, work, and recreation. Writing, handshaking, handling papers, and a host of other daily activities can be adversely affected by hyperhidrosis. When hyperhidrosis is severe, the sweat spontaneously drips from an individual's hands. Topical agents and systemic drugs provide only temporary or partial symptomatic relief.[1-3,10] In contrast, the success rate of sympathectomy for the permanent relief of palmar hyperhidrosis is 90% or higher.[1-9,11]

Severe axillary hyperhidrosis and bromhidrosis (axillary malodor) can also be treated effectively with sympathectomy. Alternative treatments include topical antiperspirants and excising the axillary sweat glands. Axillary innervation is mainly related to the T3 and T4 ganglia.[4]

Sympathectomy is a reasonably effective method for the treatment of reflex sympathetic dystrophy.[2,5,9] Patients typically present with posttraumatic pain and trophic changes.

Medical therapy (i.e., analgesics, antiinflammatory drugs, physical therapy, or centrally acting drugs such as carbamazepine, amitriptyline, gabapentin, etc.) tends to be ineffective in relieving the symptoms adequately or on a long-term basis. Patients with reflex sympathetic dystrophy are only considered for surgical sympathectomy if they experience significant pain relief from percutaneous stellate ganglion blocks with a local anesthetic. The blocks are used to verify that the patient's sympathetic nervous system is involved in the etiology of the symptoms.

Sympathectomy also may be used as a salvage technique to treat ischemic syndromes (e.g., Raynaud's disease), in which the ischemia is severe enough to threaten the loss of the patient's hands.[2,5,9] Unfortunately, however, sympathectomy is often just a temporizing method because ischemic diseases usually progress even after the procedure has been performed. Nonetheless, sympathectomy sometimes can be used acutely to prevent the amputation of the hands of a patient with severe ischemia.

The sympathectomy used to treat hyperhidrosis, reflex sympathetic dystrophy, or ischemic syndromes of the upper extremities removes the second sympathetic ganglia through the fourth or fifth sympathetic ganglia. The sympathetic chain with the ganglia is excised sharply en bloc. If present, the accessory nerve of Kuntz (an additional division of the sympathetic trunk arising from the level of T1, T2, or T3) must also be resected to ensure that the sympathectomy will be effective.[12] The stellate ganglia is preserved to prevent Horner's syndrome, and doing so does not compromise the effect of the sympathectomy in the arms. Some surgeons have advocated resecting the inferior third of the stellate ganglia, but this resection is usually unnecessary.

Sympathectomy also can effectively relieve pain among patients with advanced pancreatic carcinoma.[13] The procedure, however, differs from the sympathectomy for the upper limbs. Pain can be palliated by dividing the *greater and lesser splanchnic nerves* as they emerge from the *left sympathetic chain and the vagus nerve* (truncal vagotomy). The greater splanchnic nerve originates from the T5 to T9 sympathetic ganglia; the lesser splanchnic nerve originates from the T10 and T11 levels.

SURGICAL TECHNIQUE

The procedure is performed with the patient in the lateral decubitus position under general endotracheal anesthesia. A double-lumen endotracheal tube is used. If bilateral sympathectomies are required, both procedures are performed under the same anaesthetic, repositioning and redraping the patient after the sympathectomy has been completed on the first side.

The patient's arm is abducted and elevated 90° to the chest wall, and the arm is flexed 90° at the elbow. The patient's arm is padded and secured to an ether screen to provide access to the axillae and to move the scapula away from the lateral chest wall (Fig. 14–1). The patient's chest is prepared widely in case the procedure must be converted to a thoracotomy. The patient is taped securely to the operating table, rotated 40° anteriorly, and placed in a reverse Trendelenburg position to allow gravity to retract the lung away from the apex of the chest and the upper thoracic spine. Ventilation to the ipsilateral lung is stopped to provide atelectasis and exposure.

Three portals are used. The portal for the endoscope (11-mm diameter) is placed in the middle or posterior axillary line in the fourth or fifth intercostal space. The two working portals (7-mm diameter) are placed in the anterior axillary

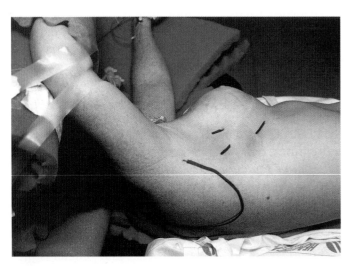

Figure 14–1. Patient positioning for a right-sided sympathectomy. The patient is in a left lateral decubitus position. The right arm is abducted, padded, and secured to an ether screen. Portals are positioned in the third, fourth, and fifth intercostal spaces. The position of the scapula was marked on the skin. A portal for the endoscope is placed in the fourth intercostal space in the posterior axillary line. Two working portals are placed ventrally in the anterior axillary line in the third and fifth intercostal spaces.

line in the third and fifth intercostal spaces. The first and second intercostal spaces must be avoided to prevent injuring the subclavian vessels. The first portal and the endoscope are inserted, and the other portals are inserted under direct visualization.

The apex of the lung is mobilized away from the spine, and the region is inspected to identify the stellate ganglia, the sympathetic chain, and any accessory sympathetic trunks. These structures are visible directly beneath the parietal pleura. The sympathetic chain lies over the rib heads. The stellate ganglion is located directly over the head of the first rib and is surrounded by a fat pad within the thoracic outlet, adjacent to the subclavian artery and veins (Figs. 14–2, 14–3, and, 14–12).

The sympathetic chain usually courses superficially to the segmental and intercostal arteries and veins in the region. Several large tributaries of the second, third, and fourth intercostal veins often merge over the vertebral body of T3 or T4 to form the superior intercostal vein, which empties into the azygos vein (Fig. 14–3). The first intercostal vein usually drains directly into the brachiocephalic vein. The first and second segmental and intercostal arteries arise from the supreme intercostal artery, which is a branch of the costocervical trunk of the subclavian artery. All other segmental thoracic arteries arise directly from the aorta. Because the sympathetic chain is positioned superficial to the vessels, it usually can be excised without sacrificing any blood vessels. The surgeon, however, should look for and ligate any *anomalous* blood vessels that run superficial to the sympathetic chain.

To remove the sympathetic chain, the surgeon will find that the dissection is most easily begun at the level of T4–T5 and continued rostrally. The pleura is grasped and tented up adjacent to the sympathetic chain caudal to the ganglia of T4. The pleura is incised with scissors directly over the sympathetic trunk (Figs. 14–4 and 14–5). The pleural incision is extended rostrally to the T1 rib head and stellate ganglia using endoscopic scissors or a pleural dissector (Fig. 14–6). The accessory sympathetic nerve of Kuntz is identified, mobilized, and excised (Figs. 14–6 and 14–7). Below the T4 ganglion, the sympathetic trunk is grasped with a tissue forceps and transected with scissors. The trunk is grasped with forceps, elevated away from the vessels on the surface of the spine, and the chain is undermined by sharp and blunt dissection with microscissors. The rami that communicate with each ganglion have a rich microvascular supply. Consequently, the rami undergo bipolar cauterization before they are transected with scissors. Monopolar cauterization should be avoided so that thermal energy or electrical current is not transferred to the nerves or spinal cord. The multiple rami to each ganglion are transected to mobilize the sympathetic trunk en bloc (Fig. 14–8). The trunk is transected just caudal to the stellate ganglion, which lies over the first rib. The specimen is removed as a single piece and sent for histopathological analysis (Figs. 14–9 and 14–10).

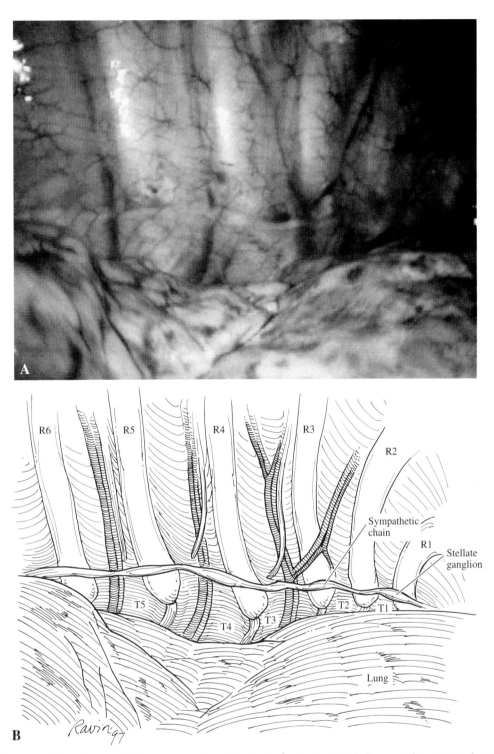

Figure 14–2. **(A)** Intraoperative view and **(B)** corresponding illustration of a right-sided sympathectomy. The sympathetic chain is positioned beneath the parietal pleura, overlying the rib heads and segmental blood vessels. R = rib, T = thoracic level.

The effectiveness of the sympathectomy can be judged intraoperatively by measuring the palmar skin temperature bilaterally. A unilateral increase of 1 to 3°C or more occurs when an adequate sympathectomy has been achieved.[4,8,11] If the palmar skin temperature does not change after the sympathetic chain has been excised, an aberrant accessory sympathetic trunk (the nerve of Kuntz) may exist and must be identified and removed. Alternatively, the inferior third of the stellate ganglia may need to be excised.

When the sympathectomy is completed, bipolar cauterization is used to obtain meticulous hemostasis from the pleural and spinal surfaces (Fig. 14–11). If the pleura is thick enough, it can be closed with endoscopic suturing. A small diameter apical chest tube is inserted through one portal to facilitate reinflation of the lung. The lung is inspected during reinflation to ensure that the parenchyma was not violated and the lung has no air leaks. The portals are removed and the incisions closed with subcuticular sutures.

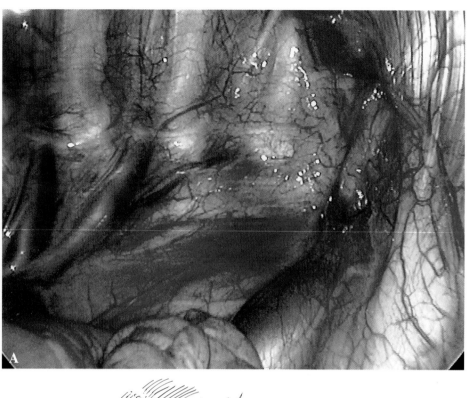

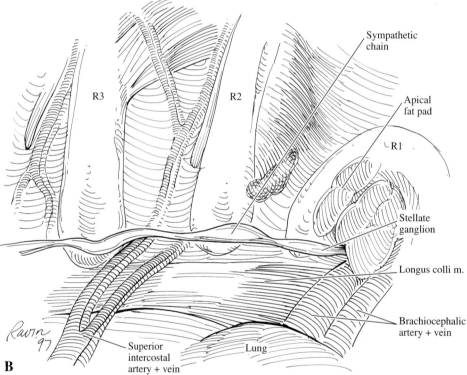

Figure 14–3. **(A)** Intraoperative view and **(B)** corresponding illustration of a right-sided approach from an apical view. The stellate ganglion and an accompanying fat pad overlie the head of the first rib. Adjacent to the stellate ganglion medially are the subclavian artery and the junction of the brachiocephalic and subclavian veins. The first intercostal vein drains into the brachiocephalic vein. The supreme intercostal artery arises from the costocervical trunk of the subclavian artery and branches into the first and second intercostal arteries. The second, third, and fourth intercostal veins merge to form the superior intercostal vein, which drains into the azygos vein. R = rib.

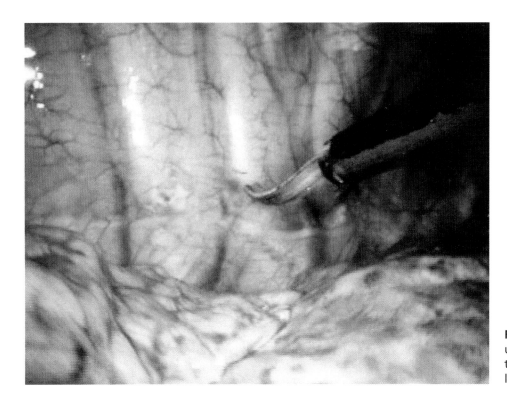

Figure 14–4. Endoscopic scissors are used to incise the pleura adjacent to the thoracic sympathetic chain at the T4 level.

Chest tubes can be avoided or they can be removed immediately after the lung is reinflated (i.e., in the recovery room or the operating room) so long as hemostasis is complete and the lung is uninjured. Avoiding an indwelling chest tube eliminates postoperative pleuritic chest pain. Usually, patients can be discharged within 24 hours of the procedure if their condition permits.

When a sympathectomy is performed on the left side, the approach and portal positions are similar to the right-sided approach. The differences in the anatomy between the right and left hemithorax should be kept in mind (Fig. 14–12, 14–13, and 14–14). The left subclavian artery and the thoracic duct are structures that should be avoided at the thoracic apex when a left-sided sympathectomy is performed.

SURGICAL OUTCOMES

Palmar hyperhidrosis is the most common surgical indication for thoracic sympathectomy. The prevalence of palmar hyperhidrosis is higher among Asians than among other ethnic groups. The largest surgical series have been reported from the Far East. The success rate of endoscopic sympathectomy for relieving palmar hyperhidrosis is a remarkable 95 to 100% (Table 14–1).[1–9,11] Excising the sympathetic chain and achieving an intraoperative palmar temperature increase of 3° or more provide the best immediate and long-term clinical outcomes and minimize the risk of recurrent hyperhidrosis.[4] If the increase in palmar temperature is less than 1°C, the sympathectomy was ineffective.[4,8] Postoperatively, patients occasionally have several transient episodes of sweating in one or both hands. Such

episodes should not alarm the patient because they typically cease after a few days.[4]

Sympathectomy for palmar hyperhidrosis has secondary benefits, which have been referred to as *dividend* benefits. Two-thirds of patients will also obtain relief from their plantar hyperhidrosis.[4] Axillary hyperhidrosis and bromhidrosis will also improve or be relieved in 80% of patients if the T3 and T4 ganglia are surgically excised.[4] The mechanism of relief of the plantar hyperhidrosis has not been determined, although several hypotheses exist.[1,2]

Sympathectomy for hyperhidrosis is associated with several complications that patients should be informed of before surgery is performed. Thirty to 75% of patients with hyperhidrosis will experience a postoperative *compensatory* hyperhidrosis that involves increased sweating of the chest, abdomen, legs, and/or back.[3,4,8,14] Typically, the symptoms are mild to moderate, but they can be severe in 5 to 10% of cases. The symptoms of generalized compensatory hyperhidrosis occur despite complete relief of the palmar hyperhidrosis. Fortunately, the compensatory hyperhidrosis tends to improve or resolve within 6 months of surgery.[8] This phenomenon probably represents a manifestation of the patient's generalized autonomic hyperactivity and continued autonomic dysfunction.

Horner's syndrome and gustatory sweating (facial sweating elicited by the smell or taste of food) have been reported after sympathectomy, but they rarely occur.[1–7,11,14] The mechanisms underlying gustatory sweating are unknown; however, aberrant nerve regeneration and aberrant signal pathways have been postulated. Horner's syndrome can be prevented during a sympathectomy by preserving the stellate ganglion.

TABLE 14–1 Thoracoscopic Sympathectomy for Palmar Hyperhidrosis

Author (Reference) Year	No. Patients	No. Sympathec-tomies	Relief of Palmar Hyperhidrosis No. (%)	Failure Rate No. (%)	Dividend Benefits			Complications		
					Plantar Hyperhidrosis Relief No. (%)	Axillary Hyperhidrosis Relief No. (%)	Compensatory Hyperhidrosis No. (%)	Gustatory Sweating No. (%)	Horner's Syndrome No. (%)	
Kao et al.[4] 1994	300	600	287 (96)	13 (4)	210 (70)	19/24 (79)	150 (50)	3 (1)	0	
Lee and Hwang[8] 1996	82	164	164 (100)	0	41 (50)	—	50 (61)	0	0	
Robertson et al.[5] 1993	22	—	22 (100)	0	—	—	3 (14)	0	1 (5)[†]	
Johnson et al.[9] 1996	26	52	26 (100)	0	—	—	—	—	2 (8)[†]	
Lin[7] 1990	21	42	42 (100)	0	3 (14)	—	1 (5)	—	0	
Kux[6] 1977	63	124	63 (100)	0	—	51 (81)	28 (44)	2	0	

[†]transient

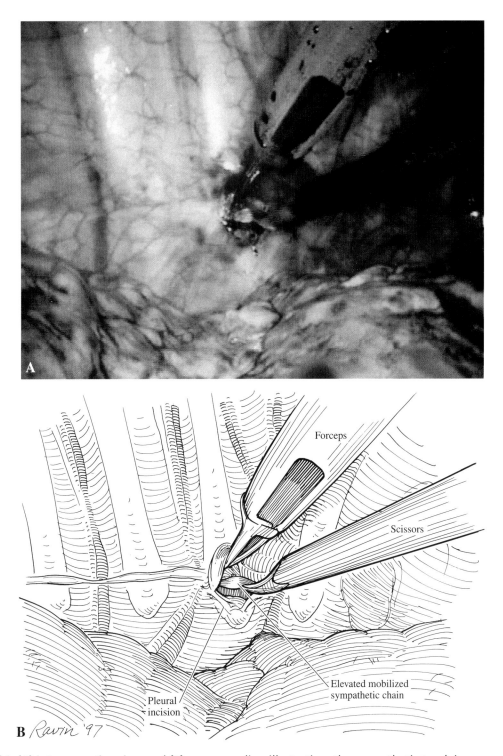

Figure 14–5. In this **(A)** intraoperative view and **(B)** corresponding illustration, the sympathetic trunk is grasped and elevated with an endoscopic Debakey forceps and mobilized from the surface of the spine with sharp dissection.

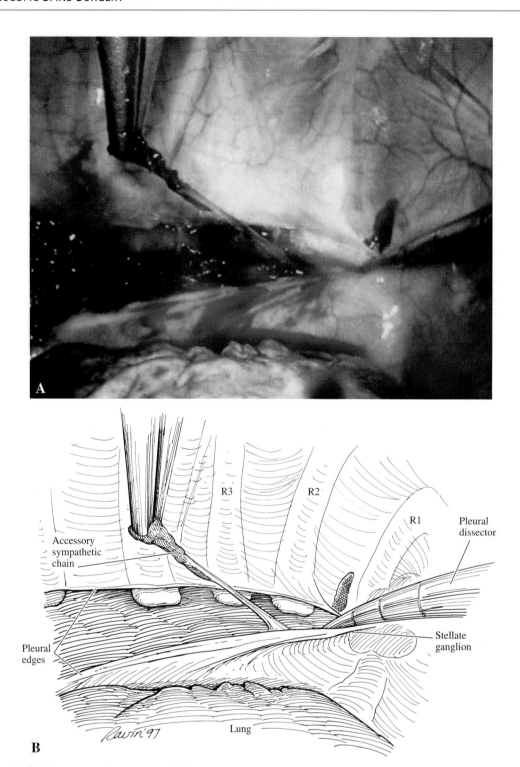

Figure 14–6. In this **(A)** intraoperative view and **(B)** corresponding illustration, the pleural incision is extended rostrally to the stellate ganglion adjacent to the first rib. A pleural dissector is used to elevate and incise the pleura. The accessory nerve of Kuntz is identified adjacent to the main sympathetic trunk and mobilized with sharp dissection. R = rib.

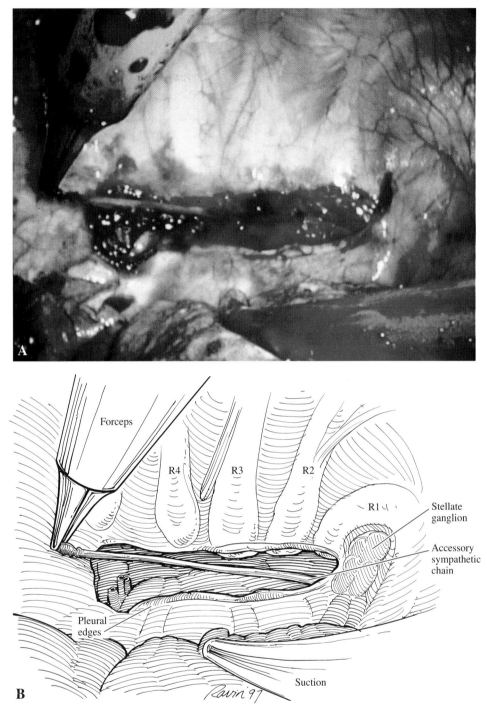

Figure 14–7.   In this **(A)** intraoperative view and **(B)** corresponding illustration, the nerve of Kuntz is grasped with a forceps, mobilized, and excised before the sympathetic trunk is removed. R = rib.

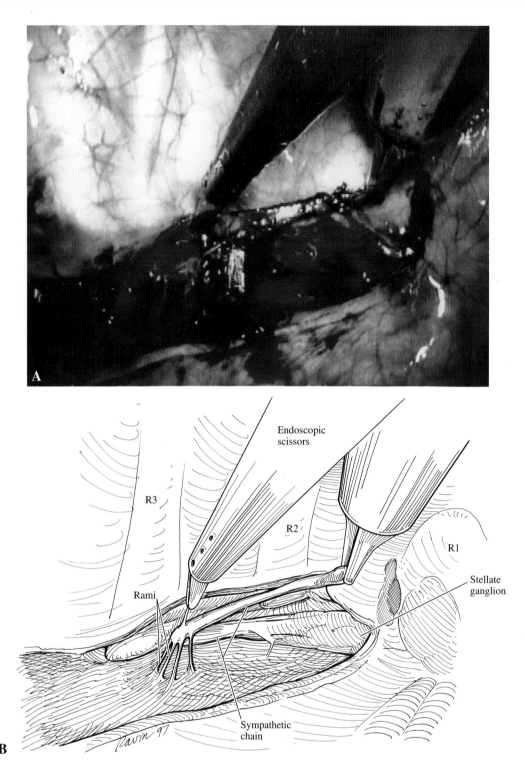

Figure 14–8. In this **(A)** intraoperative view and **(B)** corresponding illustration, the sympathetic trunk is mobilized with sharp microdissection. The trunk is grasped with a forceps and the rami to each ganglion are transected with scissors. R = rib.

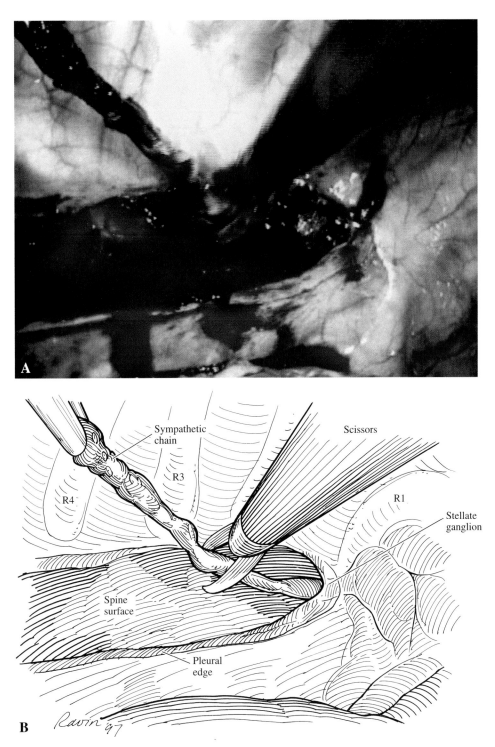

Figure 14–9. In this **(A)** intraoperative view and **(B)** corresponding illustration, the sympathetic trunk is transected with endoshears at the caudal border of the stellate ganglion. R = rib.

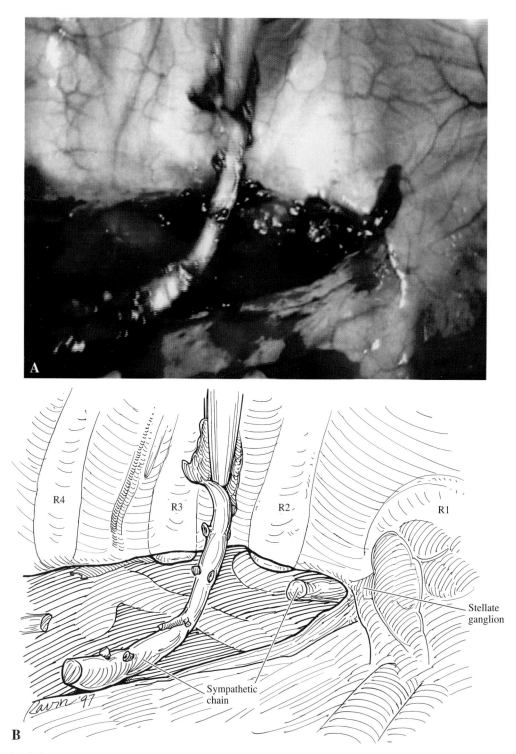

Figure 14–10. In this **(A)** intraoperative view and **(B)** corresponding illustration, the sympathetic chain is removed en bloc. The specimen may be sent for histological analysis if desired. R = rib.

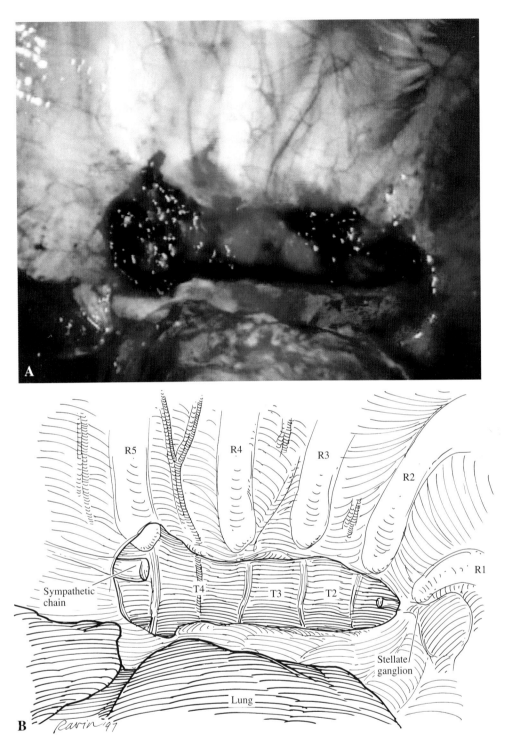

Figure 14–11.   In this **(A)** intraoperative view and **(B)** corresponding illustration, the final appearance of the surgical site after meticulous hemostasis was achieved with bipolar cauterization. R = rib, T = thoracic level.

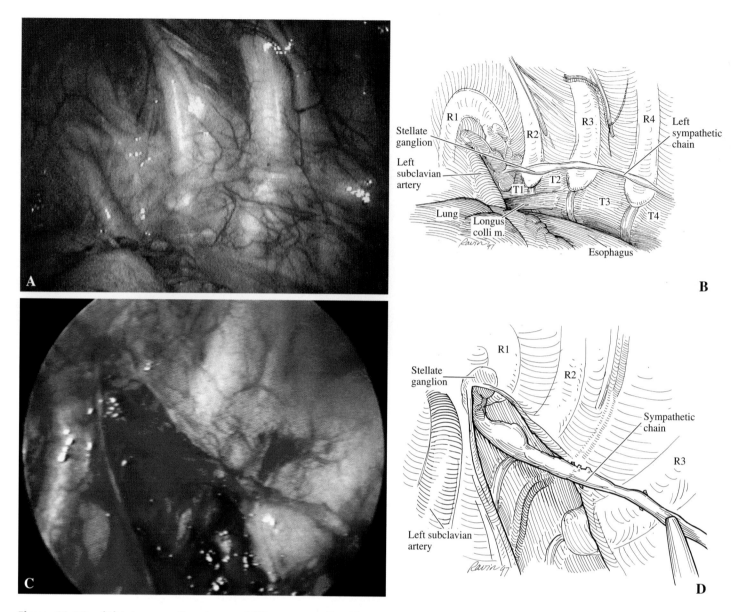

Figure 14–12. **(A)** Intraoperative view and **(B)** corresponding illustration of the anatomy of the left upper hemithorax. In this **(C)** intraoperative view and **(D)** corresponding illustration, the left sympathetic chain is mobilized and detached from its rami. The chain will be transected just caudal to the stellate ganglion.

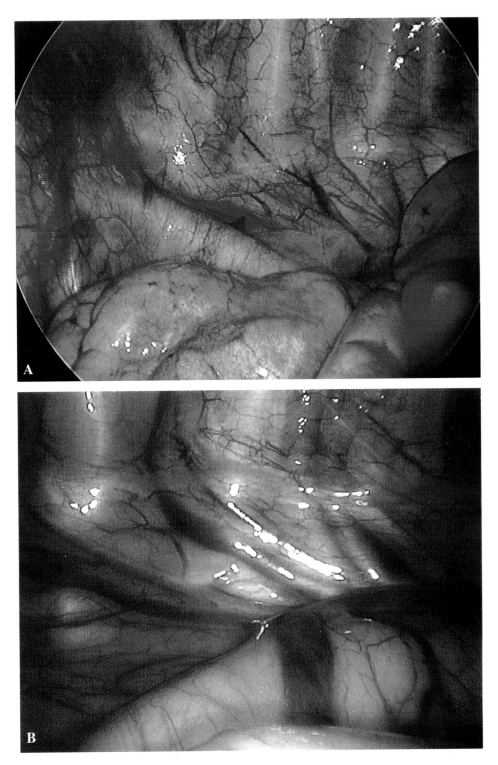

Figure 14–13. Anatomy of the left upper thoracic cavity. **(A)** An apical view demonstrates the subclavian artery, the stellate ganglion, and the left sympathetic chain. **(B)** Close-up view of the sympathetic chain more caudally. The aortic arch, the highest intercostal vein, and the rib and spine surfaces are visible.

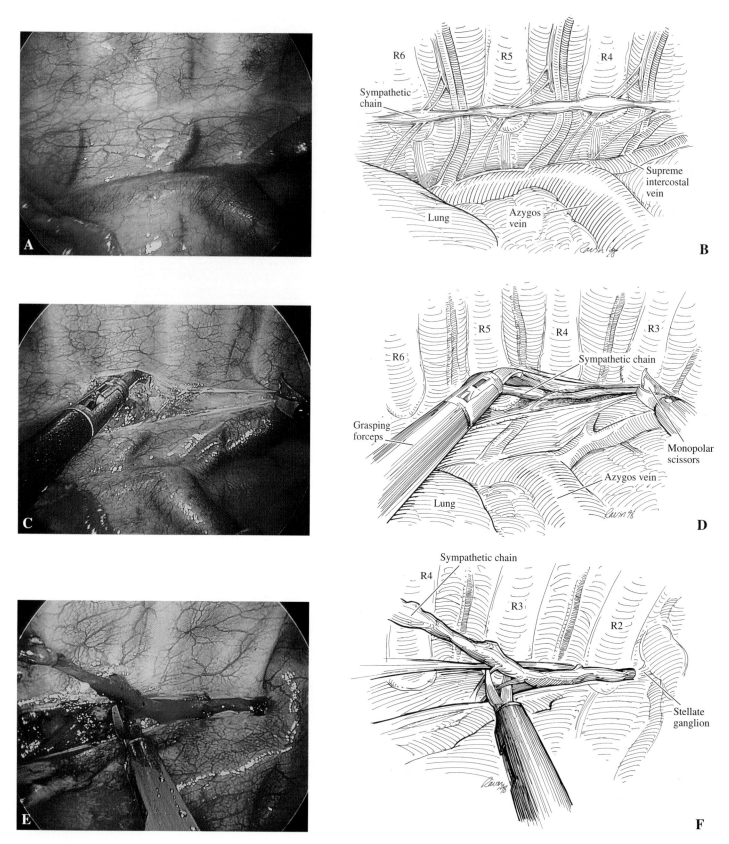

Figure 14–14. **(A)** Intraoperative photograph and **(B)** corresponding illustration showing thoracoscopic view of the sympathetic chain ganglion glistening beneath the pleura. The supreme intercostal vein and azygos arch are clearly visible. **(C)** Intraoperative photograph and **(D)** corresponding illustration showing grasping forceps being used to elevate the pleura from the sympathetic chain while the pleura is opened with monopolar scissors. **(E)** Intraoperative photograph and **(F)** corresponding illustration showing dissection of the sympathetic chain. Proceeding from the caudal edge of the incision, the sympathetic chain is dissected free and the rami communicante are cut at each level. The sympathectomy includes the second through fourth ganglia, stopping just below the stellate ganglion to avoid inducing Horner's syndrome.

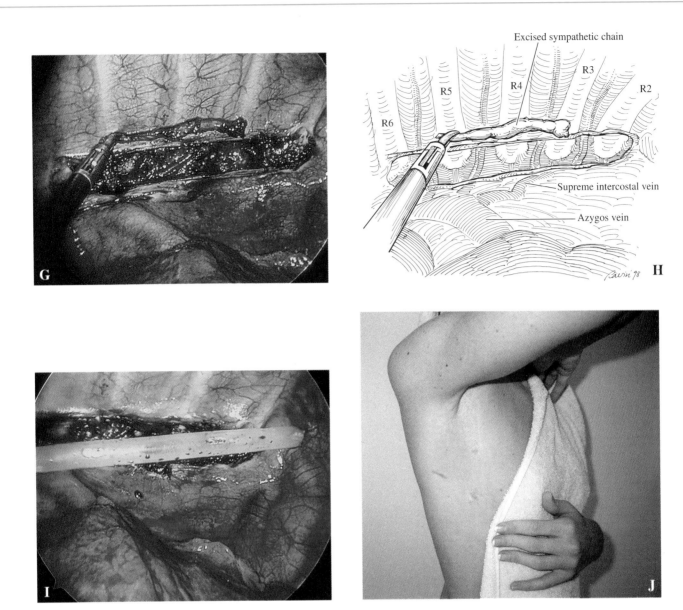

Figure 14–14.   *(continued)*   **(G)** Intraoperative photograph and **(H)** corresponding illustration showing the sympathetic chain being excised. The resection bed is visible. After the sympathetic chain has been removed, the bed is cauterized for secure hemostasis. **(I)** Before closure, a chest tube is inserted under endoscopic visualization to allow reinflation of the lung. The chest tubes are removed immediately before the patient leaves the operating room. The patient was discharged after an overnight stay in the hospital. **(J)** The appearance of the patient's small scars two weeks after surgery. [A through I with permission from Barrow Neurological Institute.]

CONCLUSION

Thoracoscopy for sympathectomy provides an excellent method to access, fully visualize, and completely excise the thoracic sympathetic chain or its tributaries using small incisions in the intercostal spaces. This technique requires less muscle dissection for access than any of the open techniques and provides better visualization of the anatomy.

Thoracoscopic alternatives to sharp excision of the sympathetic chain include laser photoablation, cautery ablation, or clip ligation.[4,6–8,11,13] We prefer to excise the upper sympathetic chain definitively on the affected side and to confirm the specimen histologically. Thoracoscopy increases the clinical utility of sympathectomy because it reduces approach-related morbidity and facilitates recovery. This technique provides a reliable way of achieving the desired effect of sympathectomy.

REFERENCES

1. Cloward RB: Hyperhydrosis. *J Neurosurg* 1969; 30(5):545–551.
2. Ray B: Sympathectomy of the upper extremity. Evaluation of surgical methods. *J Neurosurg* 1953; 10:624–633.
3. Shih CJ, Wang YC: Thoracic sympathectomy for palmar hyperhidrosis: Report of 457 cases. *Surg Neurol* 1978; 10(5):291–296.
4. Kao M-C, Tsai J-C, Lai D-M, et al: Autonomic activities in hyperhidrosis patients before, during, and after endoscopic laser sympathectomy. *Neurosurgery* 1994; 34(2):262–268.
5. Robertson DP, Simpson RK, Rose JE, et al: Video-assisted endoscopic thoracic ganglionectomy. *J Neurosurg* 1993; 79(2):238–240.
6. Kux M: Thoracic endoscopic sympathectomy in palmar and axillary hyperhidrosis. *Arch Surg* 1978; 113(3):264–266.
7. Lin CC: A new method of thoracoscopic sympathectomy in hyperhidrosis palmaris. *Surg Endosc* 1990; 4(4):224–226.
8. Lee KH, Hwang PYK: Video endoscopic sympathectomy for palmar hyperhidrosis. *J Neurosurg* 1996; 84(3):484–486.
9. Johnson JP, Ahn SS, DeSalles AD, et al: Thoracoscopic sympathectomy. *J Neurosurg* 1996; 84(2):348A.
10. Stolman LP: Treatment of excess sweating of palms by iontophoresis. *Arch Dermatol* 1987; 123(7):893–896.
11. Kao MC: Video endoscopic sympathectomy using a fiberoptic CO_2 laser to treat palmar hyperhidrosis. *Neurosurgery* 1992; 30(1):131–135.
12. Kuntz A: Distribution of the sympathetic rami to the brachial plexus: Its relation to sympathectomy affecting the upper extremity. *Arch Surg* 1927; 15:871–877.
13. Worsey J, Ferson PF, Keenan RJ, et al: Thoracoscopic pancreatic denervation for pain control in irresectable pancreatic cancer. *Br J Surg* 1993; 80(8):1051–1052.
14. Shelley WB, Florence R: Compensatory hyperhidrosis of sympathectomy. *N Engl J Med* 1960; 263:1056–1058.

CHAPTER **15**

Anterior Release of Spinal Deformities

Alvin H. Crawford, M.D.

Within the last few years, the field of video-assisted thoracoscopy (VATs) has grown to considerable proportions. In September 1991, an article in the medical science section of the *New York Times* espoused VATs as a "new surgical route into the chest."[1] The technique represented a revolutionary advance because surgical instruments guided by an endoscope could access the chest without breaking ribs, and inch-long incisions (portals) could be used rather than an 8- to 10-inch incision. The endoscope was linked to a video camera and inserted through portals, through which other instruments could also be inserted. The camera optics provided the necessary magnification. On March 23, 1992, *Time* magazine identified endoscopic surgery as the "Kindest Cut of All," whereby palm-sized video cameras, miniaturized tools, and minute incisions were starting to take the "ouch" out of surgery (i.e., the use of minimally invasive technology for video-assisted approaches to surgical problems).[2]

Thoracoscopy has been used to treat lung lesions for 70 to 80 years.[2] Only recently has the technology been applied to spinal surgery. In the early 1990s, Michael Mack[3] and John Regan[4] initiated clinical trials for spinal thoracoscopy at the Texas Back Institute. At about the same time, Frank Eismont[5] performed animal studies and Ronald Blackman[6] performed animal, cadaveric, and clinical studies. In 1993, this technology was presented at the Scoliosis Research Society meeting in Dublin, Ireland,[4] and also at the North American Spine Society (NASS) meeting in San Diego, California.[7] A summary of spinal thoracoscopy subsequently appeared in *USA Today* on November 1993.[8] Advances in video technology with multi-chip cameras have significantly improved the surgeon's ability to identify structures in the chest through very small incisions or portals. Video endoscopy has been instrumental in allowing spinal surgeons to perform endoscopic anterior releases

for spinal deformity. Bone grafts from the iliac crest or ribs can be placed into the intervertebral disc space through a narrow endoscopic portal. Compared to the 9- to 12-inch incisions associated with thoracotomy, the cosmetic outcome of VATs for the treatment of scoliosis is enhanced tremendously.

In December 1993, we began to perform VATs for the anterior release of severe spinal deformities in children and adolescents at the Children's Hospital and Medical Center in Cincinnati, Ohio. The potential benefits of this procedure include diminished postoperative pain and ventilatory compromise, briefer hospitalizations, reduced health care costs, improved wound care, an earlier return to preoperative activities, reduced shoulder dysfunction, and a reduced risk of infection in patients because of the decreased duration of surgery and the small wound exposure.

INDICATIONS AND CONTRAINDICATIONS IN CHILDREN AND ADOLESCENTS

The indications for VATs are the same as those for patients who require an open anterior spinal release surgery (Table 15–1): (1) rigid idiopathic scoliotic deformities of

TABLE 15–1 Indications for Video-Assisted Thoracoscopy for Spinal Deformity

Rigid idiopathic scoliotic deformities (≥ 75° curves)
Prevention of crankshaft phenomenon in skeletally immature children
Rigid kyphotic deformities (> 70°)
Neuromuscular spinal deformities
Progressive deformity from metabolic disease
Hemivertebrae resection
Severe rib hump deformities
Pseudarthrosis of anterior interbody fusion

approximately 75° or more, with correction to less than 50° on side-bending radiographs, (2) prevention of the crank-shaft phenomenon in a skeletally immature child with a curvature greater than 50°, (3) kyphotic deformities greater than 70°, (4) treatment of neuromuscular spinal deformities in patients with high-risk pulmonary status, (5) progressive deformity and metabolic disease, (6) a severe rib hump deformity uncorrected by spinal instrumentation, (7) neurofibromatosis in patients with intrathoracic tumors in addition to a significant spinal deformity, (8) resection of congenital hemivertebral deformities, and (9) pseudarthrosis after anterior intervertebral fusion. We now use thoracoscopy to treat *all* spinal problems previously approached through an open thoracotomy.

The aim of spinal deformity surgery is to straighten the spine or to obtain normal physiological curvatures safely. It is desirable to correct a deformity in both the sagittal and coronal planes. The surgeon should attempt to balance the position of the head and trunk over the pelvis (i.e., achieve sagittal balance) and to stabilize the spine permanently by performing an adequate arthrodesis.

The ability to correct a large curve in the safest manner is paramount in the management of young children. Rigid curvatures greater than 70° can be corrected more safely and with better cosmetic outcomes if the annulus fibrosis, intervertebral disc, and anterior longitudinal ligament are removed to release the anterior spinal soft tissues. Before 1993, we used thoracotomy exclusively for anterior releases, which mobilize the vertebrae, decrease the rigidity of the spine, facilitate interbody fusion, and permit safer and greater correction of the deformity. Currently, we prefer VATs for performing anterior releases because it is associated with fewer complications than thoracotomy.

In young children, anterior approaches are also required for ablating the cartilaginous end plates and for anterior intervertebral bone grafting. These ablations are needed to enhance the stability of spinal fusions and to prevent the crankshaft phenomenon from developing.[9] The crankshaft phenomenon occurs in skeletally immature children when the posterior spine is solidly fused yet continued growth of the anterior vertebral bodies causes the deformity to progress uncontrollably. Surgeons have been reluctant to perform a thoracotomy in children for anterior release and intervertebral fusion because of the postoperative pain, high incidence of respiratory complications, and the residual 9- to 12-inch scar on a patient who is undergoing surgery for "cosmetic" purposes. These reservations have caused surgeons to brace large deformities inappropriately or to observe patients until they have attained skeletal maturity. VATs allows an extensive anterior release of the spine to be performed without the morbidity or cosmetic effects of thoracotomy. Consequently, it is a major advance in our surgical armamentarium.

There are also several contraindications for VATs: (1) an inability to tolerate single-lung ventilation, (2) severe or acute respiratory insufficiency, (3) high airway pressures with positive pressure ventilation, (4) pleural symphysis, and (5) empyema. A previous thoracotomy or thoracostomy is only a relative contraindication. We have successfully performed thoracoscopy in patients who previously had undergone thoracotomy. The resection of adhesions, however, is time consuming. In addition, the risk of developing an air leak from the lung or an infection is higher.

OPERATIVE TECHNIQUE

VATs is an extremely demanding technical procedure that requires extensive training, practice, and experience. The ideal way to obtain experience with this procedure is to practice with animals, models, and cadavers in training laboratories, to be proctored, to perform hybrid procedures (endoscopic and open), to observe thoracoscopic procedures at active clinical centers, and to teleconference surgeries for interactive discussions. Study groups to help design instruments and suggest other improvements are also necessary. We have found goat and sheep to be the best animal models for thoracoscopy. However, the porcine model (which appears to be readily available and less expensive) can also be used. Ultimately, credentialing will likely be necessary to ensure that surgeons are trained properly and have attained the skills needed to perform thoracoscopic spine surgery safely.

Team Coordination

VATs for spinal deformity is performed by a team of surgeons, anesthesiologists, nurses, and surgical technicians who undertake many complementary tasks. The anesthesiologist must be able to use a fiber-optic bronchoscope as well as to intubate and deflate one lung selectively. This task is best achieved with a double-lumen endotracheal tube, although bronchial blockers may be necessary in smaller children.

Operating Room Setup

The setup of the operating room is variable. Some surgeons prefer to work on the same side of the table facing the patient anteriorly (with the patient in the lateral decubitus position). Other surgeons prefer to work opposite each other and to view the intrathoracic contents by placing monitors directly across from them (Fig. 15–1). Endoscopic instrumentation includes angled thoracoscopes (capable of 15x magnification) as well as specialized thoracoscopic spinal instruments (i.e., rongeurs, curettes, periosteal elevators, electrocautery devices, and suction devices, Fig. 15–2).

Procedure

Routine intraoperative monitoring for thoracic procedures (i.e., an arterial pressure line, a central venous catheter, pulse oximeter, and end-tidal CO_2 monitoring) is initiated.

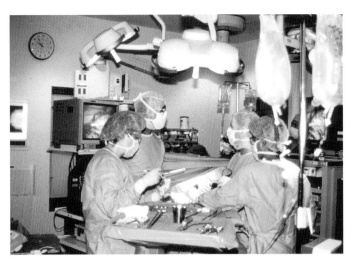

Figure 15–1. The operating room setup for thoracoscopy as used at Children's Hospital, Cincinnati, Ohio. This view looks from the foot of the table directly toward the head of the table. Monitors are positioned bilaterally near the head of the table.

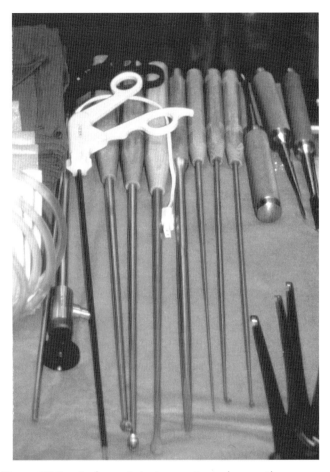

Figure 15–2. Endoscopic instruments are longer than conventional spinal instruments. The shorter conventional instruments are in the top right corner of the Mayo stand. The endoscopic instruments are on the left. The instruments have either thin (5-mm diamater) or wide (1-cm diameter) shanks. The instruments with wider shanks are mostly used for bone dissection as well as laparoscopic spinal surgery.

General anesthesia is administered, and a double-lumen endotracheal tube or bronchial blocker is inserted. The patient is placed in the lateral decubitus position. The anesthesiologist deflates the lung before the patient is draped and allows 20 minutes to obtain complete resorption atelectasis. Because most thoracic spinal deformities are curved toward the right side, the patient is placed in the left lateral decubitus position with a kidney rest support; the patient's right side is positioned up. The arm is extended at the shoulder to allow portals to be placed into the axilla. The Mayo stand is situated so that the monopolar cauterization, suction devices, and the light source are fully accessible from both sides of the table.

The borders of the scapula, twelfth rib, and iliac crest are identified and outlined with a surgical marker (Fig. 15–3). The first portal is most frequently placed at or about the T6 or T7 interspace in the posterior axillary line (Fig. 15–4). The most common configuration for the portals is a reversed "L." To insert the portals, we prefer to make the incision through the dermis with a scalpel. Electrocautery is used to incise through the subcutaneous tissue and intercostal muscles into the chest cavity. The incision is made over the top of the rib to avoid the intercostal nerve and vessels. There tends to be less bleeding when the Bovie® electrocautery device is used. It is important to coagulate the blood vessels around the portals because surgery is impeded if blood continuously drips from a portal site. It can interfere with keeping the lens of the endoscope clean and inhibit intrathoracic visualization during the surgery. A 15-mm trochar is placed, and a 10–mm, 30°-angled rigid telescope is inserted through it. The 30° endoscope allows direct viewing of the intervertebral disc spaces without impeding the surgical instrumentation or obscuring the operative field. Until it is needed, the end of the telescope is kept in warm saline to prevent it from fogging when the chest is entered.

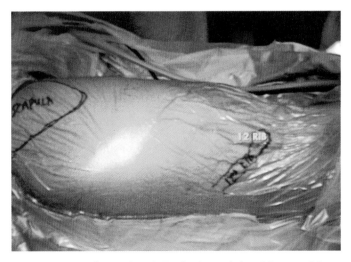

Figure 15–3. The patient is in the lateral decubitus position. The scapula and the 12th rib are marked on the skin. The extended arm allows greater access to the superior axilla. The axilla is draped out of the field. The iliac crest is also accessible for harvesting bone grafts.

The thoracoscope is introduced and the lung is observed as it deflates. The intrathoracic cavity should be assessed panoramically to determine the topography of the anatomy as well as other portal sites that would provide the most direct working approach to the intervertebral discs (Fig. 15–5). Rotating the patient anteriorly into a Trendelenburg (for the lower thoracic spine) or reverse Trendelenburg (for the upper thoracic spine) position causes the collapsed lung to fall away from the spinal surface and obviates the need to retract the lung manually.[10] The superior thoracic spine can usually be visualized well without retraction once the lung is deflated completely. Below T9–T10 the diaphragm usually must be retracted. To avoid pulmonary injury, the fan retractor should be visualized endoscopically whenever it is opened, closed, manipulated, or adjusted.

Palpating or percussing the chest wall and visualizing the movement endoscopically from within the chest aid in positioning the working portal sites. We use rigid as well as flexible thoracoscopic portals for the endoscope and for inserting instruments. Flexible thoracoports cause less intercostal neuralgia. Occasionally, more than one instrument may be placed through a single flexible portal. The camera and viewing field are different from those used by thoracic surgeons: the field of view is rotated 90° from standard VATs. The orientation of the spine and dissection is most easily viewed and recognized when the spine is projected horizontally.

Once the spinal anatomy has been identified, it is important to select the levels to perform annulotomy and discectomy. The ribs are counted visually and by palpating with a blunt instrument. The superior intercostal vein usually empties into the azygos arch near the T3 or T4 interspace. To confirm the localization of the exact level, a spinal needle can be inserted into an intervertebral disc and a radiograph obtained.

The vertebral column is approached by incising and mobilizing the pleura. We prefer to open the parietal pleura with a longitudinal incision along the spinal surface, similar to the pleural incision used when an open thoracotomy is performed (Fig. 15–6). The intervertebral discs are identified as convex mounds on the spinal column. The vertebral bodies appear as concave "valleys" (Fig. 15–7). The segmental vessels reside in the valleys directly overlying the middle of the vertebral bodies. Multilevel anterior discectomies are necessary to correct a severe spinal deformity. Anterior release of a spinal curvature usually requires discectomy at six to eight levels.

Multilevel ligation and transection of the segmental vessels provide mobilization that vastly improves the exposure of the spinal surface and appears to be fairly safe. In a recent report of 1197 anterior release procedures from the Minnesota Spine Center, the ligation of more than 6000 vessels by cross ligation of the segmental vessels was associated with no neurological deficits.[11] However, whether the segmental vessels should be ligated and transected to allow better exposure of the spine or whether they should be

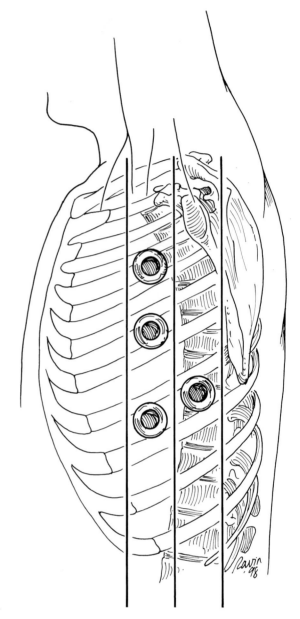

A

Figure 15–4. Alternative portal configurations for anterior release. **(A)** The first portal for insertion of the endoscope during an anterior thoracoscopic release of the spine is created along the posterior axillary line between the T6 and T8 intercostal spaces. Subsequent working portals are created along the anterior axillary line. This configuration is useful for release of kyphosis or a scoliotic deformity.

preserved is controversial. Reservations about transecting these vessels reflect concern about the risk of spinal cord infarction from devascularization. We recommend that surgeons perform the vascular mobilization with which they are most comfortable, exactly as they would with an open thoracotomy.

We use monopolar electrocauterization to incise the parietal pleura. A small Robinson catheter is placed over an extended Bovie to insulate the tip, leaving 3 to 4 mm of cutting surface to be used as a cautery scalpel (Fig. 15–8). Alternatively, endoscissors can be used to incise the pleura.

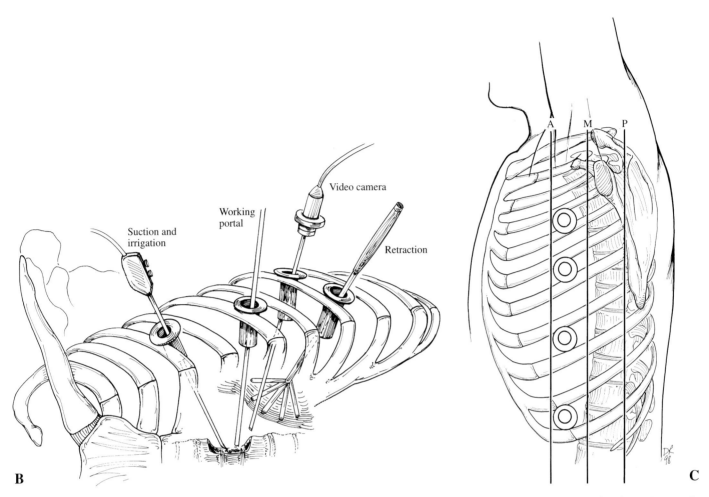

B

C

Figure 15–4. *(continued)*   **(B)** The endoscope is inserted into the posterior portal. Anterior portals are used for dissection tools and retractors. **(C)** If an extensive multilevel anterior release is needed for scoliosis, multiple portals can be placed in the midaxillary line, spanning the entire thoracic spine. The endoscope can be repositioned in different portals while the other portals are used for dissection.

The segmental vessels are coagulated with a bipolar electrocautery device or a harmonic scalpel, transected, and allowed to retract with the pleura. The pleura is elevated and retracted with thoracoscopic periosteal elevators and blunt dissectors. Any vessels that appear to be at risk for bleeding are coagulated. I prefer bipolar coagulation of segmental vessels; however, suture ligatures or endoscopic clips may be used.

After the spine has been exposed, the annulus and the anterior longitudinal ligament are incised and the discs and the vertebral end plates are excised. Spine surgeons should use the same techniques that they employ during open surgery. My technique is simple. A transverse cut is made across the vertebral body parallel to the disc, both rostral and caudal to it. A periosteal elevator is used to elevate the periosteum toward the vertebral end plate to isolate the disc. A transverse cut is made across the annulus fibrosis and continues down to the level of the nucleus pulposus. A rongeur, curettes, and periosteal elevators are used to remove the disc material and the end plates completely.

With severe deformities the spine may be rotated toward the chest wall and positioned close enough for conventional spinal instruments to be used (Fig. 15–9). The length of the

jaws of the rongeurs should be measured to the hinge so that the depth of penetration toward the posterior longitudinal ligament is known. In young children it is often possible to elevate the vertebral end plate apophysis and to excise the intervertebral disc completely back to the posterior longitudinal ligament (Fig. 15–10). The annulus and contents of the disc space can be excised in a 250° arc that extends from the ipsilateral pedicle to the contralateral pedicle. Particular attention is directed at releasing the annulus on the concave side of the curve. Using thoracoscopy, we have extended a release only as caudally as the T12–L1 disc and believe it unsafe to attempt to dissect below this level. As the rostral limit, we have been comfortable excising the T2–T3 interspace.

The contents of the disc space are removed down to the end plate in mature patients and to the cancellous bone in the skeletally immature patients. A small piece of gelfoam is then inserted into the disc cavity for hemostasis (Fig. 15–11). After each release, the spinal column should be stressed with moderate force to determine if mobility has been achieved. A complete anterior release should improve the mobility of the spine substantially (Fig. 15–12). Some surgeons prefer this complete anterior release to enhance

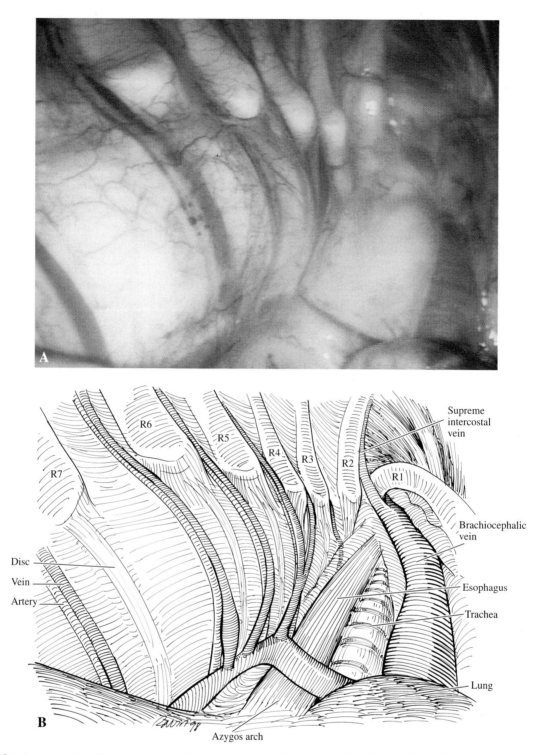

Figure 15–5. **(A)** Intraoperative photograph and **(B)** corresponding illustration showing a right-sided thoracoscopic approach provide a panoramic view of a child's spine with significant angular spinal deformity and dysplasia. The rib heads are abnormal. The azygos venous system and the brachiocephalic vein are anterior to the spine. Approaching the curvature from the *convex* surface is facilitated because the segmental vessels are widely separated and the disc spaces are widened. On the *concave* surface of the spinal curve, the vessels and the disc spaces are clustered closely together, interfering with exposure and dissection of the spine. R = rib.

correction of a deformity and to expose the cancellous bone without placing bone grafts in the intervertebral disc spaces. Intervertebral bone grafts with morcellized bits of iliac crest bone, portions of ribs, or allograft placed into the disc spaces can enhance the arthrodesis.

When the procedure is completed, all disc fragments and debris are removed from the thoracic cavity. The pleura can be sutured or left open (Fig. 15–13). All efforts are made to obtain complete hemostasis. The pleural fluid or irrigant should be inspected carefully for any cloudiness to detect injury to the thoracic duct. A chest tube is placed through the most posteroinferior portal. The thoracoscope is used to observe placement of the chest tube along the vertebral column to avoid inserting it into one of the intervertebral

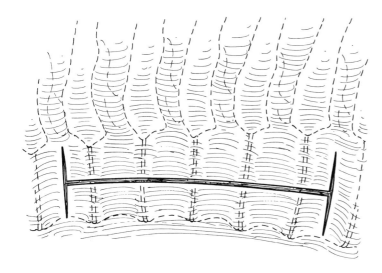

Figure 15–6. The pleural incision for a multilevel anterior release extends longitudinally over the spine surface to expose all the required spinal levels.

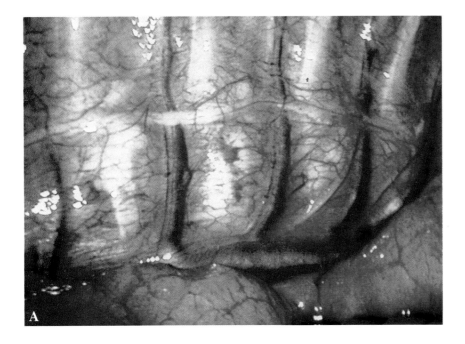

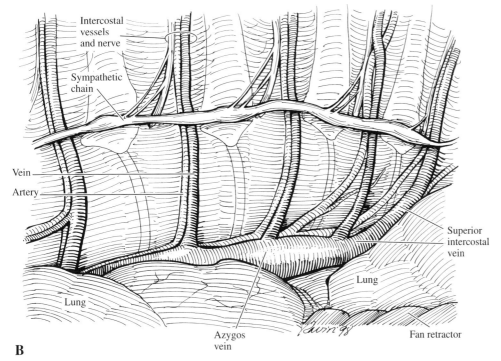

Figure 15–7. **(A)** Intraoperative photograph and **(B)** corresponding illustration showing the upper thoracic spine where the superior intercostal veins enter into the azygos vein. Note the mounds and the valleys along the vertebral column. The convex bulges are the intervertebral discs (mounds), and the concave valleys are the surfaces of the vertebral bodies. The segmental vessels cross the spine over the middle of the vertebral bodies and continue laterally as the intercostal vessels. The sympathetic chain crosses horizontally just above the head of the ribs.

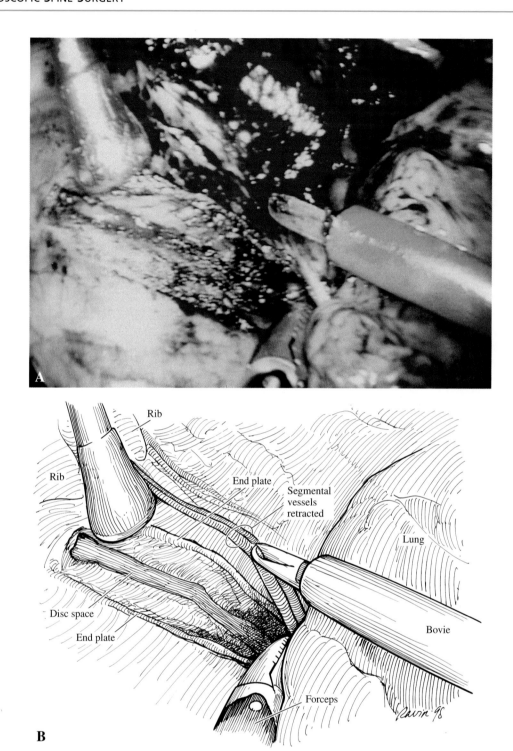

Figure 15–8. **(A)** Intraoperative photograph and **(B)** corresponding illustration showing a Robinson catheter placed over an extended Bovie to insulate its tip. The parietal pleura has been incised and an annulotomy performed. The disc space is positioned between the suction tip and the Bovie tip. A forceps, placed below the Bovie, was used to retract the preserved segmental vessels. The nucleus pulposus was directly beneath the suction tip.

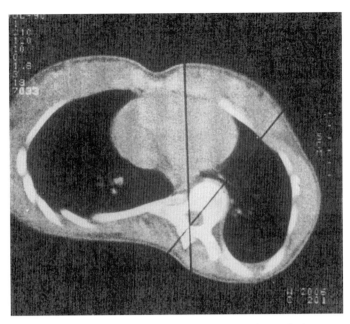

Figure 15–9. A computed tomographic cut through the midthorax illustrating the rotation of the thoracic spine caused by scoliosis. The distance from the surface of the chest wall exterior to the deformed spine is always less on the convexity. Consequently, conventional spinal intrumentation (rongeurs, curettes, elevators) sometimes can be used instead of endoscopic tools.

spaces. The chest tube is placed to water seal, and the anesthesiologist reinflates the lung to determine whether an air leak exists. Marcaine® is injected into the muscle adjacent to each port, followed by a deep-layer and subcuticular skin closure. Usually, the patient is reintubated and turned prone for a posterior spinal fusion (Fig. 15–14).

Typically, the sympathetic chain is transected at several levels, but the transection seldom causes permanent residual problems. Both parents and child should be made aware that after surgery the child might experience hot and cold phenomena (i.e., a *sympathetic release*) in the upper or lower extremities or trunk.

VATs costoplasty (i.e., convex rib resection) may be performed endoscopically to decrease the rib hump deformity (Fig. 15–15). After the costoplasty is performed, the fragments of rib can be placed in the intervertebral disc spaces to enhance fusion. Once the thoracoscopic release and fusion are completed, the child is usually turned to a prone position and reintubated. A posterior spinal fusion with instrumentation is then performed. With severe chest and spinal deformities, an anterior release may be performed first. Postoperatively, the patient may be placed in halo femoral or halo wheelchair traction to further reduce the severity of the deformity before corrective instrumentation is applied. These patients usually undergo a staged posterior spinal fusion within 7 to 10 days.

Other uses of thoracoscopy have included anterior hemiepiphyseal ablation, strut (rib) graft fusion for pseudarthrosis, correction of severe kyphosis (Fig. 15–16), and excision of intercostal neurofibromas (Fig. 15–17).

The entire endoscopic anterior release and posterior

fusion procedures require 6 to 8 hours to complete. Throughout the intraoperative period, the circulating nurse remains in close contact with the patient's family members, giving them frequent updates on the patient's condition. At the completion of surgery, the anesthetist extubates the patient before he or she is transported to the intensive care unit (ICU). The circulating nurse gives a detailed report to the ICU nurse to assist in planning the patient's postoperative care.

COMPLICATIONS

Thoracoscopy offers a safe and minimally invasive approach for performing an anterior release. Some risks, however, are involved. Potential complications from VATs are the same as those that may occur with open thoracotomy procedures.

Bleeding

When bleeding occurs, the surgeon should remain calm and remember that the surgical view is magnified 15 times. The scrub assistant should have a radiopaque sponge loaded on a sponge stick available at all times to allow the surgeon to

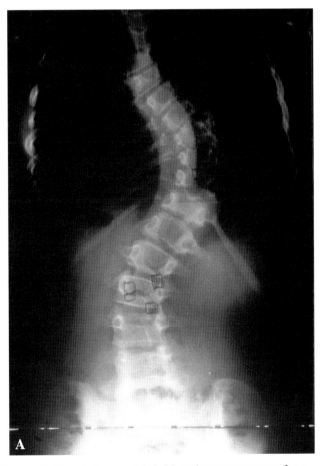

Figure 15–10. A 9-year-old child underwent surgery for a severe spinal deformity. **(A)** Preoperative standing posteroanterior radiograph demonstrates a double primary thoracic scoliotic curvature. *(Figure continued next page.)*

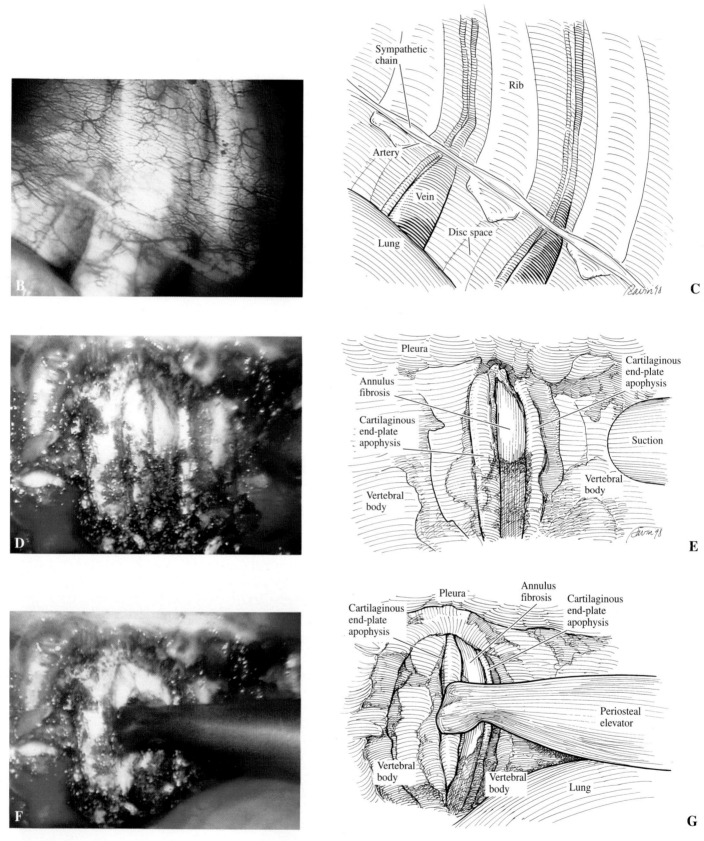

Figure 15–10. *(continued)* **(B)** Intraoperative photograph and **(C)** corresponding illustration of the thoracic spine at the time of thoracoscopy. The spine was approached from the right side because of the major curve. **(D)** Intraoperative photograph and **(E)** corresponding illustration showing that the intercostal vessels were sacrificed. Note the midforeground where the annulus fibrosis and vertebral endplates were exposed. **(F)** Intraoperative photograph and **(G)** corresponding illustration showing that the periosteal elevator has been placed between the cartilaginous end-plate apophysis and the vertebral body. The cartilaginous apophysis was elevated from the vertebral body, and the entire annulous-apophyseal complex was excised with a rongeur.

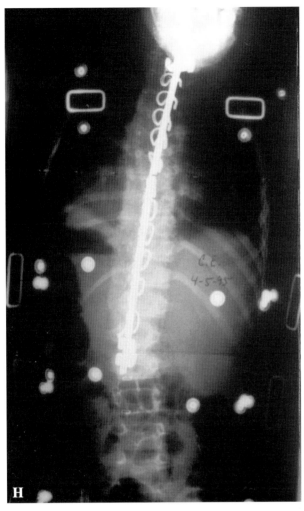
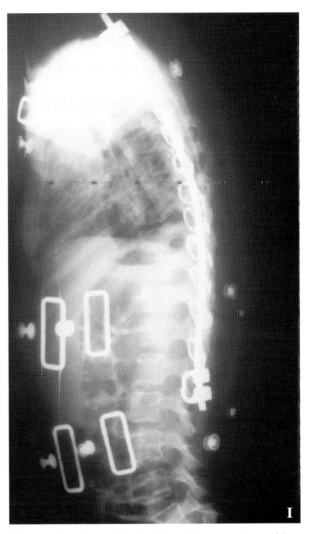

Figure 15–10. *(continued)* Postoperative **(H)** anteroposterior and **(I)** lateral radiographs depicting the correction achieved after posterior instrumentation for fixation has been placed (a clawed, sublaminar, wire-and-rod construct).

exert pressure on a source of bleeding. A suture tie must be secured to the radiopaque sponge to allow its easy retrieval. The surgeon should ensure that the sponge stick easily fits through one of the portals. Gentle direct pressure is applied to the bleeding vessel, and the field of blood is cleared using suction. Typically, an endoscopic monopolar electrocautery device with an extension tip is sufficient to achieve hemostasis. However, endoscopic bipolar forceps and/or an argon gas coagulator may be needed. Endoscopic clip appliers and a variety of hemostatic agents (e.g., absorbable gelatin sponges, topical thrombin, collagen hemostat) should also be readily available. The scrub nurse should ensure that instrumentation for performing an open thoracotomy incision is set up on the sterile back table to avoid delays and confusion in the event of an emergency.

Lung Tissue Trauma

Although the lung is deflated and retracted away from the spine, the delicate lung tissue can be damaged any time. The scrub nurse should ensure that an endoscopic suture ligature or stapling device is ready for sealing air leaks.

Dural Tear

A dural tear is recognized by the leakage of clear cerebrospinal fluid (CSF) from the spine. Fibrin glue, tissue coverage, lumbar drainage, and hemostatic agents (e.g., absorbable gelatin sponges, topical thrombin, collagen hemostat) will seal small CSF leaks. Neurosurgical consultation should be obtained if the dural tear continues to leak CSF.

Lymphatic Injury

The presence of milky or cloudy fluid in the operative field indicates a lymphatic injury to the thoracic duct or a lymphatic tributary. A lymphatic injury can be closed with an endoscopic clip applier and small surgical stainless-steel clips or with an endoscopic electrosurgical device.

Spinal Cord Injury

If SSEP monitoring reveals spinal cord compromise, corticosteroids are administered and the surgeon changes the position of the endoscopic instruments or the spine.

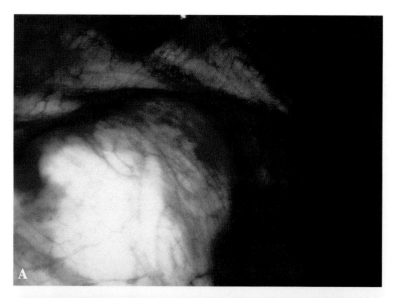

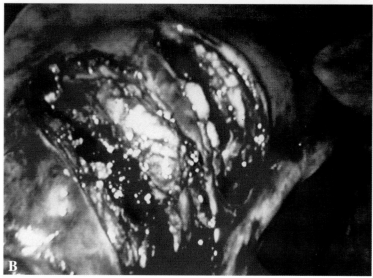

Figure 15–11. This patient underwent an anterior release with annulotomy and disc excision. The segmental vessels were preserved. **(A)** Intraoperative photograph of the deformed anterior spine viewed from a caudal perspective, toward the apex of the chest. **(B)** Intraoperative photograph showing the preserved segmental vessels. The anterior longitudinal ligament, annuli, and disc contents have been excised. Gelfoam was placed into the disc spaces to facilitate hemostasis.

Sympathectomy

Transection of the sympathetic trunk causes little or no morbidity. However, the surgeon should inform the patient and family members of the possibility of changes in temperature and skin color below the level of injury.

ADVANTAGES AND DISADVANTAGES OF VATS

The benefits of the thoracoscopic anterior release include reduced surgical time, less tissue damage, decreased blood loss, reduced postoperative pain, improved postoperative respiratory function, and shorter stays in the ICU and hospital. The potential for infection is reduced, as is shoulder dysfunction. The small incisions needed for the minimally invasive VATs approach preclude the need for rib retraction and therefore reduce postoperative pain and improve respiratory function. When the VATs procedure is completed, the surgeons aspirate residual fluid directly from the patient's pleural cavity. The subsequent amount of chest tube drainage is minimal, and chest tubes usually can be removed 24 hours after surgery. Early removal of chest tubes improves patients' mobility and hastens their convalescence. Using the VATs approach to anterior thoracic release in scoliosis surgery has shortened our mean postoperative stay in the ICU from several days to 24 hours. The smaller incisions minimize surgically associated cosmetic disfigurement. Potentially, these benefits should decrease the overall costs of the procedure. Procedure-related expenses, however, may increase because of the amount of technology and disposable tools required.

The limitations of the VATs for spinal deformities include the inability to insert corrective implants into the thoracic cage. If corrective implants could be introduced endoscopically and manipulated satisfactorily within the chest, the posterior operation could be eliminated completely. The cosmetic advantages would be even greater, and surgical morbidity related to a second operation would be eliminated.

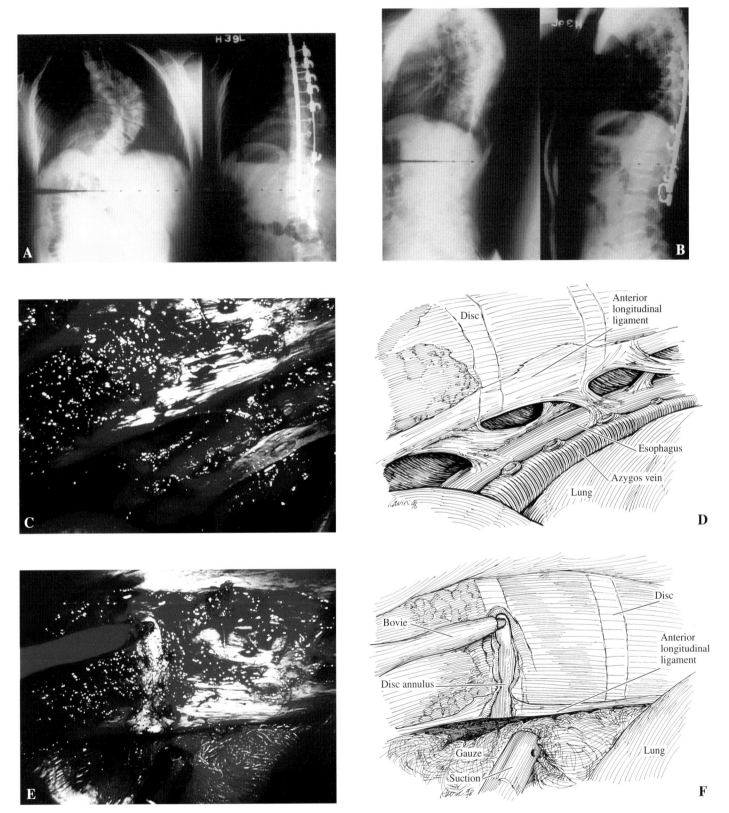

Figure 15–12.   A 17-year-old adolescent with cleidocranial dysostosis presented with a 100° curvature. He was treated by thoracoscopic anterior release and posterior spinal fusion with segmental instrumentation. **(A)** Pre- (left) and postoperative (right) anteroposterior radiographs demonstrating that the 100° curvature has been corrected to less than 25°. **(B)** Pre- (left) and postoperative (right) lateral radiographs demonstrate correction of the thoracic lordosis with segmental instrumentation. **(C)** Intraoperative photograph and **(D)** corresponding illustration demonstrating the anatomy in an adolescent. The segmental vessels have been sacrificed and the parietal pleura was retracted. The thoracic spine is positioned horizontally. **(E)** Intraoperative photograph and **(F)** corresponding illustration showing a sponge placed into the chest cavity to retract the parietal pleura from the concave surface of the spine. A Bovie was used to incise the annulus and anterior longitudinal ligament over the disc spaces. A free suture should be attached to the sponge so that it can be removed easily after it is inserted into the chest cavity. *(Figure continued next page.)*

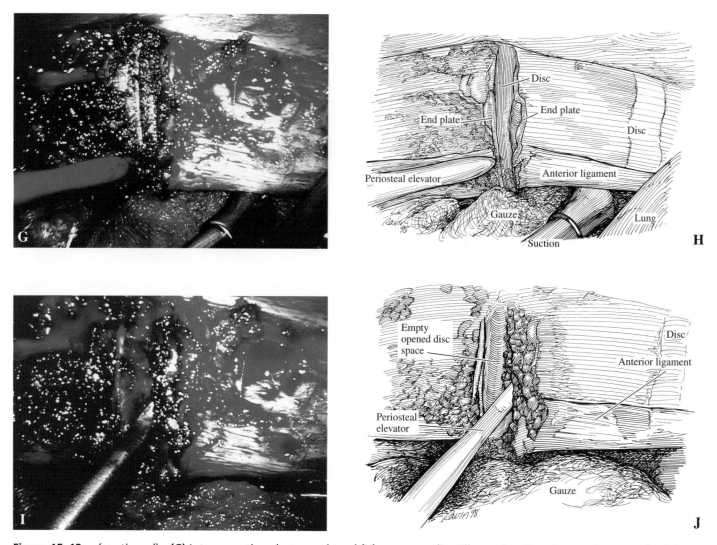

Figure 15–12. *(continued)* **(G)** Intraoperative photograph and **(H)** corresponding illustration showing the intervertebral disc space fully exposed. The end-plate apophysis, annulus fibrosis, and the intervertebral disc were fibrotic and contracted. The disc space was very narrow. **(I)** Intraoperative photograph and **(J)** corresponding illustration after the annulus has been excised. The intervertebral disc space was widely opened, and the disc material and end plates were removed with periosteal elevators, curettes, and disc rongeurs.

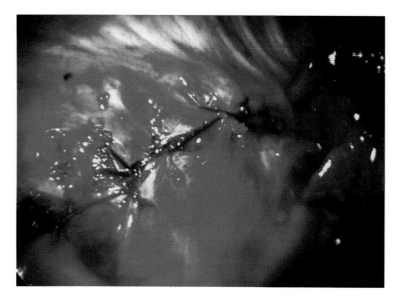

Figure 15–13. Intraoperative photograph after the parietal pleura was closed with suture after the multilevel annulectomy, disc excision, and bone grafting were performed.

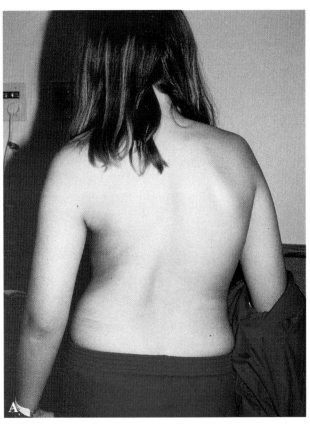

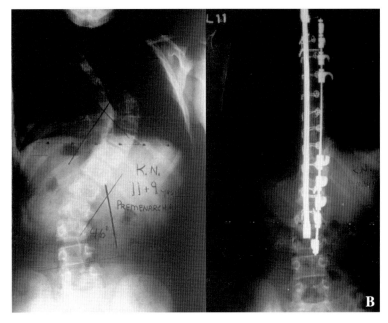

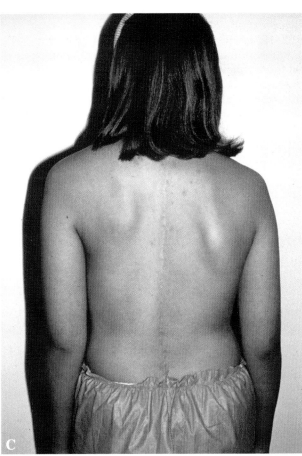

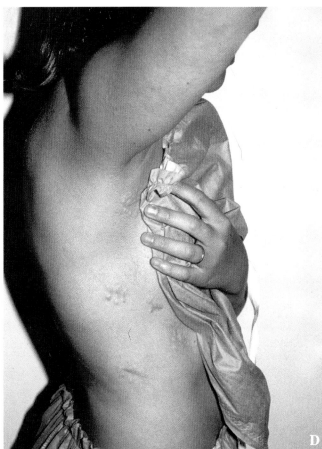

Figure 15–14.   An 11-year-old girl presented with a severe spinal deformity and underwent anterior release followed by posterior interspinous segmental instrumentation. **(A)** Photograph of the patient standing shows the severe deformity of the right chest and the shift of the trunk to the right. **(B)** Standing pre- (left) and postoperative (right) radiographs after the VATs anterior release and posterior spinal fusion with segmental instrumentation. The curvature was corrected and truncal balance was restored. **(C)** Posterior view of the girl 1 year after surgery. Clinically, the spinal deformity is improved considerably. **(D)** Compared to a 12- to 15-inch thoracotomy scar, the portal incisions along the axillary line caused minimal disfiguration.

FUTURE DEVELOPMENTS

The future of VATs in the management of spinal deformities is promising. Current techniques are versatile and offer satisfactory results. Anterior release and discectomies can be performed identically to open procedures with better visualization and access to a greater number of levels of the thoracic spine. Autologous or homologous bone can be placed into the disc space to obtain fusion and ensure a more stable spine once posterior instrumentation and fusion have been performed.

The next advance needed is the development of thoracoscopic corrective spinal instrumentation that could be applied through the portals. Emerging technology and the development of new implants and instrumentation devices ultimately should lead to the ability to correct and stabilize spinal deformities thoracoscopically.

Future needs also include the ability to use heads-up displays and "virtual reality" phenomena. Such improvements would avoid the need for the surgeon and associate to view monitors with special glasses and allow the display to be part of their direct optics. Three-dimensional (3-D) video assistance has been used. Robotics are not yet utilized as often in the thoracic spine as they have been with laparoscopy but have the potential to improve dissection, exposure, and visualization. VATs also creates a potential for navigational direction of transthoracic anatomy. Intraoperative magnetic resonance imaging of the anatomy is another possibility.

VATs is an excellent tool for teaching. Endoscopic surgical procedures can be telecommunicated via telephone lines and observed at distant conference centers. The capabilities of this technique appear unlimited, and I look forward to participating in its development.

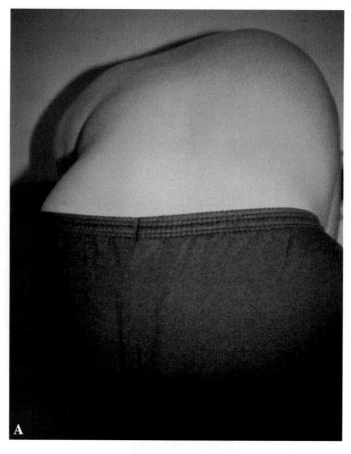

Figure 15–15.   A 16-year-old female presented with a severe double primary scoliosis and a large rib hump. Internal thoracoplasty was performed to excise portions of six ribs. **(A)** Preoperative photograph of the patient bending forward demonstrates the dramatic rib hump.

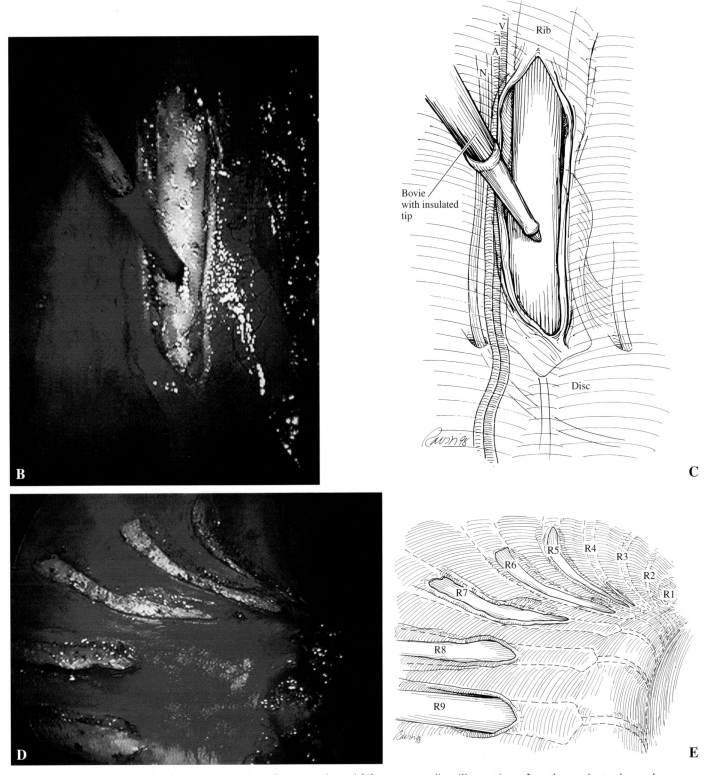

Figure 15–15. *(continued)* **(B)** Intraoperative photograph and **(C)** corresponding illustration after the periosteal membrane was incised over the rib with a Bovie electrocautery device and elevated from the rib circumferentially. The neurovascular bundles were preserved. **(D)** Intraoperative panoramic view and **(E)** corresponding illustration show the six ribs isolated before their excision. The spine, which had previously undergone an anterior release, is to the right. *(Figure continued next page.)*

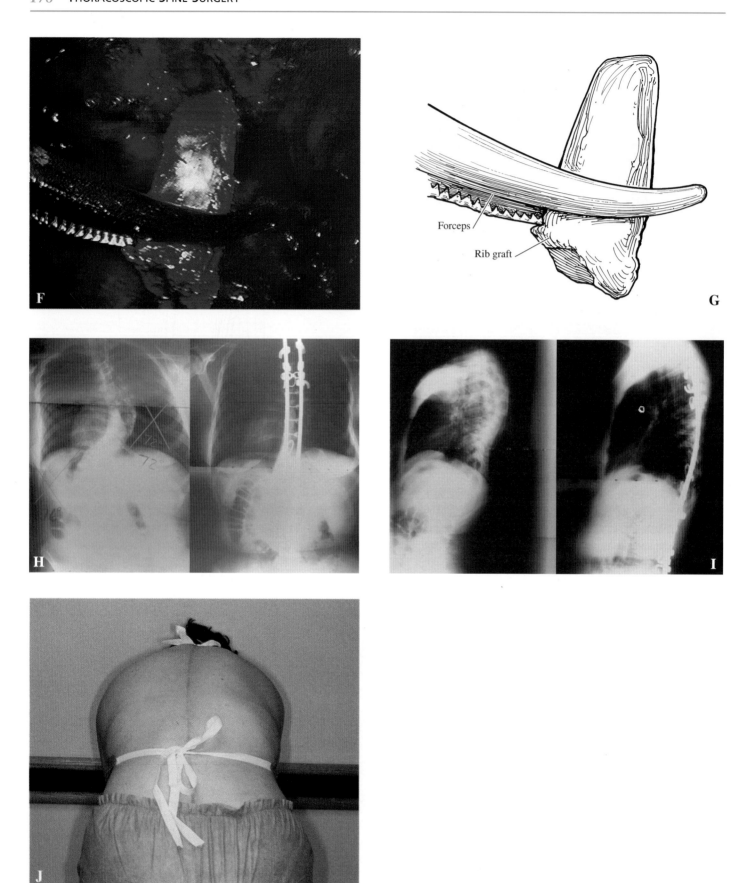

Figure 15–15. *(continued)* **(F)** Intraoperative view and **(G)** corresponding illustration after the forceps were used to remove the ribs through a 15-mm portal. The ribs were then cut into small segments, and the pieces were inserted into the disc space for intervertebral bone graft. **(H)** Pre- (left) and postoperative (right) radiographs showing excellent correction of the double primary curve. Note the gap between the ribs on the right (convex) side where the segments were excised. **(I)** Lateral pre- (left) and postoperative (right) radiographs show the correction of the thoracic lordosis. **(J)** Postoperative photograph of the patient bending forward at 6 months after surgery. The rib hump deformity is completely corrected. N = nerve, A = artery, V = vein, and R = rib.

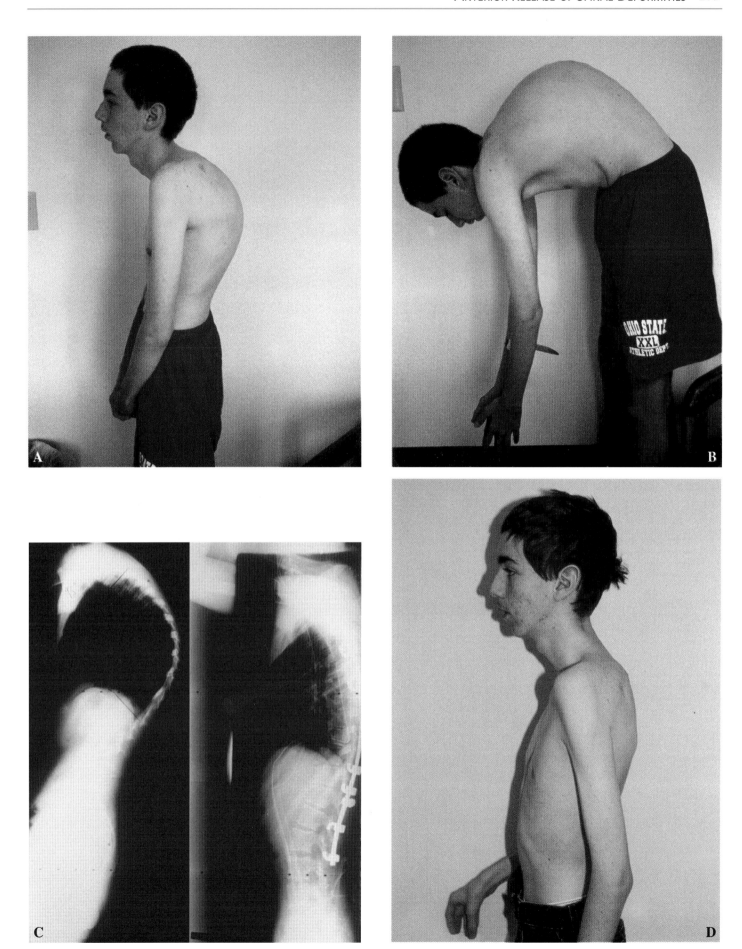

Figure 15–16.   Preoperative photographs of an adolescent with a significant kyphosis **(A)** standing and **(B)** bending. Note the protrusion of the chin and the hyperlordosis of the cervical spine. **(C)** Pre- (left) and postoperative (right) lateral radiographs show excellent correction of the kyphosis. **(D)** Postoperative photograph of the patient 6 months after surgery.

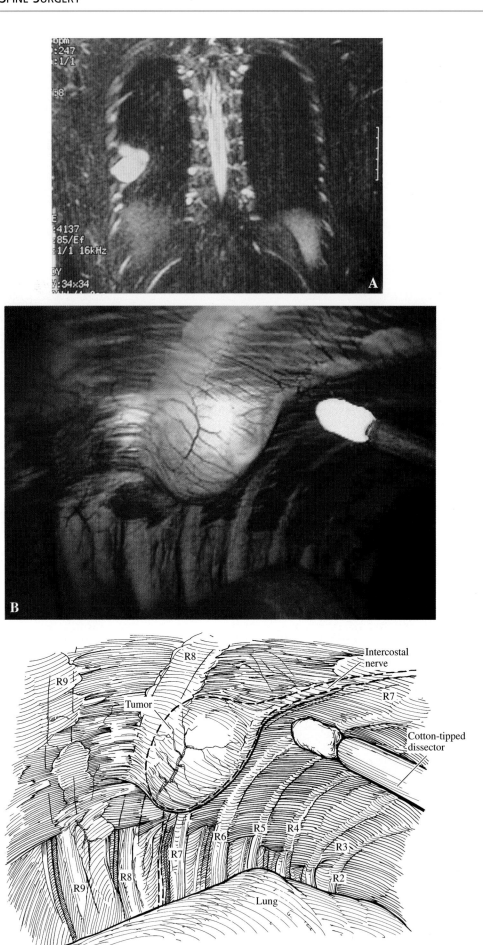

Figure 15–17. **(A)** Preoperative magnetic resonance image shows a large intercostal neurofibroma on the right side in a 16-year-old male with Type I neurofibromatosis. **(B)** Intraoperative and **(C)** corresponding illustration showing that the tumor arises distally from the seventh intercostal nerve. R = rib.

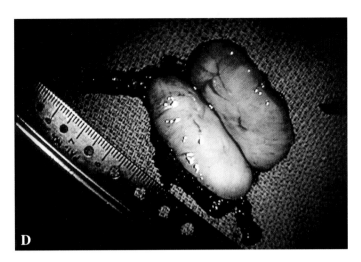 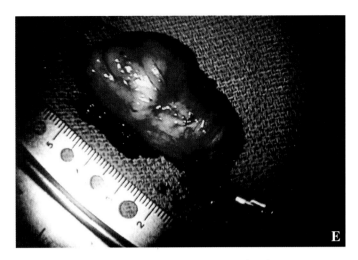

Figure 15–17. *(continued)* **(D** and **E)** Views of the tumor after excision, which was removed en bloc as a single piece.

CONCLUSIONS

Thoracoscopy is a major advance in the surgical armamentarium for treating children and adults with spinal deformities by performing anterior releases, interbody fusions, osteotomies, and hemivertebral resections. Thoracoscopy has significant advantages compared to thoracotomy. It provides better visualization, wider exposures, and greater access to multiple levels that cannot be reached through a single thoracotomy incision. It also is associated with better cosmetic outcomes, less pulmonary and shoulder dysfunction, shorter hospital stays, and faster recovery times.

ACKNOWLEDGMENT

Kind appreciation is extended to Ms. Tamara Hoffman for assistance in the preparation of this chapter.

REFERENCES

1. Medical Science: *New York Times*, September 19, 1992.
2. Nash MJ: The kindest cut of all. *Time Magazine*, March 23, 1992.
3. Jacobaeus HC: Possibility of the use of cystoscope for the investigation of the serous cavities. *Muench Med Wochenschr* 1910; 57:3090–3092.
4. Regan JJ, Mack MJ, Picetti GD, III: A comparison of VAT to open thoracotomy in thoracic spinal surgery. Scoliosis Research Society Annual Meeting, Dublin, Ireland, September 18–23, 1993.
5. Riley LH, Lebwohl NH, Eismont FJ: Thoracoscopic corpectomy: Description of a new technique and its outcome in canine model. Scoliosis Research Society Annual Meeting, Dublin, Ireland, September 18–23, 1993.
6. Blackman R: Multiple level anterior thoracic discectomy using an endoscopic exposure. Scoliosis Research Society Annual Meeting, Dublin, Ireland, September 18–23, 1993.
7. Regan JJ: North American Spine Society, San Diego, CA, 1993.
8. Snider M: Life section. *USA Today*, December 1993.
9. Dubousset J, Herring JA, Shufflebarger H: The crankshaft phenomenon. *J Pediatr Orthop* 1989; 9(5):541–550.
10. Mack MJ, Regan JJ, McAfee PC, et al: Video-assisted thoracic surgery for the anterior approach to the thoracic spine. *Ann Thorac Surg* 1995; 59(5):1100–1106.
11. Winter RB, Lonstein JE, Denis F, et al: The risk of paraplegia secondary to segmental vessel ligation. An analysis of 1197 consecutive anterior operations. *Orthop Trans* 1996; 19(3):616.

Thoracoscopic Spine Surgery
Edited by Dickman et al. Thieme Medical Publishers, Inc., New York © 1999

CHAPTER *16*

Endoscopic Anterior Correction of Idiopathic Scoliosis

Ronald G. Blackman, M.D. and Eduardo Luque, M.D.

For more than 35 years, the combination of anterior spinal instrumentation and fusion has been a standard approach for the correction of scoliosis. Compared to posterior fusion, an anterior approach for treating scoliosis has several advantages. First, the mobility of the lumbar spine is preserved because fewer spinal segments have to be instrumented to achieve correction. Fusion also occurs more rapidly. Excision of the growth plates anteriorly can prevent the crankshaft phenomenon from developing in young patients.[1] Additionally, an anterior release for removing anterior disc material and ligaments permits the deformed spine to be more flexible. The increased flexibility then improves the correction that can be obtained with spinal instrumentation.

A thoracotomy for the treatment of scoliosis offers limited access and oblique trajectories to many of the thoracic disc spaces. The apex of the lordotic curve can be exposed, but the disc spaces rostral and caudal to the apex are not parallel to the exposure. Consequently, the instruments used to remove the disc material and the end plates cannot enter the disc space in line or parallel with the discs as needed (Fig. 16–1). These limitations may partially explain the relatively high incidence of nonunion at the upper levels of the thoracic spine when anterior fixation is performed through a thoracotomy. To augment the access provided by a thoracotomy incision, instruments have been inserted through small additional incisions.

In 1993, we began to develop an endoscopic technique for the correction of scoliosis. For the first several years, our experience was limited to an endoscopic anterior release without inserting instrumentation. Instruments were introduced through small incisions. Moving the endoscope and the surgical instruments above and below the apex of the lordotic curve permitted the ideal, parallel, in-line approach needed for optimal removal of disc material and the cartilaginous end plate. Removing the rib, as in a standard thoracotomy, was unnecessary. It was hoped that this approach would improve the correction of a spinal deformity and be associated with less pain, shorter hospitalization times, smaller scars, and more acceptable cosmetic outcomes.[2]

Traditionally, many of the surgical procedures for correcting thoracolumbar scoliosis have involved an anterior release and subsequent placement of posterior spinal instrumentation and fusion. However, when patients underwent an anterior endoscopic and open posterior fusion performed for congenital scoliosis, their hospital stay appeared to decrease compared to patients undergoing thoracotomies, as did their recovery time and return to full activity.

A multilevel anterior endoscopic discectomy was performed in 40 patients with scoliosis to increase mobility of the spine, to improve the amount of correction of the deformity, and to achieve interbody fusion.[3] A posterior fusion with instrumentation was performed to enhance correction and to reduce the lordosis for fusion. Correction consistently improved a significant amount beyond the bending Cobb angle. The total correction achieved in these stiff lordotic curves averaged 64%. When the pulmonary function in patients undergoing endoscopic anterior release with posterior fusion was compared to that of patients undergoing posterior fusion alone, no differences were found. Posterior fusion appeared to be the major factor influencing patients' decreased pulmonary function after surgery. Furthermore, subjectively, four or five 2-cm incisions had a better appearance than one long thoracotomy scar.

During our experience with more than 60 endoscopic spine procedures for anterior release of scoliosis, it became obvious that discectomy was only half of the procedure. If the deformed spine could be made more flexible and also corrected through the same four to six endoscopic portal incisions, the disadvantages associated with posterior fusion could be eliminated. After another year of developing techniques and instruments, we performed our first endoscopic scoliosis correction in January 1997. This report is based on the experience gained from the first 20 patients (15 females, 5 males; age range, 10 to 26 years) who underwent endoscopic placement of the Blackman-Luque Anterior Spinal System (Sofamor Danek, Memphis, TN).

PREOPERATIVE MANAGEMENT

Endoscopic anterior release and fixation requires a multidisciplinary surgical team. The spine surgeon, thoracic surgeon, anesthesiologist, and nursing team all play vital roles in the flow of the procedure and obtaining successful outcomes.

Preoperatively, the levels for fixation are identified from upright and bending spine radiographs. The fixation usually encompasses six to eight levels between the fifth thoracic and the first lumbar vertebrae. In selected cases, we reached the second lumbar vertebral body through this approach.

Necessary instruments include a 30-degree and a 45-degree angled, 10-mm endoscope, a three-chip video camera, a selection of long curettes, pituitary rongeurs, Kerrison rongeurs, standard endoscopic surgical instruments, and a few instruments specific to the procedure (Table 16–1, Fig. 16–2). The screws are designed to fit through an 11.5-mm diameter portal. Most of the instrumentation will also fit through a portal this size. The rod reducer and the compressor fit through the incisions, but the plastic portal must first be removed.

Anesthesia plays a major role in obtaining a successful outcome. Single-lung ventilation is mandatory. The anes-

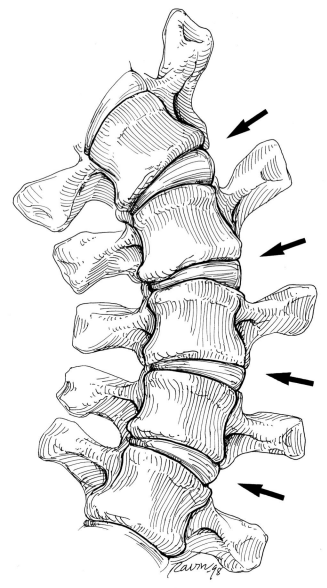

Figure 16–1. In the scoliotic thoracic spine, the trajectories for placing tools directly into the different disc spaces vary. A single thoracotomy incision does not permit full access to the disc spaces rostral and caudal to the apex of the deformity. The arrows represent the required angles for each discectomy.

TABLE 16–1 Instruments Needed for Anterior Correction of Scoliosis

Complete set of small curettes, Cobb type elevators (10 instruments)

Rongeurs (neutral and angled)

Heavy duty rib cutter

Rongeur-type (modified) rod holder (end and side cutouts)

Tap

Two "L" rod pushers

One "L" rod pusher flat top

Wooden handle screwdriver (dumbbell shape)

Screwdriver (flat blade)

Lohman clamp (rongeur locking handle)

Three-prong fork (for directing K-wire)

Metallic shaft 1/4-inch head screwdriver

Torque screwdriver handle

Rod compressor

Flex driver

Rod reducer

Screwdriver with thread to hold top screw

Bone graft introducer

Adjustor screwdriver

Special "K" wires (50 cm long)

Rod measurer

thesiologist should use a double-lumen endotracheal tube or a bronchial blocker. The "downside" (i.e., ventilated side) mainstem bronchus can also be intubated selectively. Intubating the mainstem bronchus in a small patient, particularly on the left side (the typical side), requires considerable skill.

The spine is usually approached from the right along the convex surface of the deformity. Keeping the endotracheal tube in place when the patient is turned is also difficult. If the lung is not fully deflated, often the tube position must be adjusted by the anesthesiologist when the patient is on his or her side. Consequently, the table should not be flexed or the patient's position changed once the surgical exposure has been satisfactorily achieved.

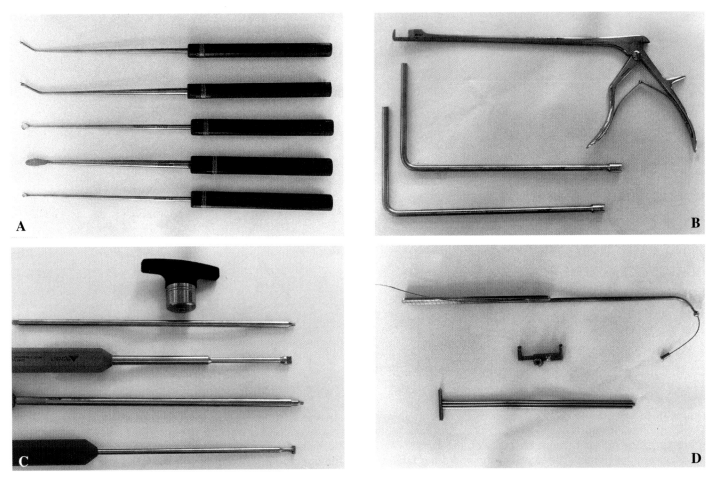

Figure 16–2.   Instruments for anterior endoscopic fixation for scoliosis. **(A)** Endoscopic ring curettes and Cobb periosteal elevator. **(B)** Endoscopic rib cutter (*top*). Two L-shaped rod pushers (*bottom*). **(C**, *top to bottom*) Torque screwdriver handle, hexagonal screwdriver top, flat-bladed screwdriver, threaded screwdriver for top-capture screw, and dumbbell-shaped screwdriver tip. **(D**, *top to bottom*) Rod measurer, rod compressor, and a three-pronged guide for K-wire drilling. Additional tools used for this procedure (not depicted) include rod grasping tools, rod holders, taps, flat-tipped rod pusher, Lohman clamp-rongeur, disc rongeurs, rod reducer, bone-graft introducer, and 50-cm long K-wires.

SURGICAL TECHNIQUE

The patient is positioned in a lateral decubitus position on the operating table with the concave side of the curve down. The chest and back are prepared in sterile fashion and draped. Included in the draping is the scapula, which may need to be retracted to provide access to the fourth and fifth thoracic vertebrae. The spine surgeon stands posterior to the patient's back (Fig. 16–3).[4] Posterior to the posterior axillary line, usually in the sixth or seventh intercostal space, the initial 1.5-cm incision for inserting the endoscope is made. The diaphragm is usually caudal to these levels. The remaining portals are positioned in the posterior axillary line in a trajectory that is coaxial with the screws.

The surgeon must ensure that the lung is deflated and that no lung adhesions exist. The surgeon inserts a finger into the pleural space to feel for lung adhesions before any portals are inserted into the incision. The surgeon's finger is the best initial probing tool because this is the only part of the procedure done "blindly." Once the first portal is placed, additional portals are placed while visualized with the endo-

scope. These 1.5-mm diameter portals are usually in the midaxillary line. The only exception is placement of an anterior caudal portal so that the diaphragm can be swept anteriorly to expose the diaphragmatic crus between T12 and L2 if these vertebra are to be instrumented.

Discectomy

The endoscope can be positioned to visualize the entire thoracic spine from the thoracic apex caudally to the diaphragm. The level of the disc can be determined by counting the ribs sequentially from caudally to the apex (Fig. 16–4), but the anatomic level should also be confirmed radiographically.

The pleura is incised longitudinally with a hook cautery along the entire surface of the spine to be fused (Fig. 16–5). The discs are identified, cleaned of overlying tissue with a cotton-tipped dissector, incised with an electrocautery blade, and excised using periosteal elevators, pituitary rongeurs, and curettes. The disc material is removed, the anterior longitudinal ligament and annulus are sectioned, and the end plate is ablated in a manner similar to open

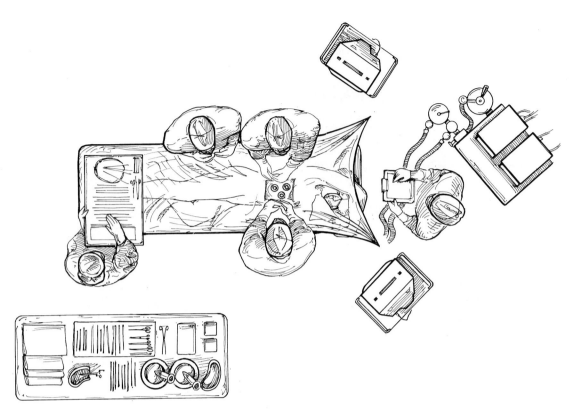

Figure 16–3. Operating room setup for thoracoscopic anterior release and instrumentation for correction of thoracic scoliosis. The surgeon stands posterior to the patient to facilitate angling the hardware (screw trajectories) anteriorly away from the spinal cord. The portal incisions are made on the surface of the chest collinear with the intended trajectories of the screws. Monitors are positioned at the head of the operating table to view the operation.

surgery. The segmental vessels are not disturbed at this time. In cases of kyphosis, only the anterior longitudinal ligament needs to be sectioned. For most other procedures, the anterior part and the opposite side of the anterior longitudinal ligament and annulus are preserved to serve as an envelope for the bone graft. Correcting scoliosis by this approach is a *shortening* procedure; therefore, the entire anterior longitudinal ligament does not need to be resected. As far as the surgeon can visualize, the annulus fibrosus is removed laterally and anteriorly. Only a limp ligament is left. The discectomy is completed leaving the rib head intact. The cartilaginous end plates are removed (Fig. 16–6). Bone bleeding is controlled by electrocauterization and by packing the end plates with Surgicel™ (Johnson & Johnson, Arlington, TX; Fig. 16–7). Each disc is sequentially prepared in this fashion.

A branch of the lesser or greater splanchnic nerve crosses the disc space caudal to the T5 vertebrae. The splanchnic nerves arise from the T5 to T11 sympathetic ganglia (Fig. 16–8). The splanchnic nerves can be transected without causing complications.

If the procedure is only an anterior release and fusion, the Surgicel™ is removed and the bone graft and/or allograft gel is packed into the disc spaces to promote fusion. If no hardware is used, the pleura can be closed using a monofilament absorbable 00 suture. This technique, however, is time consuming, technically difficult, and requires

special instruments. Either the suture passer commonly used in the shoulder (Linvatec®; Largo, FL) or the U.S. Surgical Autosuture® (U.S. Surgical Corp., Norwalk, CT) tool can be used. The pleura is usually flimsy and does not hold suture well. It probably is unnecessary to close the pleura, although no studies have shown whether doing so decreases pleural adhesions or is otherwise helpful.

Placement of Instrumentation

The next stage involves inserting the corrective spinal instrumentation. The most accurate way to insert the screws is under combined fluoroscopic radiograph and endoscopic visualization. The screws are inserted just anterior to the head of the rib at each level. Initially, the position of the screws will not align perfectly because the spine is deformed, rotated, and malaligned. The position of the screws resembles a "V" adjacent to the apex of the deformity. Inserting a straight rod onto the screws decreases the rotation of the spine. Placing the screw adjacent to the rib head also helps direct the screw trajectory safely across the vertebral body. To avoid penetrating the spinal canal posteriorly, the screw trajectory should be 20 degrees anteriorly.[5]

It is difficult to assess if the trajectory of the screw is correct by looking endoscopically into the pleural cavity at the contour of the surfaces of the vertebral body. A cannulated

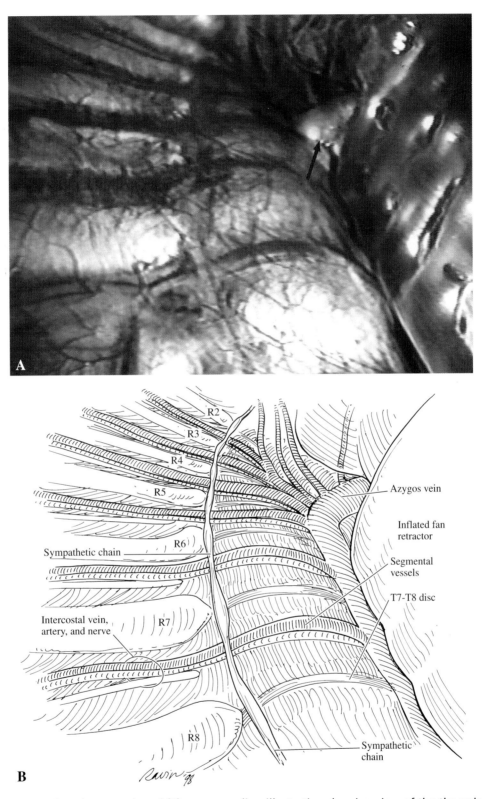

Figure 16–4. **(A)** Intraoperative photograph and **(B)** corresponding illustration showing view of the thoracic spine (right-sided exposure). The lung was deflated and retracted medially with a fan retractor. The azygos vein is visualized as it empties into the superior vena cava at the level of T4. R = rib.

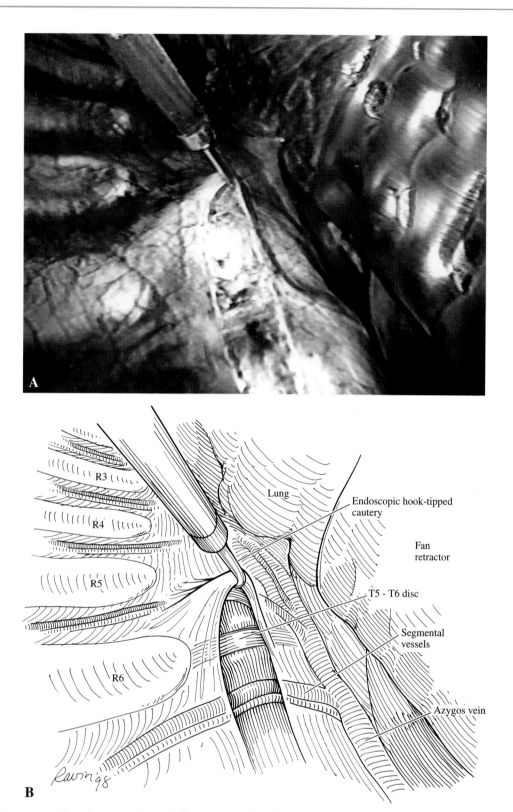

Figure 16–5. **(A)** Intraoperative photograph and **(B)** corresponding illustration showing an endoscopic hooked-tip cautery being used to elevate the pleura away from the segmental vessels while the pleura is incised. The segmental vessels are preserved until the screws are inserted. R = rib.

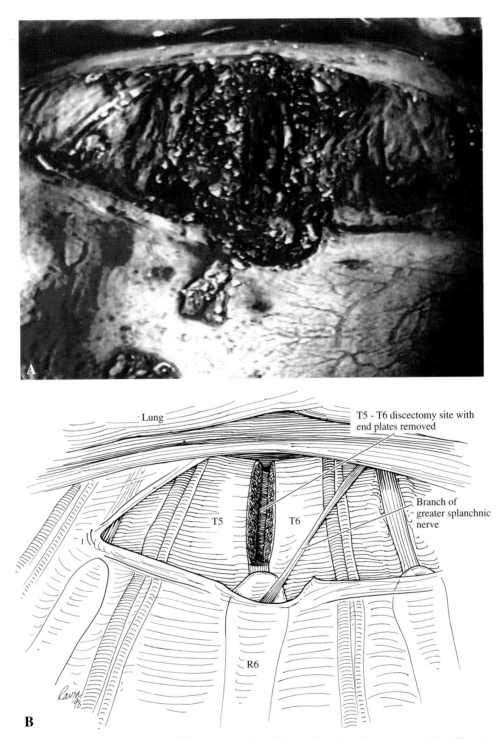

Figure 16–6. **(A)** Intraoperative photograph and **(B)** corresponding illustration showing a completed discectomy. The lateral annulus was incised and most of the disc material and the cartilaginous end plates were removed. The rib head and the posterior longitudinal ligament were preserved. T = thoracic vertebrae and R = rib.

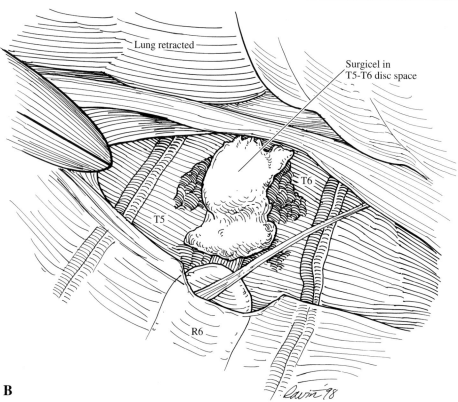

Figure 16–7. **(A)** Intraoperative photograph and **(B)** corresponding illustration showing the bleeding bone surfaces in the discectomy site being packed with Surgicel™ (Johnson & Johnson, Arlington, TX) for hemostasis. T = thoracic vertebrae and R = rib.

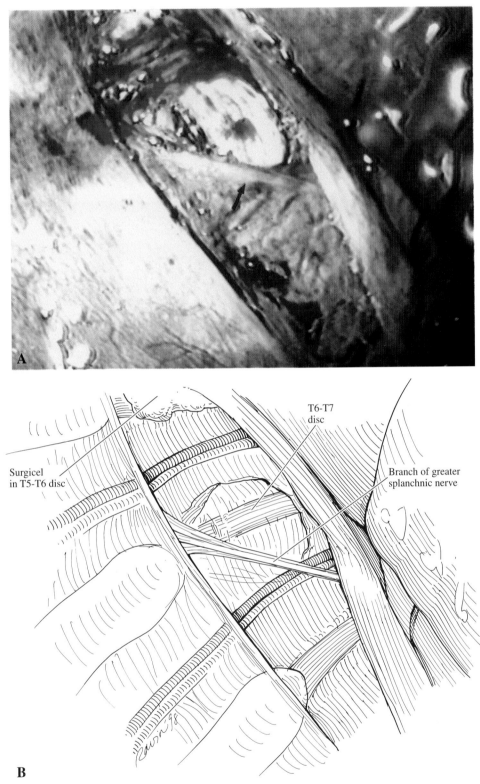

Figure 16–8. **(A)** Intraoperative photograph and **(B)** corresponding illustration showing a branch of the greater splanchnic nerve crossing anteromedially along the surface of the spine at the T6–T7 disc space.

screw and cannulated instruments, which are inserted over the Kirschner wire, are used to facilitate the procedure. The operating room personnel wear lead aprons. The C-arm is positioned at the operating table using an anteroposterior cross table view. The segmental vessels are left intact up to this point because they form an anatomical landmark for inserting the screws at the middle of the vertebral body. The segmental artery and vein at the lateral surface of the vertebral body are mobilized, ligated, cauterized, and then divided (Fig. 16–9). There appears to be almost no risk of spinal cord infarction if the segmental vessels are ligated at the midvertebral body on the convex side of the curve.[6] Ligation at this level preserves collateral blood flow to the spinal cord via the intercostal vessels.

Alternatively, the vessels can be mobilized and preserved. The thin film of tissue holding the vessels in place is cut. The vessels are mobilized by passing a tonsil clamp or right angle under them and retracting the vessels. We avoid this maneuver because there is a risk of lacerating the vessels or wrapping them in the screw threads.

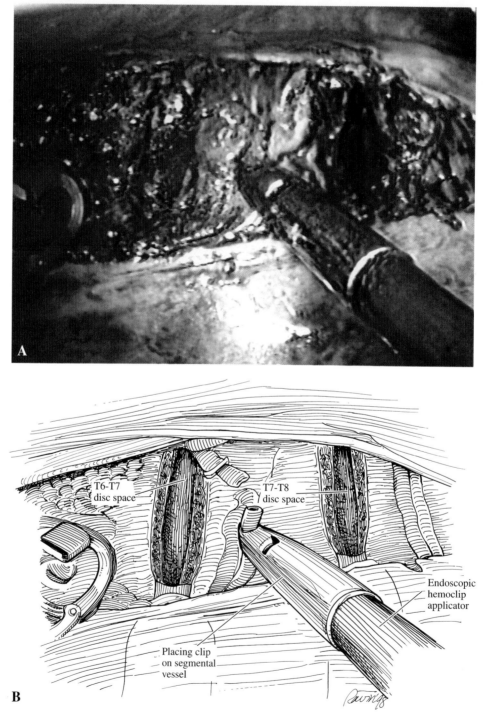

Figure 16–9. **(A)** Intraoperative photograph and **(B)** corresponding illustration showing the segmental vessels being clipped. The segmental vessels are mobilized, cauterized, ligated, and divided to provide access to the vertebral bodies to insert the screws.

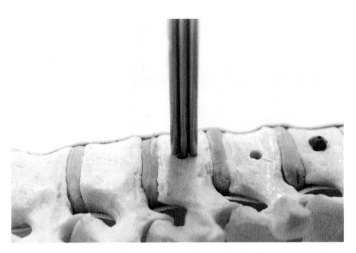

Figure 16–10. The three-pronged K-wire drill guide in place on a spine model. Each of the three channels can hold a K-wire to allow a variety of wire positions.

The space just anterior to the head of the rib is cleaned, and the three-pronged starter guide is positioned on the vertebral body with the center prong at the midpoint of the vertebra. The guide is also angled so that it is parallel to the end plates at each level. The guide is also angled 10 to 20 degrees anteriorly from the head of the rib to avoid the spinal canal.

Fluoroscopy with the C-arm confirms that the trajectory and placement of the screw are correct. A Kirschner (K-wire) is inserted through the three-pronged starter guide and drilled into the vertebral body (Figs. 16–10 and 16–11). Visualizing the K-wire on the image intensifier confirms its correct placement (Fig. 16–12). If the K-wire is too caudal or cephalad, another one can be inserted using the other hole of the starter guide. The first K-wire is then removed. The K-wire and screw trajectory are visualized using the endoscope to confirm their trajectory relative to the anterior surface of the spine (Fig. 16–13). A lateral radiographic view can also be used to confirm the trajectory.

Once the K-wire is placed, the pilot hole is tapped in the vertebral body (Fig. 16–14). Care is taken to prevent the tap from binding the K-wire and driving it past the opposite cortex. This maneuver is best done by holding the proximal tip of the K-wire with a forceps at the junction of the K-wire/tap handle. When the tap is removed, the K-wire is also held to prevent it from dislodging from the vertebral body. The tap is slightly undersized and should penetrate halfway into the vertebral body. The screw is then inserted over the K-wire. A cannulated screwdriver is used to insert the screw into the vertebral body (Fig. 16–15).

Ideally, the tip of the screw should just penetrate the opposite cortex (Fig. 16–16). The length of the screws increases in 5-mm increments. A screw can therefore penetrate 1 to 4 mm beyond the cortex. Before the C-arm is removed, the position of each screw is assessed to verify that they penetrate the opposite cortex. If one or two screws are not placed bicortically, it is not a major concern. The

side walls of the screw heads are adjusted so that they are aligned to insert the rod (Fig. 16–17). The screw heads are oriented at each level. To approach each screw at the correct angle, one skin incision can be used to work both above and below a rib. Two approaches are then provided by one skin incision. If the angle of screw trajectories is too great or too small, the rod will not reduce the deformity satisfactorily (Fig. 16–18).

After the screws are placed, the preparation of the fusion bed is completed. The end plates are further destroyed with a curette. Particles of cancellous bone are left in place between the end plates. Finally, additional morcellized rib grafts or allograft gel is placed in the disc spaces. The rib graft can be harvested at any point during the procedure by one of two methods. A piece of rib evident through the skin incision at the portal site can be harvested. Alternatively, a piece of rib can be harvested endoscopically using an endoscopic rib cutter.

The length of the rod is then determined. A measuring instrument with a cable running down its shaft is inserted into the chest through a portal. The cable fits onto the top screw and is then guided down to the bottom screw. The length between the screws can be measured directly by reading the scale on the shaft of the tool (Fig. 16–19).

A 4.5-mm diameter rod is cut to length and smoothed with a high-speed burr if rough. The slightly flexible rod is inserted into the chest cavity and usually kept straight. It is manipulated onto the bottom screw and held in place by a top-fitting "capture" screw. Distally, only a small amount of rod is exposed to avoid damaging the diaphragm. The rod is successively reduced onto each of the screws, and the top capture screws are applied. A rod pusher is used to push the rod snugly onto the screw head to maintain the reduction. Its internal diameter fits the screwdriver tightly so that the screwdriver and capture screw together can be passed down the center of the rod pusher. The capture screw is applied to lock the rod to the screw head. These instruments significantly reduce the chances of cross threading (Figs. 16–20 and 16–21).

The rod is fully reduced onto the screws and held in place by either the "L" pusher or the rod reducer. Compression is applied between each of the screws using a compressing tool (Fig. 16–22). Compression should be applied as each set of adjacent screws is attached to the rod. The ratchet compressor fits between the two screw heads on the rod. Turning the gear and ratcheting the two screws together provide good tension and compression. After each set of adjacent screws is compressed, the top capture screws are tightened to their final position using a torque screwdriver set internally at 75 pounds (Fig. 16–23).

The sulcus between the pleura and the lung is suctioned to make sure there is no bleeding. A No. 20 chest tube is inserted to drain fluid and blood from the chest cavity. Wounds are closed in layers, and the patient is positioned supine and extubated.

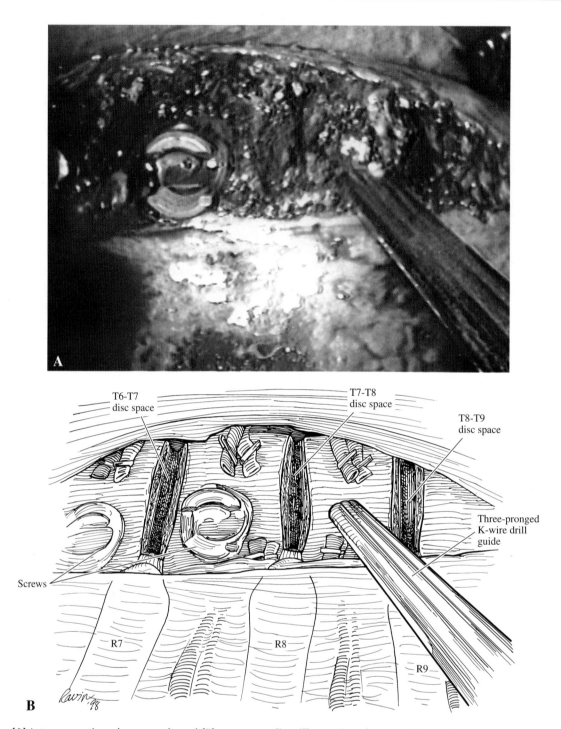

Figure 16–11. **(A)** Intraoperative photograph and **(B)** corresponding illustration showing the endoscopic surgical view of the three-pronged K-wire drill guide.

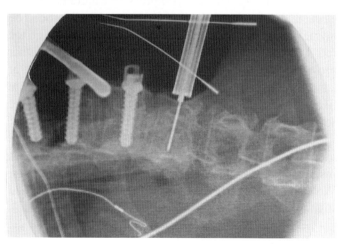

Figure 16–12. Fluoroscopic imaging is used to observe the trajectory and depth of the K-wires and the screws as they are inserted into the spine.

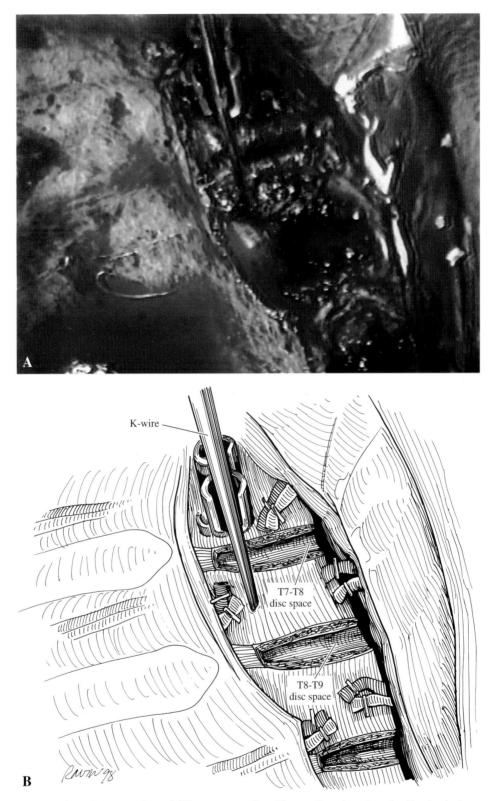

Figure 16–13. **(A)** Intraoperative photograph and **(B)** corresponding illustration showing the K-wire being positioned within the vertebral body.

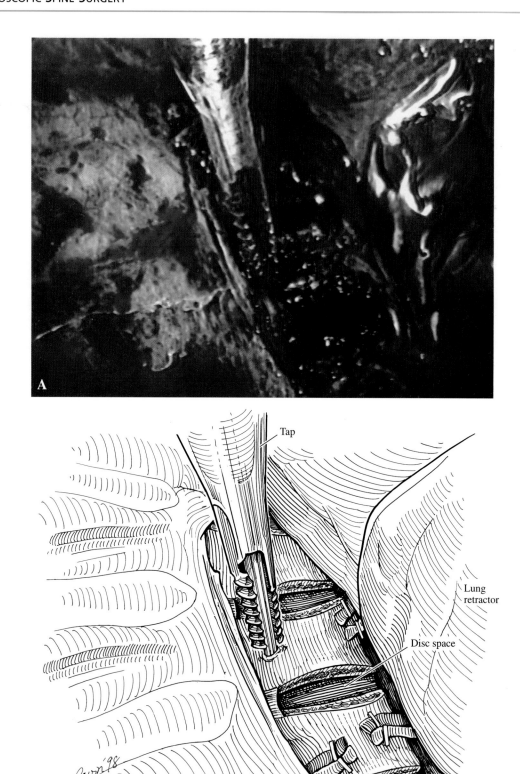

Figure 16–14. **(A)** Intraoperative photograph and **(B)** corresponding illustration of the cannulated tap cutting the thread pattern into the pilot hole in the vertebral body.

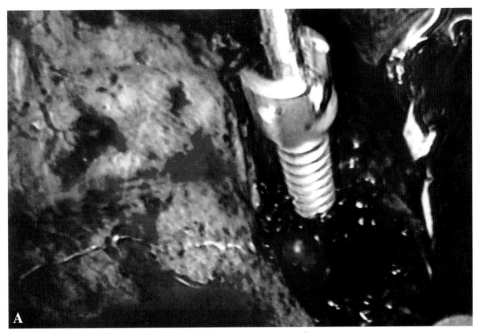

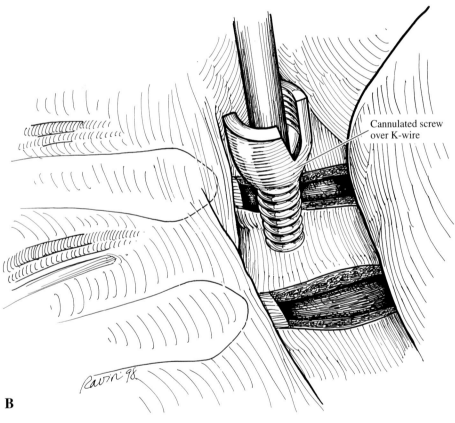

Cannulated screw
over K-wire

Figure 16–15. **(A)** Intraoperative
photograph and **(B)** corresponding
illustration showing the cannulated
screw being threaded over the K-wire
and inserted into the vertebral body
using a cannulated screwdriver.

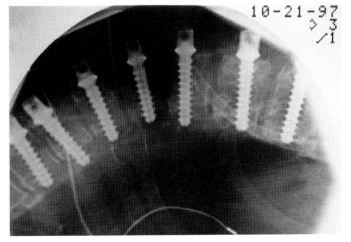

Figure 16–16. Intraoperative fluoroscopic image showing
the bicortical vertebral body fixation screws positioned
parallel to the end plates of each vertebrae.

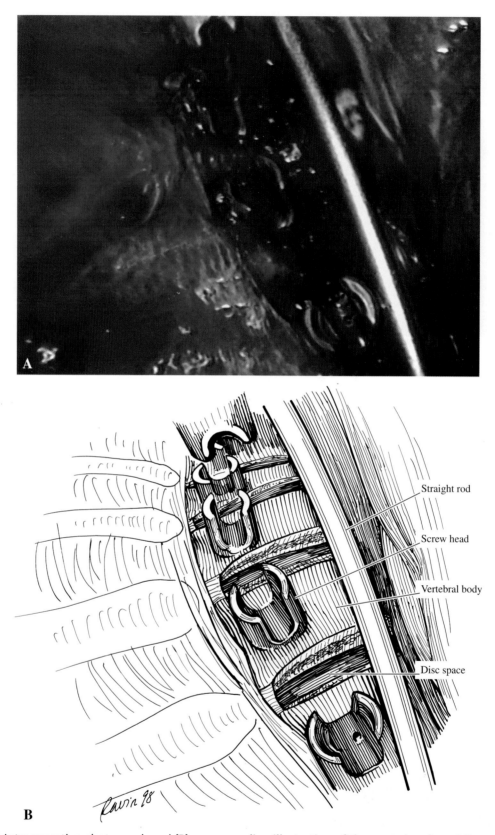

Figure 16–17. **(A)** Intraoperative photograph and **(B)** corresponding illustration of the screw heads and the rod. The screw heads form a V-shaped alignment on the surface of the spine before the scoliotic deformity is reduced. The heads of the screws are aligned in the same orientation to fit the straight rod onto the screws.

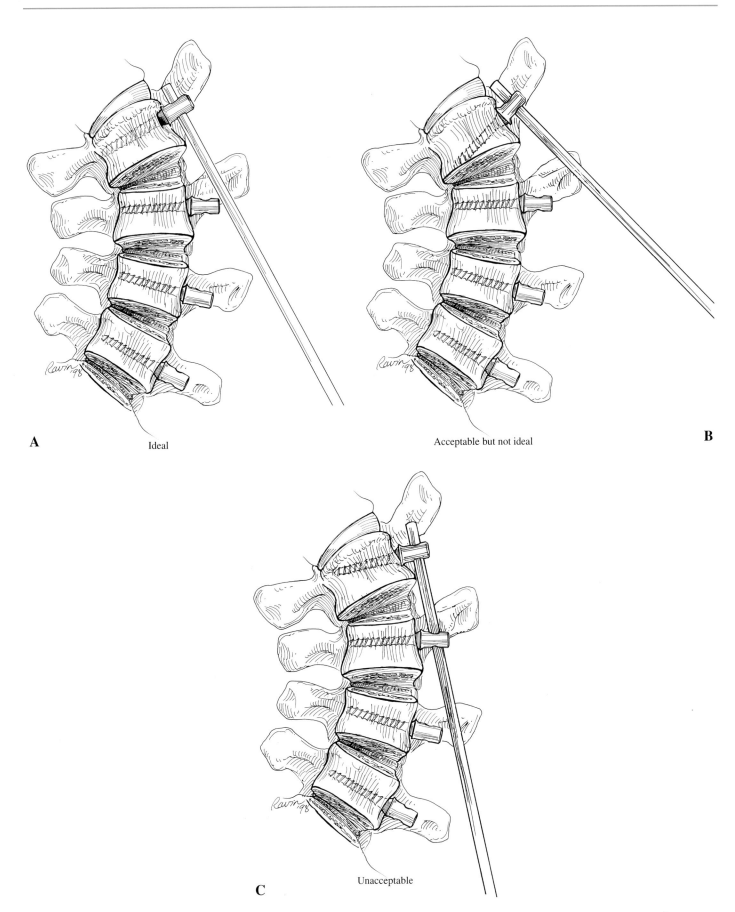

A   Ideal

B   Acceptable but not ideal

C   Unacceptable

Figure 16–18.   The position of the screws within the vertebral bodies is a critical determinant of the ability to correct the deformed spine. The screws should be parallel to the end plates. **(A)** When the screws are exactly parallel to the end plates of each vertebrae in the deformed spine, the rod is in an ideal position to correct the deformity. **(B)** If the screws are inserted with too steep an angle, it is difficult to insert the rod and excessive stress is exerted on the screws at the distal end of the fixation. **(C)** If the screws are inserted into the vertebral bodies with a rostral trajectory, the rod will not correct the scoliotic deformity.

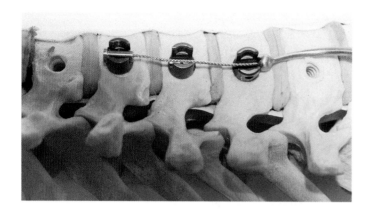

Figure 16–19.   The length of the rod is measured using a tool that has a flexible cable to fit over the screw heads. The length measured is read using a calibration on the handle of the tool, which is outside the chest.

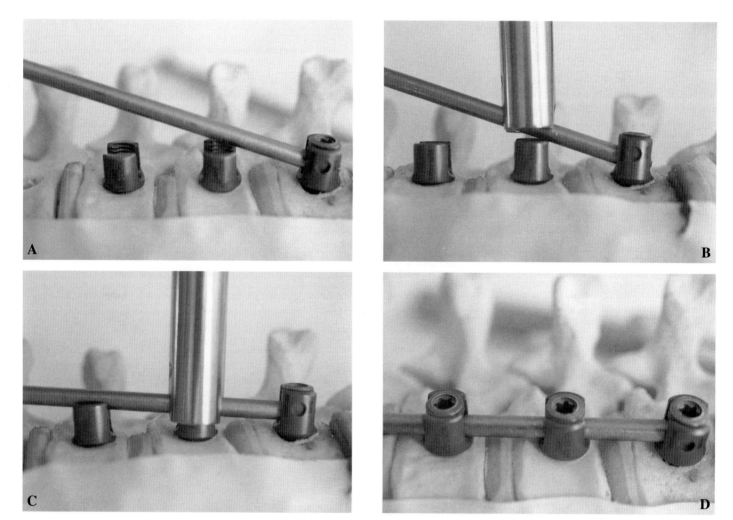

Figure 16–20.   Insertion of the rod and reduction of the spinal deformity. **(A)** The rod is connected to the distal screw first and secured in position with a locking nut. **(B)** The hollow rod-reducing tool is placed over the rod adjacent to the screw head. **(C)** Downward force is applied to reduce the rod onto the screw head. The top-fitting locking screw and its driver fit through the shaft of the reducing tool to lock the rod and screw together. **(D)** Final view of the construct showing the rod locked to each of the screws with a top-fitting capture screw.

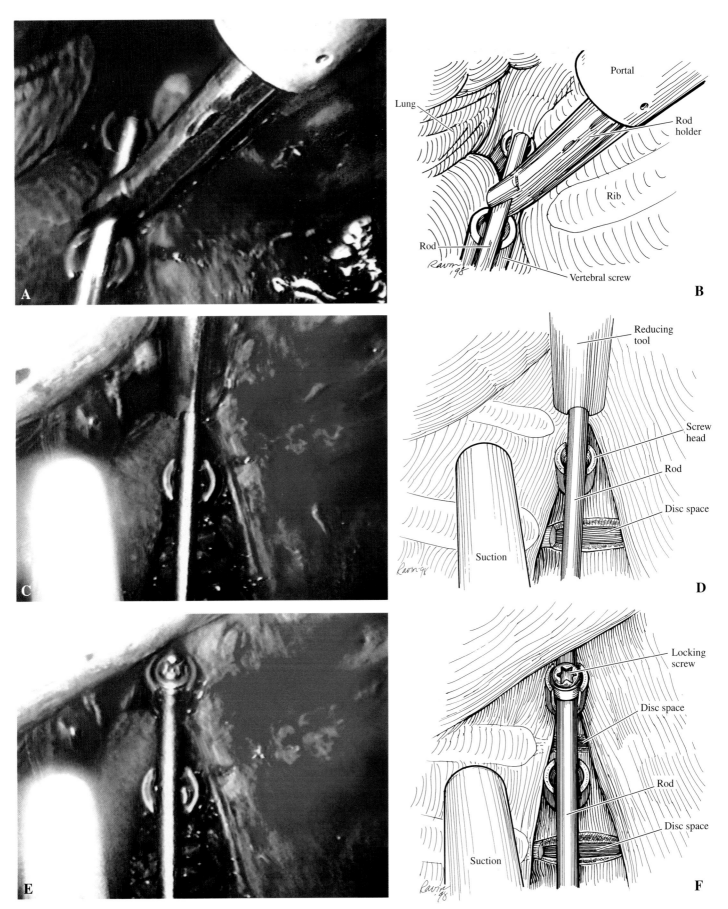

Figure 16–21. Instrumentation and deformity reduction. **(A)** Intraoperative photograph and **(B)** corresponding illustration showing insertion of the rod onto the head of the distal screw. **(C)** Intraoperative photograph and **(D)** corresponding illustration showing alignment of the rod, screw head, and top capture screw using the reducing tool. **(E)** Intraoperative photograph and **(F)** corresponding illustration showing the top capture screw after it was tightened to lock the rod and fixation screw together.

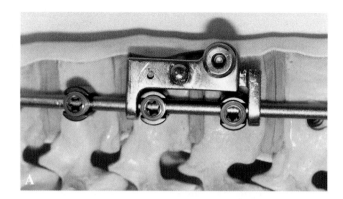

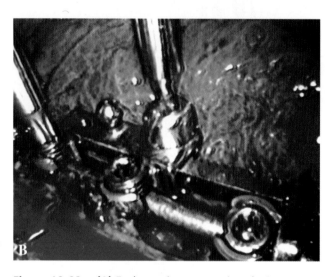

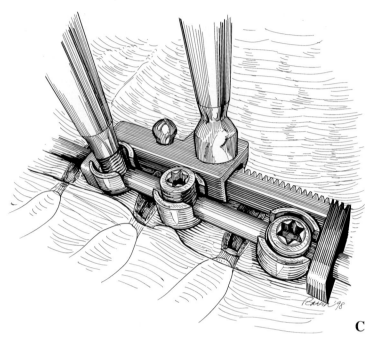

Figure 16–22. **(A)** Endoscopic compression device on a spine model. The ratcheted compressor reduces the deformity to its desired position before final tightening of the locking screws. **(B)** Intraoperative photograph and **(C)** corresponding illustration of the compressor being used. This tool requires dexterity and practice to manipulate it successfully.

POSTOPERATIVE MANAGEMENT

Postoperative management after an endoscopic correction of scoliosis is similar to the care provided after open thoracotomy. Typically, the chest tube is removed within 36 to 48 hours; the output must be less than 30 ml/8 hours or less than 100 ml/day. Patients can begin ambulating the day after surgery; most are out of bed by the second day. A front-opening Boston brace with a left underarm extension that is made and fitted before surgery is applied. The patient wears the brace before surgery to become accustomed to it so that its feel is familiar. It is then worn full-time for 4 months after surgery. On the third to fifth postoperative day, patients are usually discharged home (Fig. 16–24).

RESULTS

In our experience with endoscopic anterior instrumentation, curves have ranged from 41 to 98 degrees, with the majority falling between 60 and 65 degrees (Tables 16–2 and 16–3). Most curves were relatively stiff as demonstrated by bending films. The mean correction of the curve was 61%, which was 30% greater than the correction achieved with bending radiographs. In most patients, their rib hump deformities improved significantly (Figs. 16–25, 16–26, 16–27, and 16–28). Percent greater than bending was included because one would expect to achieve correction, at least, to the degree of preoperative bending. A correction greater than that achieved with bending can be attributed to surgical technique. There was no difference in the percent correction of the curve when the first 10 cases were compared to the second 10. Measuring the top and bottom magnitude of the curve is inadequate because the greatest correction occurs at the apex of the curve. The apical vertebra shifted (translated) significantly toward midline, thereby rebalancing the spine. We rarely extended the instrumentation below T12 to spare the mobility of the lumbar spine.

Once home, all our patients were ambulatory and most were able to resume light activities within 10 days. Activities like walking around the block and even visiting classmates in school were rapidly resumed. By the fourth week, adolescents usually returned to school and the adults to

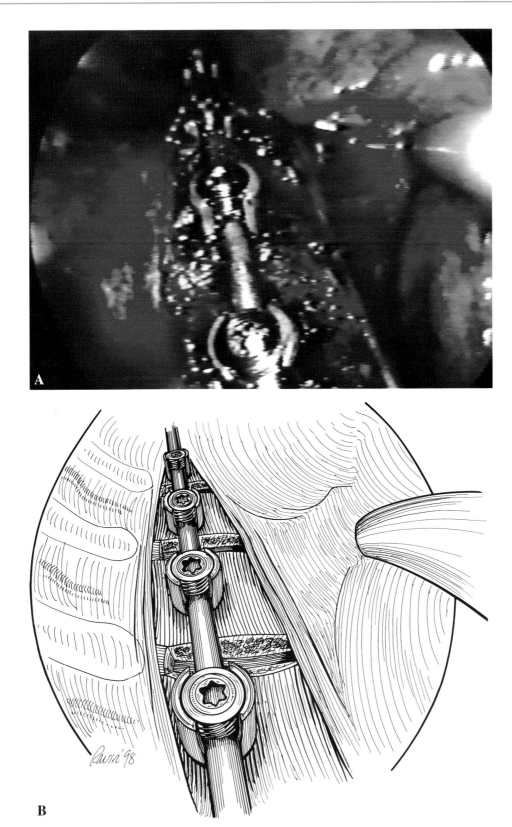

Figure 16–23. **(A)** Intraoperative photograph and **(B)** corresponding illustration of the rod attached to each of the screws with excellent reduction of the scoliotic deformity.

TABLE 16–2 Thoracoscopic Reduction and Fixation of Scoliosis: Extent of Deformity Reduction

Pt.	Age/Sex	Preop Curve (degrees)	Bending (degrees)	Postop Curve (degrees)	Percent Correction[a] (%)	Actual Correction (degrees)	Correction >Bending[b] (%)
1	15/F	52	12	15	71	37	-25
2	15/F	62	40	18	71	44	55
3	13/F	47	37	21	55	26	43
4	13/F	50	28	36	28	14	-29
5	10/M[c]	98	88	40	59	58	55
6	14/F	57	38	15	74	42	61
7	14/F	57	42	30	47	27	29
8	14/F	58	23	15	74	43	35
9	13/F	66	36	22	67	44	39
10	14/M	47	33	16	66	31	52
11	15/F	65	45	31	52	34	31
12	13/M	50	30	25	50	25	17
13	17/F	46	20	16	65	30	20
14	17/F	90	50	35	61	55	30
15	18/M	41	16	18	56	23	-13
16	16/F	87	50	35	60	52	30
17	26/F	60	43	27	55	33	37
18	19/M	52	33	29	44	23	12
19	12/F	49	18	7	86	42	61
20	15/F	53	32	15	72	38	53

[a] Average for all patients is 61%.
[b] Average for all patients is 30%.
[c] Juvenile scoliosis; all other patients had idiopathic scoliosis.

TABLE 16–3 Summary of Spinal Curvature Data Before and After Endoscopic Release

Curvature	Mean (degrees)	Range
Preoperative		
Actual	59°	41 to 98°
Reduction with bending	36°	12 to 50°
Postoperative	23°	7 to 40°
Percent correction	61%	28 to 86%
Actual correction	36°	14 to 58°
Correction > bending correction	30%	−29 to 61%

work between 6 and 8 weeks. Many patients were off intravenous narcotics within 48 hours of surgery, and some required no pain medications after discharge.

Complications

Intraoperatively, the most common problem that we encountered was related to anesthesia. Of the 20 cases, three had to be aborted because adequate oxygen saturation levels could not be maintained. In one case, a patient had copious bronchial secretions. When she was turned onto her side, the secretions accumulating and draining into the downside (ventilated) lung blocked her airway. Another patient had an acute asthmatic attack before surgery, and her peak flow volume was still low. After the

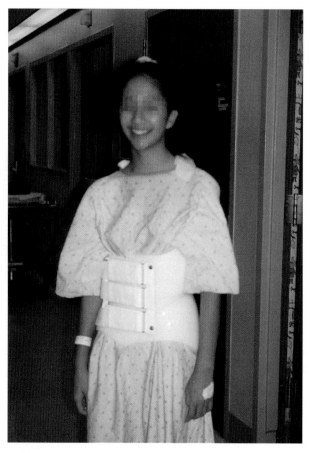

Figure 16–24. A patient wearing her brace on the fourth postoperative day just before her discharge from the hospital.

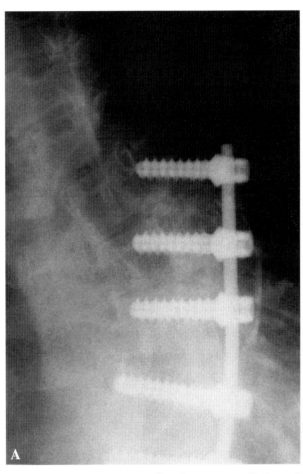

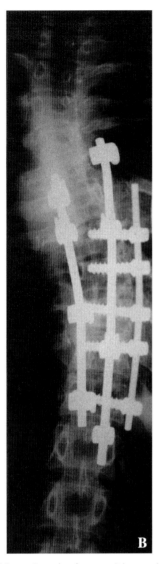

Figure 16–25. **(A)** The uppermost fixation screw pulled out from the spine when this patient had a vomiting episode after surgery. The correction of the deformity was lost. **(B)** The patient was reinstrumented with posterior spinal instrumentation after the upper anterior screw was removed endoscopically.

initial skin incision, she went into acute bronchospasm, her oxygen saturation dropped, and the procedure was stopped. In the third case (personal communication, Dr. George Picetti III, 1998), the anesthesiologist failed to appreciate the nuances of single-lung ventilation and used an endotracheal tube that was too small and could not transport enough gases. The patient's pCO_2 climbed to intolerable levels, and the procedure was terminated. In this case, the discectomy had been performed, but no instrumentation was placed.

Most complications were mild or moderate. Fixation was lost in two patients. After the screws were inserted in a 12-year-old boy who had neuromuscular scoliosis and poor quality bone, we realized that fixation with anterior instrumentation was a poor choice for treatment. While the rod was being connected, all the screws pulled out. The anterior hardware was removed, and the patient underwent a posterior fixation and fusion without incident. In another case, an adult had a vomiting episode that caused the upper

screws to pull out after discharge to home. The upper screws were removed endoscopically 1 month later. A short thoracic fusion was performed through a posterior approach, and her curvature was recorrected (Fig. 16–25).

A 10-year-old boy had a minor hardware-related complication, but correction of the deformity was not lost. He had a 98-degree curve that bent to 88 degrees with a final correction to 45 degrees (personal communication, Dr. George Picetti III, 1998). Five screws were placed over six levels. Intraoperatively, one screw toggled loose and was removed before the rod was seated. Intercostal neuralgia occurred in five patients. All had transient hyperaesthesia just below the breast. Six weeks after surgery all were asymptomatic.

Blood loss during the procedure was minimal, ranging from 50 to 150 ml. Chest tube drainage, a mixture of serous fluid and blood, averaged approximately 350 ml after surgery. However, patients who had a rib resection for graft harvest had more chest tube drainage (occasionally up to

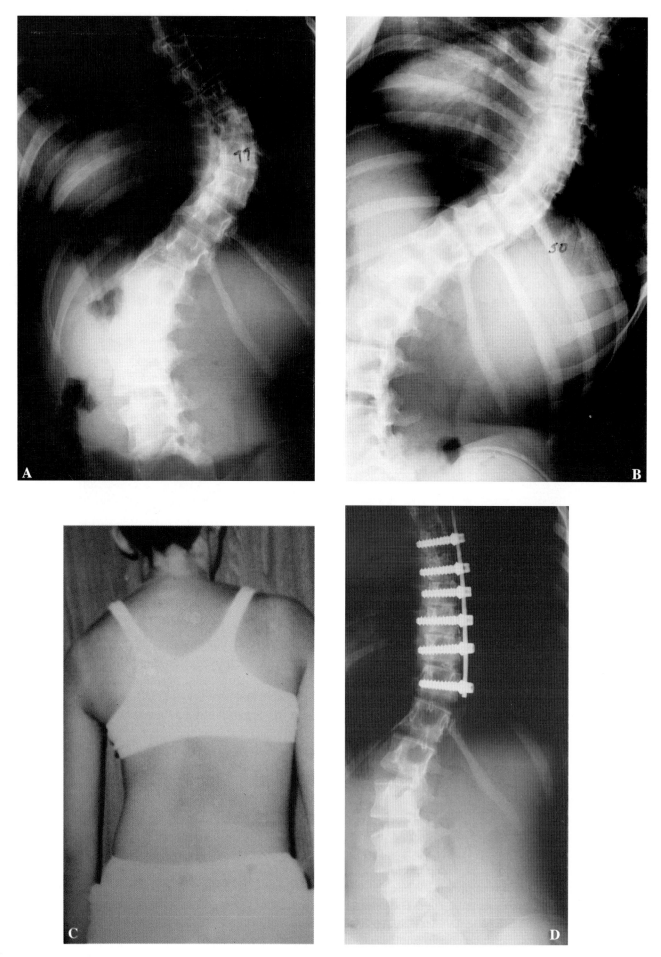

Figure 16–26. Preoperative **(A)** anteroposterior (AP) and **(B)** bending AP radiographs of a 16-year-old female with a 77-degree King II curve. **(C)** Patient's preoperative appearance. **(D)** Postoperative AP and *(Figure continued next page.)*

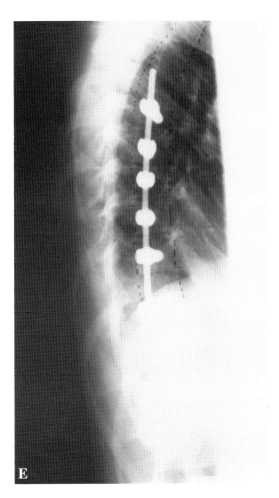
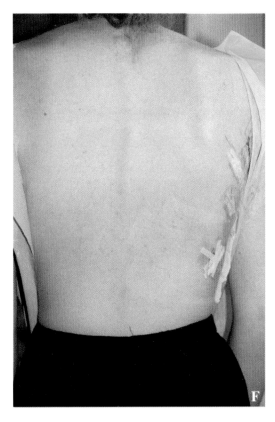

Figure 16–26. *(continued)* **(E)** lateral radiographs. **(F)** Patient's postoperative appearance after the thoracic curve was instrumented, substantially correcting the deformity. Cosmetically, she has rebalanced her curve. Note that the apex of the curve has shifted toward the midline, straightening the apex.

1000 ml). No patients received a transfusion of donated autologous blood after surgery.

DISCUSSION

Our early series had many technical glitches: the rod was too short, the screws were not quite right or malaligned, and the capture screw dissociated from the main screw. Experience and modification of the hardware and tools have minimized these problems. We now have the technical ability to insert six or eight screws endoscopically into the thoracic vertebrae, connect them with a rod, compress the screws, and significantly correct the thoracic curve exclusively through several small incisions in the intercostal spaces. The follow-up is still too brief for a definitive evaluation of the technique. Potentially, the rods could break, the screws could pull out, or fusion could fail to occur. It is also uncertain whether the short fusion will hold up over time or need to be extended.

Endoscopic correction of an anterior deformity is a logical evolution of surgical technique for patients who would otherwise require a multiple-level thoracic discectomy and anterior release. Thoracoscopic instrumentation to correct scoliotic deformities with screws and rods increases the length of the surgical procedure by 2 to 3 hours. It requires no more time than does turning the patient over and performing a posterior instrumentation procedure. Endoscopic instrumentation can be used to correct thoracic curves between T5 and L1. If the diaphragm is low-lying, L2 can also be instrumented.

It is too early to determine whether the long-term outcomes associated with this technique will remain good. The preliminary results, however, compare favorably to those reported in the literature and to our results reported at the North American Spine Society in 1996.[3] We previously demonstrated that posterior fixation and fusion combined with an anterior release also yielded a mean correction of 61%. Curve correction by various methods averages between 50 and 65%. Newton compared open anterior

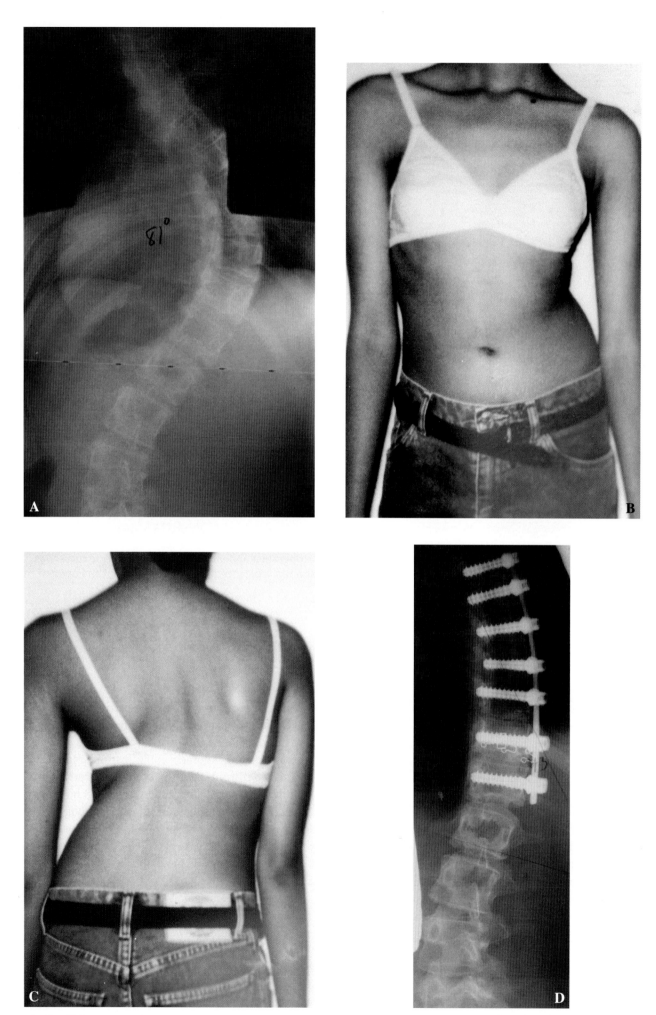

Figure 16–27. **(A)** Preoperative anteroposterior radiograph of a 15-year-old female with a flexible curve of 81 degrees. Patient's **(B)** anterior and **(C)** posterior preoperative appearance. **(D)** Postoperative radiograph shows correction of the curve to 35 degrees.

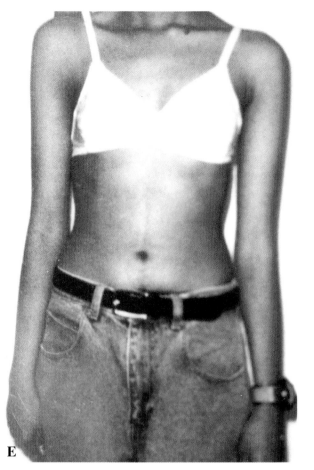
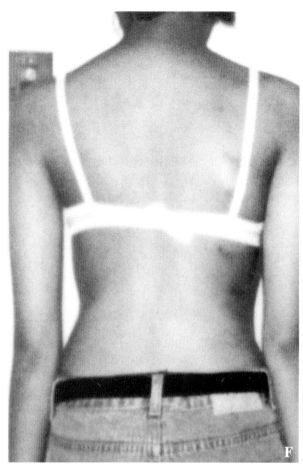

Figure 16–27. *(continued)*   Patient's **(E)** anterior and **(F)** posterior postoperative photographs indicate that the apical vertebrae are shifted toward the midline to better balance the spine. The patient's rib hump deformity improved substantially.

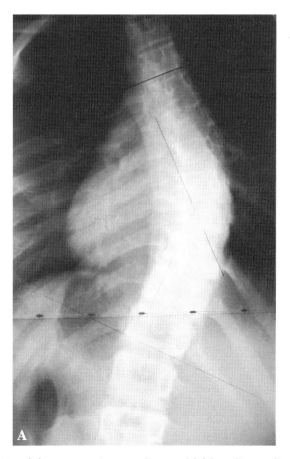
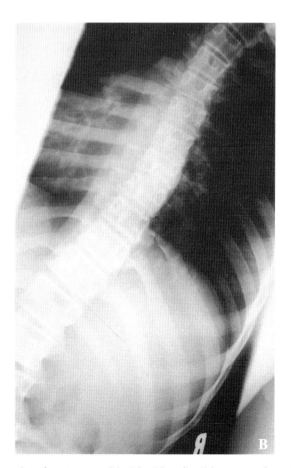

Figure 16–28.   (A) Preoperative standing and **(B)** bending radiographs of a 12-year-old girl with a flexible curve of 49 degrees. *(Figure continued next page.)*

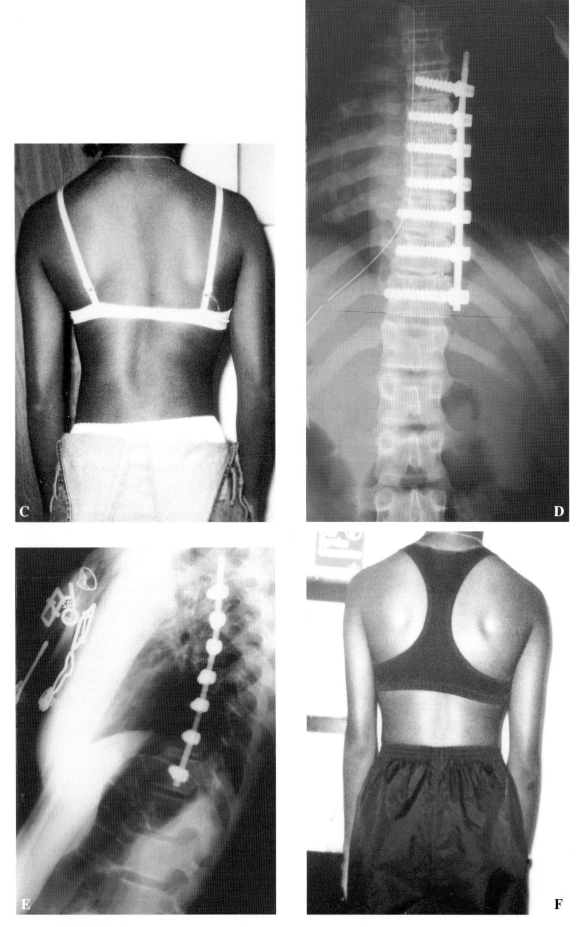

Figure 16–28. *(continued)*   **(C)** Patient's preoperative photograph. After surgery, the curve was corrected to 18 degrees with bending; the final postoperative correction was 7 degrees, as shown by postoperative **(D)** AP and **(E)** lateral radiographs and **(F)** photograph.

release and posterior fusion against endoscopic anterior release with posterior fusion and noted corrections of 56 and 60%, respectively.[7] Betz found a mean correction of the main curve of 64% with anterior instrumentation and 62% with posterior instrumentation.[8] In posteriorly instrumented patients, Richards attained a 54% correction yet 14% was lost over 2 years.[9]

CONCLUSIONS

Endoscopic correction of scoliotic thoracic spinal deformities is feasible using anterior screw-rod systems, an anterior release, and interbody fusion. Although our initial results are promising, long-term follow-up data are needed. Whether performed open or endoscopically, an anterior fixation has several advantages. The crankshaft phenomenon is prevented and fusion occurs rapidly. The translation of the apical vertebra is considerable. Consequently, the balance of the curve improves and normal motion segments are preserved. To this list of benefits, the endoscopic technique of instrumentation adds the advantages of smaller scars, less postoperative pain, and decreased duration of hospitalization. It may also improve the correction of rotation.

REFERENCES

1. Dohin B, Dubousset JF: Prevention of the crankshaft phenomenon with anterior spinal epiphysiodesis in surgical treatment of severe scoliosis of the younger patient. *Eur Spine J* 1994; 3(3): 165–168.
2. Blackman RG, Picetti G, III, O'Neal K: Endoscopic thoracic spine surgery. In White AH, Schofferman JA (eds): *Spine Care: Operative Treatment.* St. Louis: Mosby; 1995:1012–1015.
3. Blackman RG, Picetti G, III, and O'Neal K: Results of anterior endoscopic release and posterior fusion (abstract). North American Spine Society (NASS), 1995.
4. Picetti G, III, Blackman RG, O'Neal K: Alternative technique for thoracoscopic releases in pediatric patients. In Regan JJ, McAfee PC, Mack MJ (eds): *Atlas of Endoscopic Spine Surgery.* St. Louis: Quality Medical; 1995:230–231.
5. Ebraheim NA, Xu R, Ahmad M, et al: Anatomic considerations of anterior instrumentation of the thoracic spine. *Am J Orthop* 1997; 26(6):419–424.
6. Winter RB, Lonstein JE, Denis F, et al: Paraplegia resulting from vessel ligation. *Spine* 1996; 21(10):1232–1233.
7. Newton PO, Wenger DR, Mubarek SJ, et al: Anterior release and fusion in pediatric spinal deformity. A comparison of early outcome and cost of thoracoscopic and open thoracotomy approaches. *Spine* 1997; 22(12):1398–1406.
8. Betz RR, Clements DH, Harms J, et al: Comparison of anterior versus posterior instrumentation for correction of thoracic idiopathic scoliosis. *Scoliosis Research Society Annual Meeting,* Ottawa, Canada, 1996.
9. Richards BS, Herring JA, Johnston CE, et al: Treatment of adolescent idiopathic scoliosis using Texas Scottish Rite Hospital instrumentation. *Spine* 1994; 19(14):1598–1605.

CHAPTER 17

Biopsy of Vertebral Lesions

Noel I. Perin, M.D.

Endoscopic techniques are extremely useful for the biopsy of lesions of the vertebral bodies, discs, and other regions of the thoracic spine. Lesions between T2 and T12 can be accessed using standard thoracoscopic techniques. Most radiologists are reluctant to pass a needle in the thoracic spine percutaneously for fear of causing a pneumothorax. When needle aspirations are performed, the yield from the procedure tends to be low.

INDICATIONS

Endoscopic biopsy can be used to establish a tissue diagnosis and to plan further surgical procedures. It can also be used to resect metastatic tumors that involve the thoracic vertebral bodies when a vertebrectomy or lesionectomy is performed. Another common indication for endoscopic biopsy is diagnosis of the causative organisms in cases of vertebral osteomyelitis and discitis. Biopsy is especially useful for diagnosing tuberculous infections of the vertebral body and disc space and other chronic infections caused by unidentified organisms. Endoscopic biopsy can be used when, despite appropriate antibiotic treatment, an infectious process progresses as evidenced by an increasing sedimentation rate, worsening pain, and destruction of bone on radiologic images. In such patients, endoscopic biopsy can be used to drain abscesses and to remove necrotic devitalized bone (sequestrum) and the nidus of infection. When the spinal cord is compromised by pus or tumor, endoscopy can be used to obtain a biopsy for diagnosis and to decompress the spinal cord. Endoscopic biopsy can also be used to diagnose paraspinal mass lesions. In the upper thoracic spine, especially at T2–T4 on the left side, posterior percutaneous needle techniques are associated with the potential to injure the aortic arch vessels.

CONTRAINDICATIONS

There are relative and absolute contraindications for performing an endoscopic biopsy of vertebral and paravertebral lesions. The general contraindications for any thoracoscopic procedure are the inability to tolerate single-lung ventilation because of acute respiratory insufficiency, severe chronic obstructive pulmonary disease, and high airway pressure with positive pressure ventilation. A history of empyema or pleurodesis is an absolute contraindication. A previous thoracoscopy or thoracotomy on the ipsilateral side can be a relative contraindication.

THORACOSCOPIC ANATOMY

Before starting these procedures, the surgeon should be completely familiar with the local anatomy. A thoracoscope passed through a portal placed in the posterior axillary line provides a panoramic view of the entire thoracic spine and posterior chest cavity (Fig. 17–1). The orientation and anatomic relationship of the structures visualized on the video monitor should not differ from those observed during an open thoracotomy for the same procedure. The anterior structures appear at the top of the screen and the posterior structures at the bottom of the screen. If the apical or basal regions of the chest cavity are to be visualized through one of these portals, the anatomy on the video screen is usually clearly visible. Familiarity with the normal intrathoracic anatomy from different thoracoscope portal positions is essential for surgery to be successful.

Once the lung has been collapsed, the contents of the thorax, spinal column, and ribs should be inspected within the chest cavity. The sympathetic trunk is visible coursing over the heads of the ribs beneath the parietal pleura. The azygos

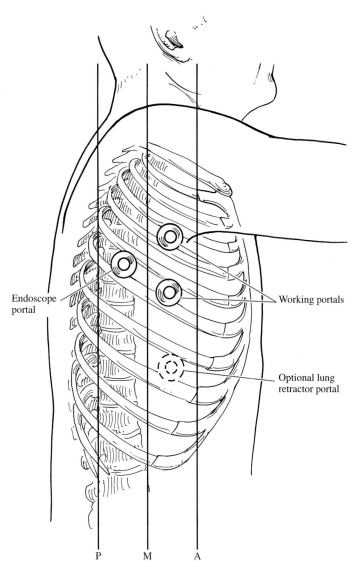

Endoscope
portal

Working portals

Optional lung
retractor portal

P   M   A

Figure 17–1. Portal configurations for midthoracic spinal biopsy. The number and location of portals needed depend on the level of the spine to be accessed. A posterior portal is used for the endoscope. Two working portals are placed in the anterior axillary line. An additional portal may be inserted if a lung retractor is needed.

vein runs along the anterior border of the spinal column on the right side, and the descending aorta is positioned antero-lateral to the vertebral bodies on the left side. To localize the spinal level, the ribs should be counted from the apex down to the basal areas. The pad of fat at the apex of the chest cavity overlies the subclavian vessels and the first rib, which is seldom visible endoscopically. The highest rib that is readily visualized is the second rib. The diaphragm can be visualized inferiorly and must be retracted inferiorly and laterally to access the inferior thoracic spine. The disc spaces appear as elevated convex bulges of the spinal column beneath the parietal pleura. The radicular vessels lie in the concave troughs midway between the disc spaces over the lateral surface of the vertebral bodies. From T2 to T10, the ribs articulate with the adjacent end plates at the level of the disc spaces. At T1, T11, and T12, the ribs articulate caudal to the disc spaces directly with their respective vertebral body. The head and neck of the rib overlie the pedicle.

PREOPERATIVE PLANNING

Diagnostic Imaging

Preoperative chest radiographs and computerized tomography (CT) scans are obtained to exclude the possibility of any chest wall or lung pathology. A CT or magnetic resonance (MR) imaging study of the proposed biopsy site will identify the relationship of the spinal pathology to the great vessels and other thoracic, mediastinal vascular, and visceral structures (Fig. 17–2A and B). If the normal lung field abuts the proposed biopsy site, this area is accessible to endoscopic biopsy. Preoperative MR imaging and CT of the pathological site will determine the side for the approach. For a midline lesion of the upper and middle thoracic spine, the lesion is approached from the right side because there is more space to work on the surface of the spine behind the azygos vein than behind the aorta. For a midline lower thoracic lesion, the spine is approached from the left side because it is easier to retract the left dome of the diaphragm adjacent to the stomach than to retract the liver on the right side. When the pathology is predominantly eccentric to one side, the lesion is approached directly from the side of the pathology.

Anesthetic Considerations

The preoperative workup for thoracoscopic procedures is similar to the workup for an open thoracotomy procedure. Single-lung ventilation is essential in all thoracoscopic procedures.

A knowledge of the problems associated with the use of CO_2 insufflation is an essential anesthetic consideration. Although CO_2 insufflation is not used routinely in thoracoscopic surgery, occasionally it is employed to compress air from the isolated lung at the beginning of the procedure. When necessary, CO_2 flow rates of 1.5 to 2.0 L/min to a maximum pressure of 10 to 12 mm Hg can be used to collapse the ipsilateral lung maximally. Higher pressures in the thoracic cavity can lead to mediastinal tamponade. Double-lumen endotracheal tubes are often used to isolate the ipsilateral lung and ventilate the contralateral lung. An endobronchial tube can also be used to isolate the ipsilateral lung, for example, in young children who cannot tolerate a double-lumen tube. Postoperatively, epidural analgesia and intercostal nerve blocks are unnecessary because pain is reduced compared to that associated with open thoracotomy.

SURGICAL TECHNIQUE

Patient Positioning and Portal Placement

Patients are positioned in a lateral decubitus position identical to the position used for open thoracotomy. The patient is positioned over the "break" or the "kidney rest"

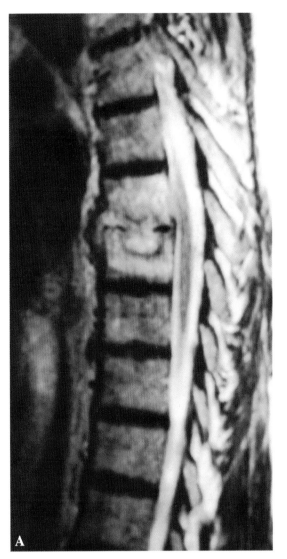
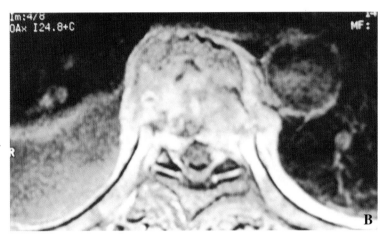

Figure 17–2. Preoperative **(A)** sagittal and **(B)** axial magnetic resonance images showing an infection of the T6–T7 disc space. The signal changes extend into the vertebral bodies adjacent to the disc and are indicative of early osteomyelitis. The pleura is thickened adjacent to the vertebrae. The position of the aorta is readily apparent on the sagittal view.

on the operating table so that the table can be flexed to open the intercostal spaces and facilitate entry into the chest cavity. Two video monitors are positioned on either side of the head when working on the mid- to upper thoracic spine— one monitor for the surgeon and one for the assistant. When the lower thoracic spine must be accessed, the monitors are placed at the foot end of the operating table. The whole chest wall is prepared and draped as for open thoracotomy. If the need arises during the endoscopic procedure, immediate thoracotomy thus can be performed. In preparation for such an event, a thoracotomy set is always opened on the sterile instrument tables before surgery begins. The anesthesiologist is asked to collapse the lung while the patient is prepared and draped for the procedure.

The initial portal is placed rostral to the sixth intercostal space to avoid injuring the diaphragm. This level varies depending on the level of the spine to be accessed. A 10-mm, longitudinal incision is made over the desired intercostal space. The dissection proceeds down through the muscles of the chest wall and intercostal muscles to the

parietal pleura. The pleural space is entered using a Kelly clamp. The clamp is opened longitudinally in the intercostal space to widen the opening. A finger is inserted into this incision and swept along the inner chest wall to lyse any lung adhesions before the trocar is introduced. The endoscope is placed via this portal and provides a panoramic view of the chest cavity and the spinal column (Fig. 17–3).

Subsequent portals are inserted under direct vision. The access portals should be placed in the anterior axillary line on either side of the projected target. The portals are placed so they are not too close to the target, thus allowing a panoramic view of the region of the target. These portals also should not be placed too closely together; otherwise, the instruments tend to duel with each other within the chest cavity. The number of portals and their location depend on the procedure and the level of the pathology.

Typically, the surgeon starts with a 0-degree angled endoscope and then switches to a 30-degree angled endoscope when working on the spine. Additional working portals may be placed as required. One portal may be

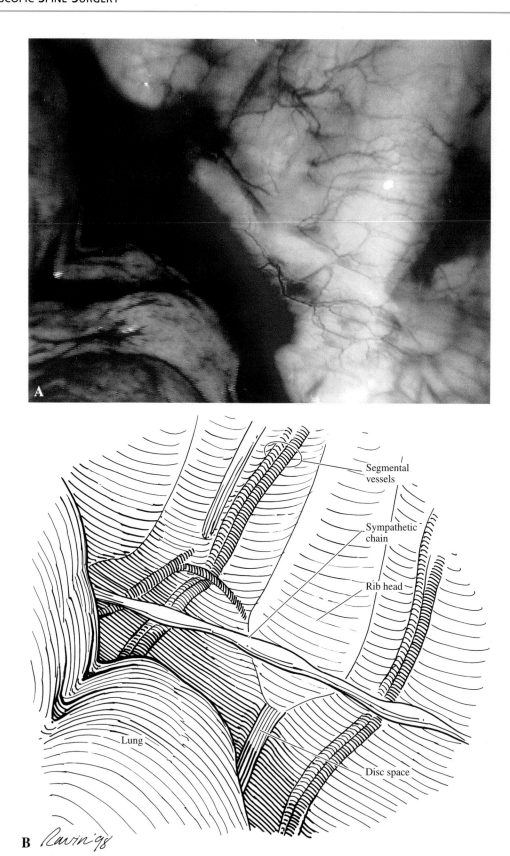

Figure 17–3. **(A)** Intraoperative photograph and **(B)** corresponding illustration showing the initial thoracoscopic view of the spine (*right side*) with the parietal pleura intact. The atelectatic lung has been retracted away from the surface of the spine. The rib heads, sympathetic chain, disc spaces, vertebral bodies, and segmental vessels are all visible.

positioned directly over the site of the pathology for drilling. In all cases, the contents of the entire chest cavity should be inspected.

Approach to Upper Thoracic Spine (T2–T5)

For apical lesions from T2 to T5, the initial endoscopic visualization portal is placed in the fourth or fifth intercostal space in the posterior axillary line just anterior to the latissimus dorsi muscle. After the chest cavity has been inspected, depending on the level to be accessed, a working portal may be placed at the anterior axillary line in the third and fifth intercostal space posterior to the lateral border of the pectoralis major muscle.

Approach to the Midthoracic Spine (T6–T9)

The initial portal is placed in the sixth or seventh intercostal space in the posterior axillary line. The endoscope is placed via this portal. A second portal is placed in the anterior axillary line above or below the first portal, depending on the location of the lesion. A third port is usually placed in the anterior or middle axillary line, inferior to the other ports, in a reverse "L" configuration. The endoscope is placed in the posterior portal, and the portals in the anterior axillary line serve as working portals.

Approach to the Lower Thoracic Spine (T10–T12)

The initial portal for the endoscope is placed in the sixth intercostal space in the midaxillary line to avoid penetrating the diaphragm or placing the portal below it. After the endoscope is introduced, the second portal is placed under direct vision at the anterior axillary line just above the diaphragmatic insertion. This portal is used for the diaphragmatic retractor. Further portals are placed in the anterior axillary line as required for working portals.

Vertebral Body and Disc Space Biopsy

The appropriate level of spinal pathology is identified visually and radiographically. A long spinal needle is passed percutaneously through the chest wall or through a portal into the disc space under direct vision (Fig. 17–4). A cross table anteroposterior radiograph is obtained to confirm the level. Once the level is identified, the parietal pleura is incised with endoscopic cautery scissors over the disc space, the adjacent vertebral bodies, and the corresponding rib (Fig. 17–5). The segmental vessels over the vertebral bodies are dissected free, ligated with hemostatic clips, and divided. The periosteum of the adjacent rib is exposed while the neurovascular bundle located inferiorly is protected. Pathology affecting the disc space and vertebral bodies without affecting the spinal canal can be biopsied without removing the rib head or pedicle (Figs. 17–6 and 17–7). The biopsy is obtained anterior to the rib head to avoid the spinal canal and spinal cord. Cultures and specimens for pathologic analysis are obtained.

If needed for exposure or for identification of the spinal canal, the rib head can be removed. The rib is divided 2 to 3 cm distal to its head using a high-speed drill or an osteotome. The head of the rib is freed from its ligamentous attachments by blunt dissection using a periosteal elevator. Once the rib is freed, it is removed in one piece. The rib is removed only if the spinal canal is to be exposed for biopsy and decompression of an epidural mass.

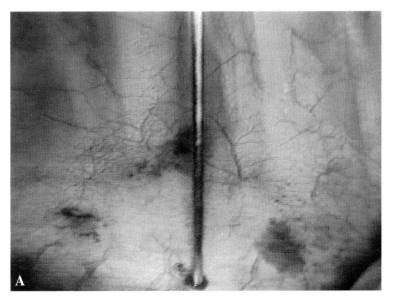
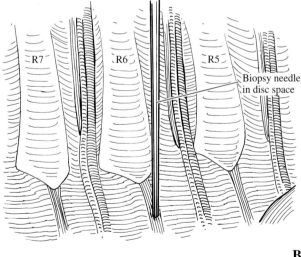

Figure 17–4. **(A)** Intraoperative photograph and **(B)** corresponding illustration showing the correct spinal level being identified radiographically after a long needle or Kirschner wire has been inserted into the disc space. The ribs can also be counted internally to aid in localization. The level, however, should be confirmed radiographically. The needle can be used to aspirate pus from the disc space if an infection is present. R = rib

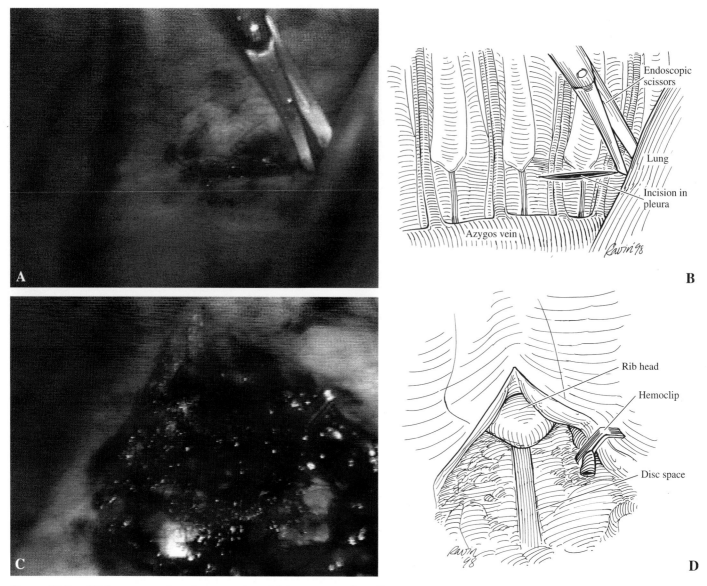

Figure 17–5. **(A)** Intraoperative photograph and **(B)** corresponding illustration showing the parietal pleura being incised over the rib head using endoscopic scissors. **(C)** Intraoperative photograph and **(D)** corresponding illustration showing that the pleura has been mobilized to expose the rib head, disc space, and vertebral bodies.

To expose the dura and the spinal canal, the soft tissue overlying the pedicle is coagulated with bipolar cauterization and the lateral surface of the pedicle is identified. A Kerrison rongeur is used to remove the pedicle of the caudal vertebral body in a rostral to caudal direction, which exposes the lateral surface of the dura. At this point, the margins of the end plate adjacent to the disc space are removed with the Kerrison rongeur, exposing the disc and the posterior longitudinal ligament along with the ventral epidural space. The epidural mass of tumor or pus can be evacuated and gently freed from the dura, thus decompressing the spinal cord.

Hemostasis is achieved with thrombin-soaked Gelfoam® and bipolar coagulation. A No. 28 French chest tube is placed into the thorax through one of the portals and guided to the apex of the chest. If excessive bleeding is anticipated, a second tube is left dependently at the base of the chest cavity. The portal incisions are closed using subcu-ticular sutures. The chest tube is usually removed within 24 to 48 hours.

Thoracoscopic Paraspinal Tumor Biopsy

Paraspinal tumors in the thoracic spine are usually benign. Neurogenic tumors can arise from the spinal ganglion or nerve sheath, the sympathetic chain, the vagus or phrenic nerves, or neural crest tissue. Neurofibromas and schwannomas can be entirely intrathoracic and extraspinal, or they may be both intra- and extraspinal. The latter are referred to as dumbbell tumors. To prevent avulsion of the root, the tumor must be released intradurally from the root of origin before the extraspinal component is removed. In a known dumbbell neurofibroma or schwannoma, the patient should undergo a posterior laminectomy and excision of the intraspinal component of the tumor first. This step is necessary to resect the intradural portion of the tumor safely.

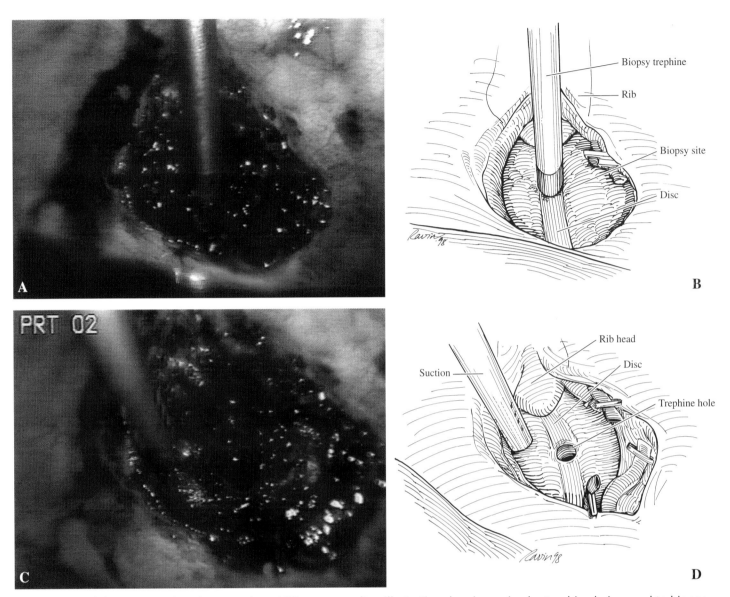

Figure 17–6. **(A)** Intraoperative photograph and **(B)** corresponding illustration showing a circular trephine being used to biopsy the disc space and vertebral body. **(C)** Intraoperative photograph and **(D)** corresponding illustration after the core of bone and disc material has been removed showing the small opening left in the surface of the disc space.

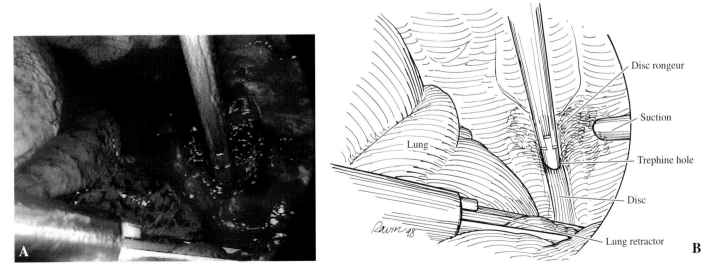

Figure 17–7. **(A)** Intraoperative photograph and **(B)** corresponding illustration showing a disc rongeur being inserted into the trephine hole to debride necrotic bone and disc material. Cultures and specimens for pathological analysis are thereby obtained.

Endoscopic access can then be used to resect the intrathoracic lesion. Once the tumor is identified within the chest cavity, adhesions of the lung to the lesion are released by sharp dissection. The parietal pleura over the tumor is opened with scissors and the tumor is biopsied for frozen and permanent sections. After the tumor is biopsied, it is dissected from the surrounding structures and removed. The tumor is placed in an endoscopic specimen pouch to avoid spilling it.

Metastatic or malignant tumors are approached differently from benign nerve sheath tumors. If bone destruction is minimal and only a tissue diagnosis is needed, a limited biopsy can be performed without also performing a resection and reconstruction, especially if the tumor is highly radiosensitive. A vertebrectomy should be performed for metastatic tumors that have destroyed the vertebral body. The vertebral body can be reconstructed with bone grafts or methylmethacrylate. If internal fixation is needed, an anterior plate can be inserted endoscopically; the patient can also undergo a subsequent open posterior segmental fixation.

CONCLUSIONS

Thoracoscopy can be used to biopsy vertebral lesions in the thoracic spine efficiently, with minimal complications and a high diagnostic yield. Thoracoscopic biopsy is relatively easy to perform and is an ideal procedure for surgeons to gain initial experience with thoracoscopic surgery.

RECOMMENDED READINGS

1. Horowitz MB, Moossy JJ, Julian T, et al: Thoracic discectomy using video assisted thoracoscopy. *Spine* 1994; 19(9):1082–1086.
2. Landreneau RJ, Hazelrigg SR, Mack MJ, et al: Postoperative pain-related morbidity: Video-assisted thoracic surgery versus thoracotomy. *Ann Thorac Surg* 1993; 56(6):1285–1289.
3. Mack MJ, Regan JJ, Bobechko WP, et al: Application of thoracoscopy for diseases of the spine. *Ann Thorac Surg* 1993; 56(3):736–738.
4. Mack MJ, Aronoff RJ, Acuff TE, et al: Present role of thoracoscopy in the diagnosis and treatment of diseases of the chest. *Ann Thorac Surg* 1992; 54(3):403–409.
5. Regan JJ, Mack MJ, Picetti GD: A comparison of video assisted thoracoscopic surgery (VATS) with open thoracotomy in thoracic spinal surgery. *Todays Theur Trends* 1994; 11:203–218.
6. Regan JJ, Mack MJ, Picetti GD, III: A technical report on video-assisted thoracoscopy in thoracic spinal surgery. Preliminary description. *Spine* 1995; 20(7):831–837.
7. Rosenthal D, Rosenthal R, de Simone A: Removal of a protruded thoracic disc using microsurgical endoscopy. A new technique. *Spine* 1994; 19(9):1087–1091.
8. Stoker DJ, Kissin CM: Percutaneous vertebral biopsy: A review of 135 cases. *Clin Radiol* 1985; 36(6):569–577.

CHAPTER **18**

Thoracoscopic Microsurgical Discectomy

Curtis A. Dickman, M.D., Daniel J. Rosenthal, M.D., and Noel I. Perin, M.D.

Thoracoscopic microdiscectomy is a reliable surgical technique that can be performed safely and with an acceptable rate of morbidity. This chapter reviews the indications, surgical techniques, and clinical outcomes associated with the procedure.

INDICATIONS FOR THORACIC DISCECTOMY

Thoracic microdiscectomy is indicated for the treatment of herniated thoracic discs that compress the spinal cord and spinal nerves. The strongest indication for surgery is injury to the spinal cord caused by compressive lesions. When myelopathy is present, the goals of surgery are to prevent further irreversible damage to the spinal cord and to improve its function. The more severe and the longer the patient has experienced the myelopathy at presentation, however, the less likely the patient is to recover neurological function.

The classical character of thoracic radicular pain from a herniated thoracic disc is a lancing, stabbing pain that begins posteriorly and radiates unilaterally (or, occasionally, bilaterally) around the chest wall in a dermatomal distribution. Although it is often associated with a concurrent myelopathy, radicular pain may occur in isolation with no spinal cord damage. The pain usually occurs with no loss of motor or sensory function at the level of the spinal root because the innervation of adjacent intercostal nerves overlaps.

Thoracic radicular pain can become disabling. When symptoms are long-standing, surgical treatment is recommended. Because radicular pain is usually less threatening to the patient's function than myelopathy, the initial treatment is nonoperative. In many cases, isolated thoracic radiculopathy pain will respond to a regimen of restricted activity, a hyperextension brace, nonsteroidal antiinflam-

matory agents, oral steroids, and/or epidural steroids. Patients who fail a full course of nonoperative management (i.e., 3 to 6 months of therapy) may be considered for surgery to remove their herniated thoracic disc.

Even when the radicular pain is long-standing, the relief offered by surgical decompression of the nerve may be excellent. One of the authors (CAD) has treated a patient who presented with 20 years of disabling thoracic radicular pain that was completely, permanently relieved after a thoracoscopic microdiscectomy.

A less well-defined indication for thoracic microdiscectomy is local axial back pain caused by a thoracic disc herniation if discrete radicular pain or myelopathy is absent. This indication is controversial. In most circumstances, we do not advocate thoracic discectomy to treat isolated back pain if there is no neurological involvement.

A large, central, broad-based thoracic disc herniation can occasionally cause a centrally located, visceral, angina-like, crushing, nonradiating chest pain. We have treated several patients with such pain from herniated thoracic discs. In these few cases that mimicked angina, the patients' comprehensive cardiac evaluations were normal, and their central visceral pain was temporarily relieved by epidural injection of steroids and a local anesthetic (Fig. 18–1). Their clinical symptoms were relieved after the herniated disc was removed.

Patient selection must be judicious because a large number of asymptomatic individuals are found to harbor incidental herniated thoracic discs when examined with magnetic resonance (MR) imaging.[1–3] Surgery should be considered primarily for patients whose spinal cord function is threatened or who have disabling, long-standing nonrefractory thoracic radicular pain. Patients with nonrefractory visceral-type pain or severe local thoracic axial pain from a herniated thoracic disc can also be considered surgical candidates in selected circumstances.

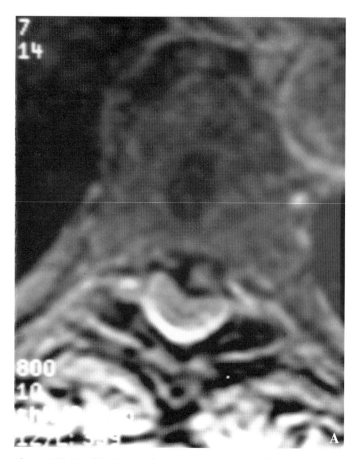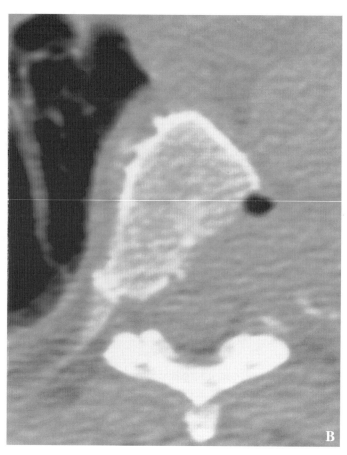

Figure 18–1. **(A)** Magnetic resonance image of a patient with a calcified, centrally located thoracic disc herniation at T5–T6 that caused angina-like pain, but who had no true radicular or myelopathic findings. **(B)** Postoperative computed tomographic scan demonstrating complete resection of the disc. The symptoms were relieved completely after thoracoscopic microdiscectomy.

SURGICAL APPROACHES TO THORACIC DISCS

In the neurosurgical literature, approaches such as the posterior transpedicular or posterolateral have often been advocated[4–12] for the treatment of thoracic discs rather than thoracotomy. The objections to thoracotomy have included the presumed morbidity associated with thoracotomy (e.g., postthoracotomy pain), the need for another surgeon during the exposure and closure, and unfamiliarity with the technique. Thoracotomy, however, also has its strong advocates[13–22] because of its superior ability to visualize and access the ventral surface of the spinal cord.

Posterior and posterolateral approaches work well if the herniated thoracic disc is located within the *lateral* half of the spinal canal or in the neural foramen, especially if the disc is a soft herniation. The limitation of posterior and posterolateral approaches is that the surgeon is blinded to the *ventral* surface of the dura. For calcified thoracic discs, large disc herniations, central discs, and broad-based discs that span the spinal canal, an *anterior* approach is needed so that the surgeon can see and protect the ventral surface of the spinal cord. It is dangerous to try to dissect a thoracic disc *blindly* without being able to visualize the interface of

the disc with the ventral dura. Thoracoscopy provides a full anterior view of the spinal cord and is associated with fewer complications than thoracotomy.[23–35]

DIAGNOSTIC IMAGING

Both MR imaging and computed tomography (CT) are helpful in planning the operation. MR imaging demonstrates the extent of neural compression and the anatomy of the paraspinal soft tissues, especially the positions of the aorta and azygos veins at the level of the pathology. This information is used to plan the side of approach. If the lesion is located centrally and the aorta is ectatic and displaced laterally, a right-sided thoracoscopic approach should be chosen. If, however, the lesion is eccentric toward the left side, a left-sided approach should be chosen. In this case, it is better to retract and mobilize the aorta judiciously when needed rather than to retract the spinal cord, which risks neurological injury.

CT is useful for depicting the extent of calcification or ossification of the lesion. If dense calcifications are present, the surgeon can anticipate removing the lesion by coring it out with a burr and then fracturing the remaining eggshell rim of the lesion and curetting it anteriorly away from the spinal cord. The bases of peduncular ossified lesions can be transected with a drill. The remaining lesion is extracted using microdissection techniques.

A preoperative radiograph of the chest is mandatory to localize the level of the pathology accurately. If the patient has an anomalous number of ribs, the spinal level could be misidentified. Large osteophytes seen on CT or plain radiography can be used as surgical or radiographic landmarks to assist with localization.

SURGICAL TECHNIQUE

The details of patient positioning, portal placement, and spinal access and exposure have been described fully in Chapters 11, 12, and 13. This chapter focuses on the most salient aspects of the technique as applied to thoracic discectomy.

The patient is positioned in a lateral decubitus position with the side of access up; the ventilated lung is positioned dependently. Before the patient is scrubbed, a C-arm is used to localize the level of the pathology. The skin is marked with ink over the pathology and at the sites where the portals are to be inserted.

After the patient's skin has been scrubbed sterilely, the portals and the endoscope are inserted. The lung is mobilized from the anterior surface of the spine. The ribs are counted internally to identify the disc space, and the pleura over the identified rib head is cauterized. To confirm the operative site, the C-arm is used to count the ribs beginning caudally at the twelfth rib. Rib identification is repeated several times to ensure accuracy. A tool or a needle is held at the disc level to confirm the localization.

The pleura is incised and mobilized over the proximal rib and disc space. Its edges are folded laterally to expose the disc space, proximal rib, and adjacent segmental vessels (Fig. 18–2). The segmental vessels that supply the foramen and rib at the pathology are mobilized. Usually, they must be ligated prophylactically with hemoclips to prevent bleeding. The segmental artery and vein are then transected sharply with endoscopic scissors. The neurovascular bundle is detached from the undersurface of the rib using subperiosteal dissection with curettes and periosteal elevators. Any bleeding from the neurovascular bundle is controlled by bipolar cauterization. If the aorta is displaced laterally, interfering with access to the disc space, several sets of segmental vessels are ligated and the aorta is mobilized and gently retracted anteriorly.

The proximal 2 cm of rib and pedicle are removed to expose the spinal canal so that the lateral surface of the dura can be visualized. The neurovascular bundle, intercostal muscles, and costotransverse and costovertebral ligaments are detached from the rib. The rib is transected, and the bone is saved in case it is needed for graft material. Typically, we do not fuse a routine thoracic microdiscectomy

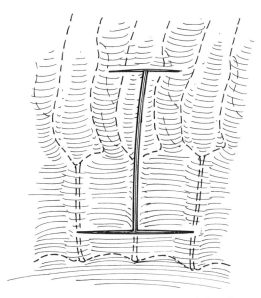

Figure 18–2. The pleura is incised and mobilized to expose the rib and the disc space.

because it does not usually destabilize the spine.[26] If, however, a corpectomy is needed for exposure, a fusion should be performed to reconstruct the vertebral body.

The pedicle caudal to the disc space is identified, and the foraminal ligaments are cut from the superior edge of the pedicle, which is removed with a Kerrison rongeur. Removing the pedicle exposes the epidural space (Fig. 18–3A). Early identification of the dura allows the surgeon to visualize the anterolateral border of the spinal canal and enables constant visual orientation to the position of the spinal cord during any subsequent dissection. This step is critical for performing the dissection safely.

The next surgical step is also critical. An empty cavity must be created in the dorsal disc space and adjacent vertebral bodies to provide room to deliver the compressive disc material away from the epidural space (Fig. 18–3B). An adequately sized cavity is mandatory for preserving neurological function. The working space permits the surgeon to *minimize* the entry of tools into the compressed epidural space. The surgeon can work using the edges of fine microsurgical tools to pull the disc material away from the spinal cord into the cavity. The cavity should be deep enough to expose the entire ventral surface of the dura across the spinal canal to the medial border of the contralateral pedicle (Fig. 18–4). To treat small or moderate thoracic disc herniations or soft disc herniations, the working cavity is shaped like a pyramid (Fig. 18–4). To expose large discs, ossified discs, or intradural discs, much more room is needed. In fact, a partial corpectomy is required (Fig. 18–5).

If the disc herniation has eroded through the dura and the disc extends intradurally, a corpectomy is used to provide adequate exposure. The intradural disc material is carefully separated from the arachnoid and pia mater with microdissectors. The dura can be closed with endoscopic suturing and sealed with fibrin glue and fascia. To prevent a cerebrospinal fluid (CSF) fistula from developing (i.e., subarachnoid-pleural fistula), the chest tube is placed to water

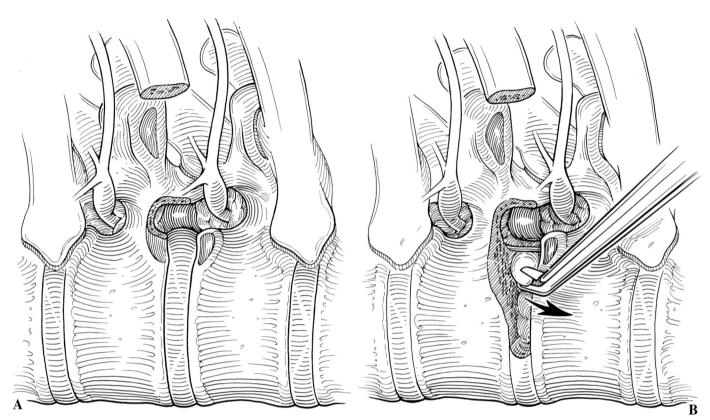

Figure 18–3. **(A)** The pedicle is removed to expose the dura. **(B)** A cavity is drilled in the vertebral body and disc space to provide room to insert the tools to remove the herniated disc. [With permission from Barrow Neurological Institute.]

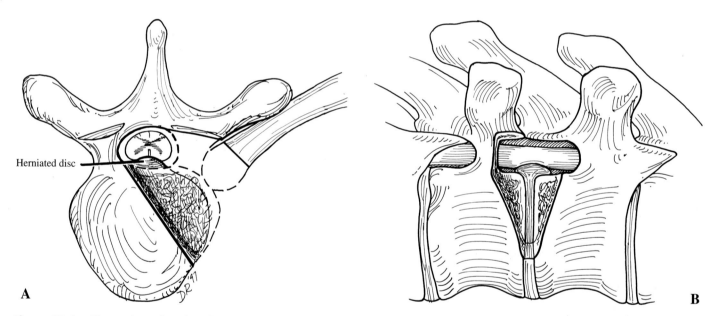

Figure 18–4. Illustrations showing the exposure of the lateral dura after the pedicle has been removed. A pyramidal-shaped cavity must be created in the vertebral bodies to expose the ventral spinal canal for the safe decompression of the spinal cord. **(A)** Axial cross section. The cavity provides room to insert surgical instruments without compressing the epidural space further. The cavity extends across the spinal canal to the contralateral pedicle. **(B)** Lateral view. A pyramidal cavity is created for small and moderate disc herniations. Normal dura is exposed cephalad and caudal to the herniated disc. [Reprinted with permission from Journal of Neurosurgery.[35]]

seal rather than suction. A lumbar drain or a lumboperitoneal shunt is used to divert CSF and reduce the intraspinal hydrostatic pressure until the dural incision has sealed postoperatively.

After the spinal cord has been decompressed, the depth of the dissection can be verified using fluoroscopy

(Fig. 18–6). Epidural hemostasis is obtained; the chest is irrigated with antibiotic solution; disc and bone debris are removed; chest tubes are inserted; the lung is reinflated; and the incisions are closed in a routine fashion. The chest tubes are left in place until their output is less than 100 ml/day—usually within 1 to 2 days.

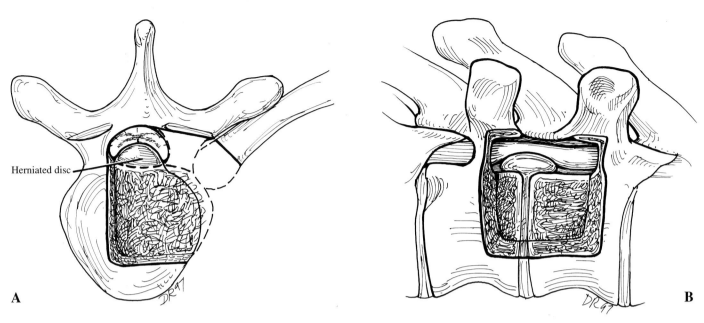

Figure 18–5. **(A)** Axial cross section and **(B)** lateral view of the corpectomy cavity that is required to expose and resect large thoracic disc herniations. This exposure is much larger than the exposure needed for small disc herniations. The large cavity provides full visualization of the dura and the pathology and permits adequate space to work. [Reprinted with permission from Journal of Neurosurgery].[35]

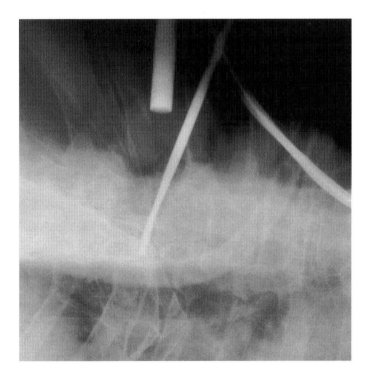

Figure 18–6. An intraoperative radiograph was used to judge the depth of dissection across the spinal canal after a T8–T9 disc herniation was resected during a right-sided approach. The endoscope is visible within the thorax. An endoscopic microdissection tool is inserted into the cavity in the disc space. Its tip is adjacent to the contralateral pedicle.

ILLUSTRATIVE CASES

Case 1: Calcified Central Thoracic Disc (T5–T6)

A 49-year-old woman had a 3-year history of progressively worsening, incapacitating dysesthetic and crushing pain that began between her shoulders and radiated anteriorly into the middle and lower chest region bilaterally. Her workup revealed no cardiac pathology. She had no signs or symp-

toms of myelopathy. Radiographic studies demonstrated a large, central calcified disc herniation eccentric to the left side of the spinal cord at the level of T5–T6 (Fig. 18–1A). She underwent, without complication, a left-sided approach for a thoracoscopic discectomy that achieved complete resection of the disc (Figs. 18–1B, 18–7 to 18–13). Postoperatively, she was intact neurologically and her preoperative pain symptoms resolved completely.

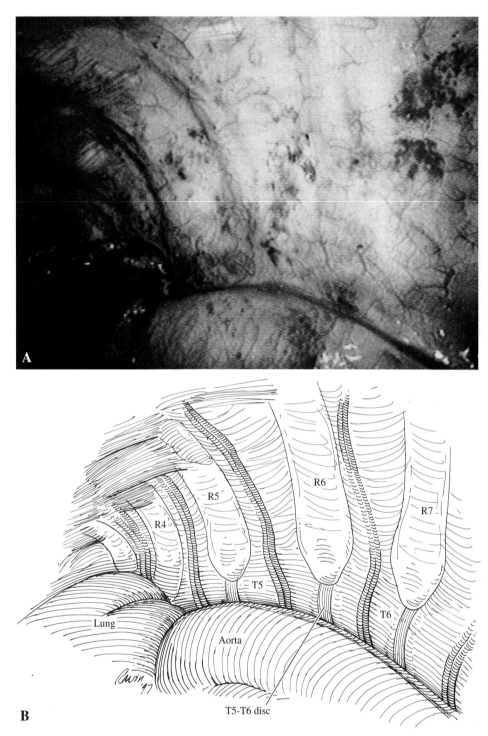

Figure 18–7. **(A)** Intraoperative photograph and **(B)** corresponding illustration showing the left-sided thoracoscopic approach used to perform this T6–T7 discectomy. This exposure provides a panoramic view of the hemithorax. The aorta is ventrolateral to the spine. The fourth through seventh thoracic vertebrae and the adjacent ribs are all visible in the operative view. R = rib.

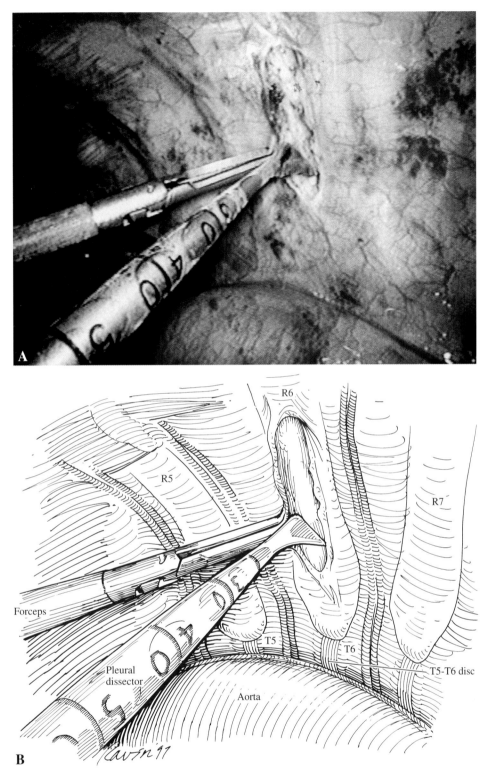

Figure 18–8. **(A)** Intraoperative photograph and **(B)** corresponding illustration showing the pleura being incised from the sixth rib, which leads the surgeon to the T5–T6 disc space. The pleural edge is held with a forceps. A pleural dissector is used to mobilize the pleura and elevate it from the surface of the spine. R = rib.

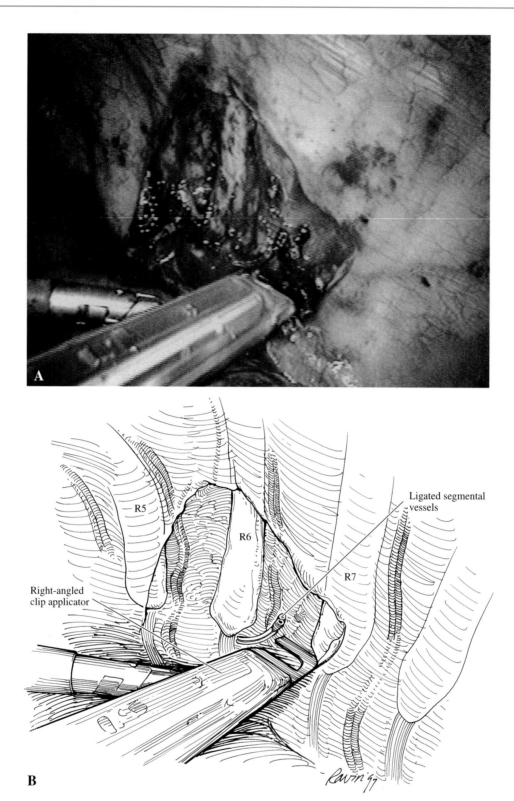

Figure 18–9. **(A)** Intraoperative photograph and **(B)** corresponding illustration showing the right-angled endoscopic hemoclip applier used to ligate the segmental artery and vein adjacent to the disc space. R = rib.

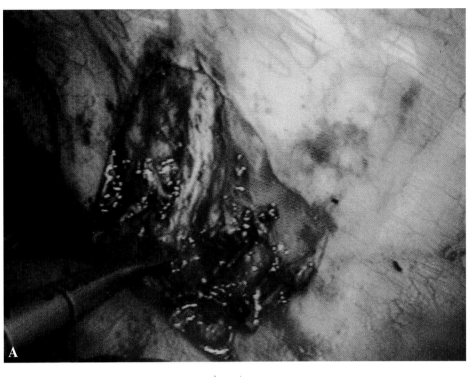

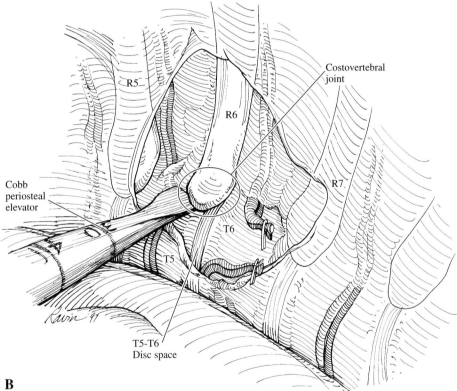

Figure 18–10. **(A)** Intraoperative photograph and **(B)** corresponding illustration showing the neurovascular bundle detached from the caudal rib margin and the intercostal muscles detached from the rib. A Cobb periosteal elevator is inserted into the costovertebral joint to cut the ligaments and to disarticulate the joint. R = rib.

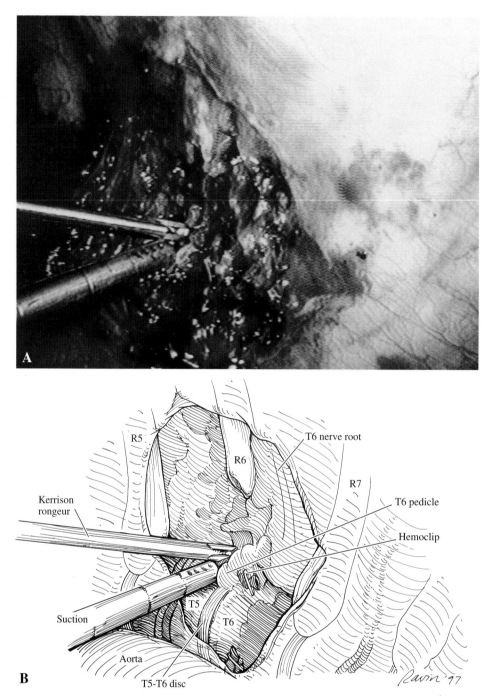

Figure 18–11. **(A)** Intraoperative photograph and **(B)** corresponding illustration showing a Kerrison rongeur being used to remove the T6 pedicle to expose the epidural space. R = rib.

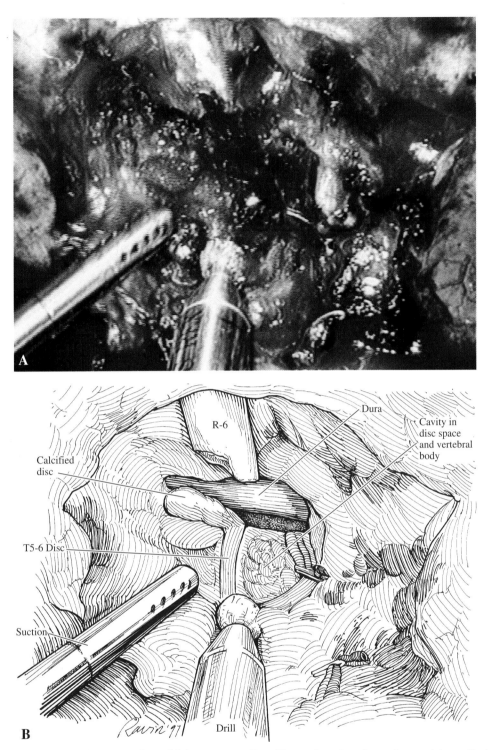

Figure 18–12. **(A)** Intraoperative photograph and **(B)** corresponding illustration showing a 2-cm wide cavity being drilled into the dorsal T5–T6 disc space and vertebral body to create adequate space to insert tools to remove the calcified herniated disc material. R = rib.

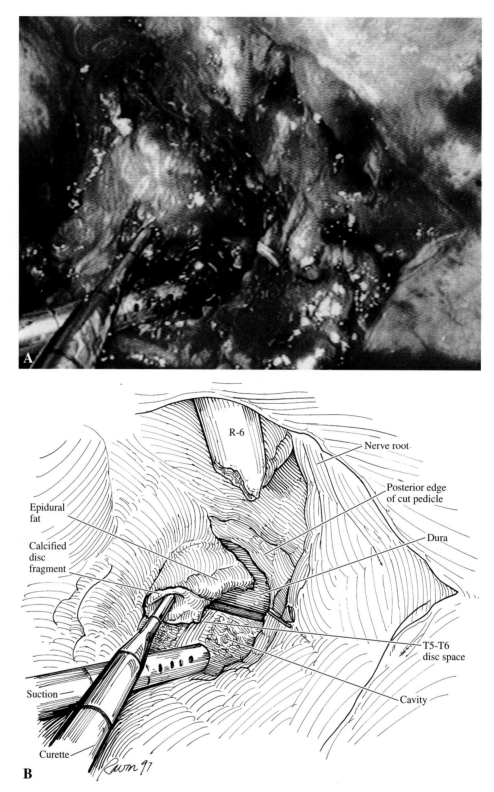

Figure 18–13. **(A)** Intraoperative photograph and **(B)** corresponding illustration showing the calcified disc material being removed from the epidural space by curetting it into the cavity with the vertebral bodies. R = rib.

Case 2: Soft Central Thoracic Disc (T8–T9)

A 53-year-old man presented with a 1-year history of progressive myelopathy. He had spastic gait, paraparesis (4/5), and diminished sensation below the T10 dermatome. A myelographic CT and MR imaging (Fig. 18–14) showed a large centrally located disc at T8–T9 compressing and deforming the spinal cord. The disc was completely removed using a right-sided thoracoscopic approach (Figs. 18–15 and 18–16). There were no postoperative complications. The patient recovered normal motor function, but had mild residual sensory loss at his 1-year postoperative evaluation. The postoperative CT scan demonstrated the amount of bone resection used to resect this herniated disc (Fig. 18–17).

Case 3: Soft Central Thoracic Disc Herniation (T7–T8)

A large, soft, central disc herniation caused a patient acute paraparesis. The herniated disc was removed using a right-sided approach (Figs. 18–18 to 18–21). No postoperative complications occurred.

Case 4: Calcified Broad-Based Disc Herniation (T8–T9)

A 47-year-old woman presented with a 3-year history of progressive myelopathy after undergoing a left-sided thoracotomy to resect a disc at the level of T7–T8. A new herniated disc at the T8–T9 level (Fig. 18–22) caused urinary incontinence, progressive spasticity, leg weakness, and sensory loss. This second herniation was removed using a right-sided thoracoscopic exposure (Fig. 18–23). Only mild focal pleural adhesions were present and they were easily detached endoscopically. A large calcified disc fragment was removed to decompress the spinal cord completely (Fig. 18–24).

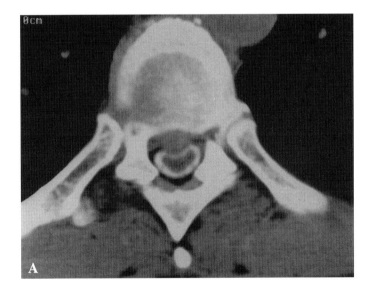 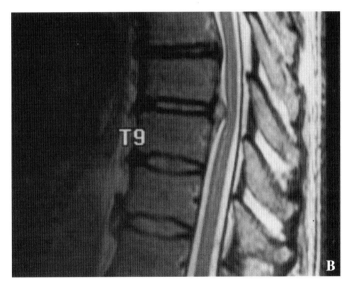

Figure 18–14. **(A)** Axial computed tomographic scan demonstrates a large central disc herniation at T8–T9 that deforms the spinal cord and occupies 30% of the diameter of the spinal canal. **(B)** A sagittal magnetic resonance image depicts the focal mass effect from the disc, which is directly adjacent to the T8–T9 disc space. The disc has not migrated rostral or caudal to the disc space.

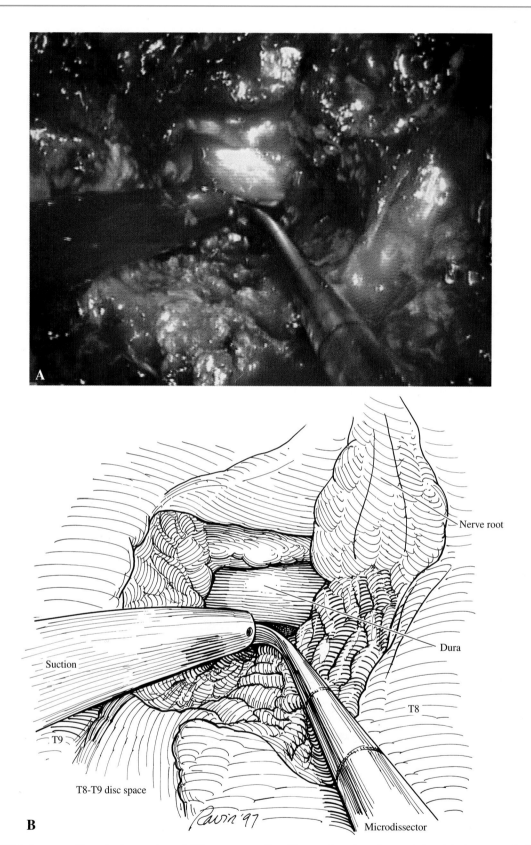

Figure 18–15. **(A)** Intraoperative photograph and **(B)** corresponding illustration showing a right-sided approach for removal of a centrally herniated T8–T9 disc. The T9 rib head and T9 pedicle were removed to expose the epidural space. A 2-cm wide pyramidal cavity was drilled into the vertebral bodies to expose the entire ventral surface of the spinal cord. A dural microdissector was placed into the epidural space after the decompression was completed to search for residual disc material.

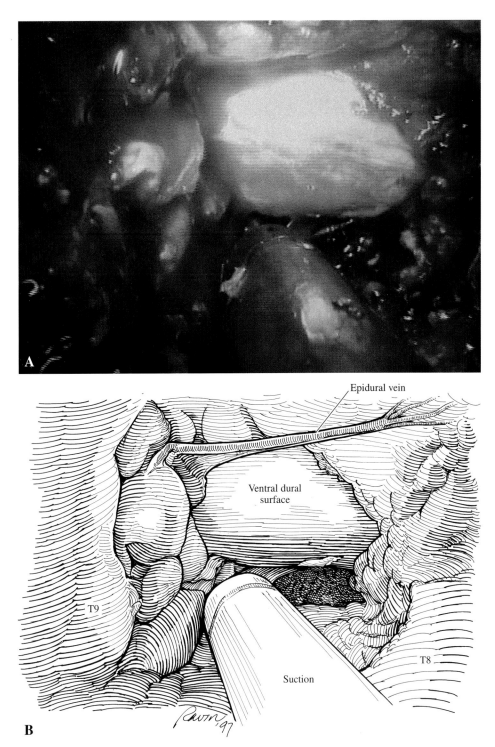

Figure 18–16. **(A)** Intraoperative magnified view and **(B)** corresponding illustration of the decompressed dura. The entire ventral surface of the dura is visible. The tip of the suction is positioned just ventral to the contralateral pedicle.

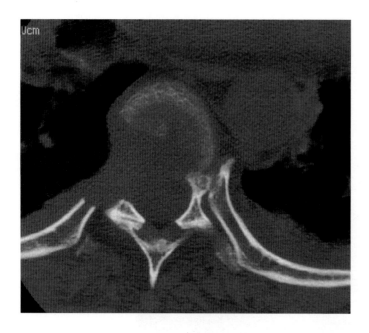

Figure 18–17. Postoperative computed tomographic scan demonstrates the pyramidal cavity created to decompress the spinal cord. The apex of the pyramid was carried completely across the spinal canal.

CLINICAL OUTCOMES ASSOCIATED WITH THORACOSCOPIC MICRODISCECTOMY

Between 1992 and 1996, the authors treated 55 patients with herniated thoracic discs thoracoscopically.[35] There were 33 males and 22 females (mean age: 48 years; range: 31 to 72 years). Thirty-six patients had become symptomatic with myelopathic signs and symptoms related to spinal cord compression; 19 patients had incapacitating thoracic radicular pain without myelopathy. The mean duration of symptoms before surgery was 13 months.

Forty-three patients underwent a single-level discectomy. However, to ensure that multilevel compressive pathology was adequately removed, 11 patients underwent a two-level discectomy and one patient underwent a three-level discectomy. These 68 discectomies were performed for 33 calcified or ossified discs and for 35 soft disc herniations. There were 65 extradural discs and three intradural extensions of the disc herniations. The mean operative time for thoracoscopic microdiscetomy was 3 hours and 25 minutes (range: 80 to 542 minutes). The mean blood loss was 327 ml (range: 124 to 1500 ml).

The operative data for a consecutive cohort of patients treated with thoracotomy ($n = 18$) or costotransversectomy ($n = 15$) for herniated thoracic discs were compared. Compared with thoracotomy, thoracoscopy required a mean of 1 hour less operative time and was associated with *less* than half the blood loss, duration of chest tube drainage, use of narcotic pain medication, and duration of hospitalization

(Table 18–1). Unlike costotransversectomy, thoracoscopy provided a direct view of the entire anterior surface of the dura, which allowed the entire discectomy to be performed under direct visualization. Endoscopic surgery offered more complete resection of the herniated discs than costotransversectomy.

The surgical complications associated with thoracoscopy included four (7%) cases of atelectasis, two (4%) cases of pleural effusion, two (4%) cases of hemothorax, nine (16%) cases of transient intercostal neuralgia, two (4%) cases of misidentified disc levels, one (2%) case of subcutaneous emphysema, two cases (4%) of retained disc fragment that required reoperation, and one (2%) case of transiently worsening myelopathy. Thoracotomy was associated with a significantly greater incidence of intercostal neuralgia that was more prolonged and disabling than the mild transient episodes of intercostal neuralgia associated with thoracoscopy (50% versus 16%, respectively). Thoracotomy was also associated with a higher incidence of postoperative atelectasis and pulmonary dysfunction than thoracoscopy (33% versus 7%, respectively; Table 18–2).

The clinical and neurological outcomes (Table 18–3) achieved with thoracoscopy were excellent (mean follow-up: 15 months). Among the 36 patients with myelopathy, 22 completely recovered normal neurological function. Five patients had functional improvement with some residual signs and symptoms of myelopathy. In 9 patients, the myelopathy was stabilized and progressed no further. Among the 19 patients with isolated thoracic radiculopathies, 15 recovered completely and the pain improved moderately in four. In no case did the radicular pain worsen.

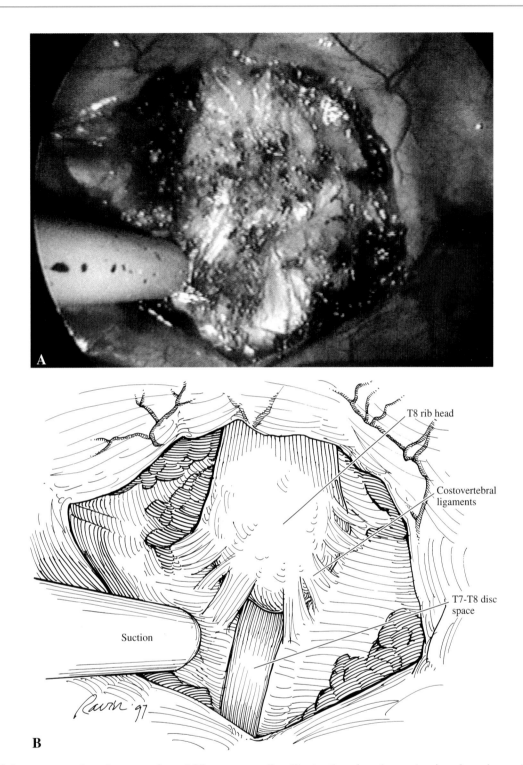

Figure 18–18. **(A)** Intraoperative photograph and **(B)** corresponding illustration showing a circular pleural opening made to expose the T8 rib head and T7–T8 disc space. The radiate ligaments (costovertebral ligaments) are visible.

TABLE 18–1 Operative Data for Thoracoscopy ($n = 55$), Thoracotomy ($n = 18$), and Costotransversectomy ($n = 15$) for Resection of Herniated Thoracic Discs

Operative Data	Thoracoscopy Mean (Range)	Thoracotomy Mean (Range)	Costotransversectomy Mean (Range)
Operative time (min)	205 (80–542)	268 (210–690)	280 (155–440)
Blood loss (ml)	327 (124–1500)	638 (250–1200)	350 (200–900)
Duration of chest tube (days)	1.5 (0–6)	3.5 (2.8–9.1)	NA[‡]
Narcotic pain medication[†]	3.7 (1.5–15)	20.4 (5–60)	3.0 (1.3–21)
Hospitalization (days)	6.5 (2–24)	16.2 (5–34)	5.0 (4–8)

NA = not applicable; [†]mg/day of intravenous, intramuscular, or epidural analgesics. [‡]Two patients had pleural violations and required chest tubes for 2 days postoperatively. [Reprinted with permission from *Journal of Neurosurgery*.[35]]

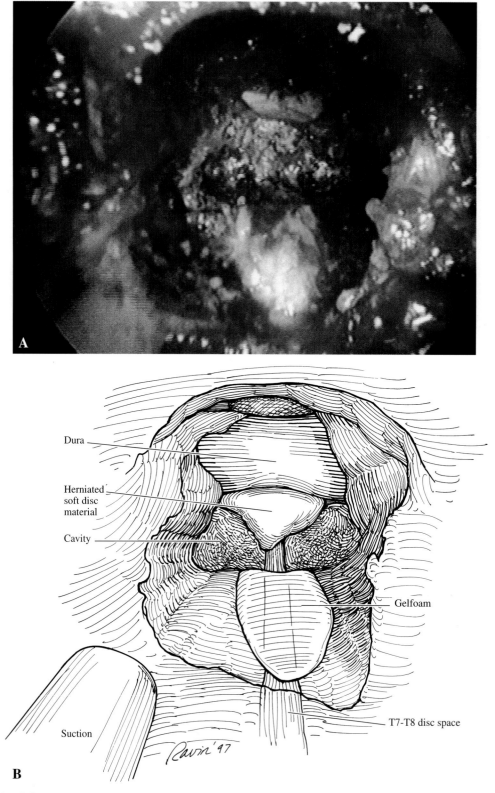

Figure 18–19.   In this **(A)** intraoperative photograph and **(B)** corresponding illustration, the T8 pedicle and rib head were removed, and a cavity was drilled into the dorsal T7–T8 disc space and vertebral bodies to expose the epidural space. The large disc herniation can be seen compressing the spinal cord.

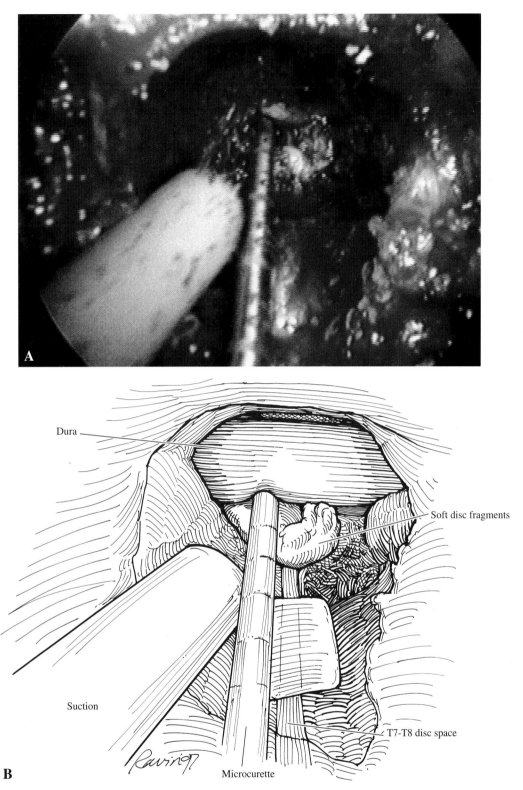

Figure 18–20.   **(A)** Intraoperative photograph and **(B)** corresponding illustration showing the spinal cord being decompressed by removing the soft disc fragments with microsurgical curettes.

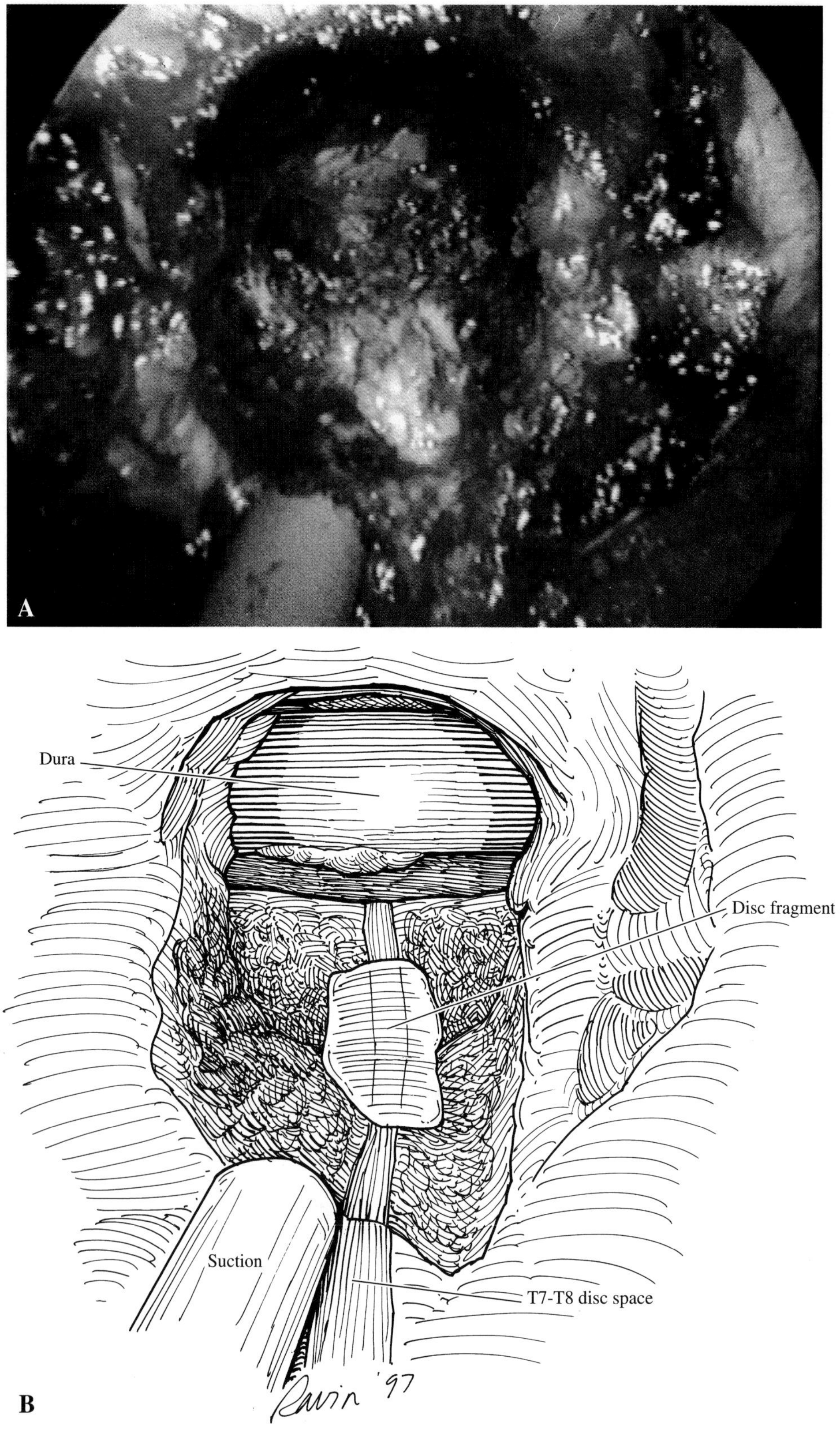

Figure 18–21.   In this **(A)** intraoperative photograph and **(B)** corresponding illustration, the large epidural disc fragment was delivered into the cavity in the vertebral body.

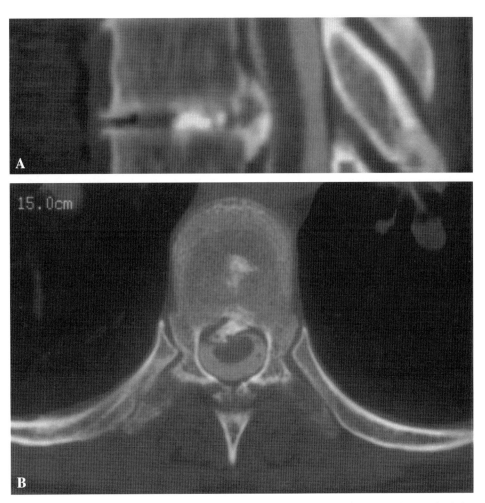

Figure 18–22. (A) Sagittal and **(B)** axial computed tomographic scans demonstrate the densely calcified, broad-based disc herniation at T8–T9, which is eccentric to the right side of the spinal canal.

TABLE 18–2 Complications Associated with Thoracoscopy ($n = 55$), Thoracotomy ($n = 18$), and Costotransversectomy ($n = 15$) for Herniated Thoracic Discs

Complications	Thoracoscopy No. (%)	Thoracotomy No. (%)	Costotransversectomy No. (%)
Atelectasis	4 (7)	6 (33)	2 (13)
Pleural effusion	2 (4)	1 (6)	1 (7)
Chylothorax	0 (0)	1 (6)	0 (0)
Hemothorax	2 (4)	1 (6)	1 (7)
Infection	0 (0)	1 (6)	0 (0)
Intercostal neuralgia	9 (16)	9 (50)	3 (20)
Subcutaneous emphysema	1 (2)	1 (6)	0 (0)
Misidentified level	2 (4)	0 (0)	1 (7)
Retained disc fragment	2 (4)	0 (0)	2 (13)
Neurological deterioration	1 (2)	0 (0)	1 (7)

[Reprinted with permission from *Journal of Neurosurgery*.[35]]

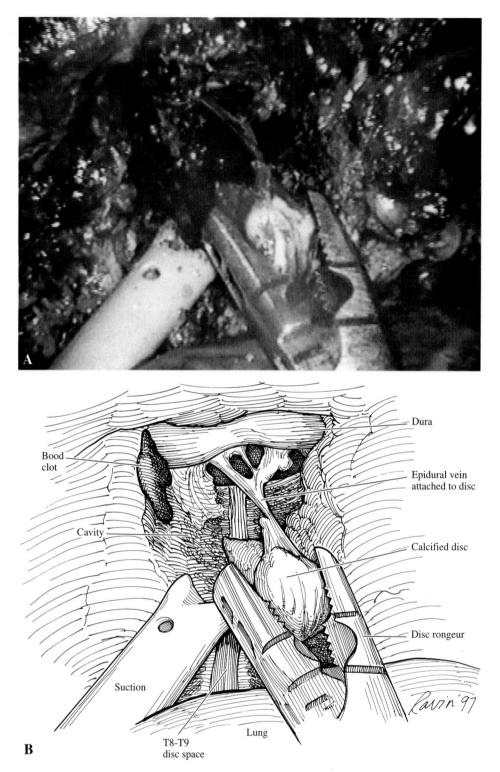

Figure 18–23. **(A)** Intraoperative photograph and **(B)** corresponding illustration of the right-sided thoracoscopic exposure used to remove the calcified disc fragment. A 2.5-cm wide cavity was drilled into the disc space and vertebrae to expose the epidural space and to provide room to work with the endoscopic tools. A complete decompression was achieved.

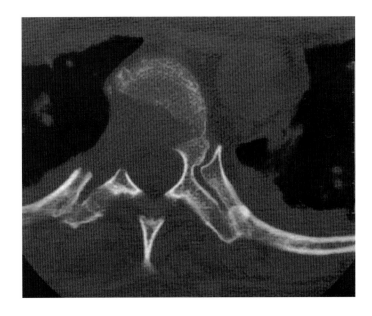

Figure 18–24. Postoperative computed tomographic scan demonstrates the pyramidal cavity that was created so the ossified disc could be resected completely.

TABLE 18–3   Outcome of 55 Patients Undergoing Thoracoscopic Discectomy Based on Frankel Grade

Preoperative Grade	Postoperative Grade				
	A	**B**	**C**	**D**	**E**
A	0	0	0	0	0
B	0	1	0	0	0
C	0	0	2	5	0
D	0	0	0	6	22
E	0	0	0	0	19

A = complete loss of neurological function; E = normal neurological function. [Reprinted with permission from *Journal of Neurosurgery.*[35]]

CONCLUSIONS

The clinical and neurological outcomes associated with thoracoscopic microdiscectomy have been excellent. Compared with posterolateral approaches to the thoracic spine, thoracoscopy provides more complete visualization and access to the ventral surfaces of the spine and spinal cord. Furthermore, midline and calcified discs can be resected more completely. Compared with thoracotomy, thoracoscopy offers identical visualization and exposure of the spine and is associated with significantly less operative morbidity. Patients experience less pain, and the duration of their hospitalization and recovery period is briefer.

REFERENCES

1. Williams MP, Cherryman GR, Husband JE: Significance of thoracic disc herniation demonstrated by MR imaging. *J Comput Assist Tomogr* 1989; 13(2):211–214.
2. Wood KB, Garvey TA, Gundry C, et al: Magnetic resonance imaging of the thoracic spine. Evaluation of asymptomatic individuals. *J Bone Joint Surg Am* 1995; 77(11):1631–1638.
3. Wood KB, Blair JM, Aepple DM, et al: The natural history of asymptomatic thoracic disc herniations. *Spine* 1997; 22(5):525–530.
4. Stillerman CB, Chen TC, Day JD, et al: The transfacet pedicle-sparing approach for thoracic disc removal: Cadaveric morphometric analysis and preliminary clinical experience. *J Neurosurg* 1995; 83:971–976.
5. Garrido E: Modified costotransversectomy: A surgical approach to ventrally placed lesions in the thoracic spinal canal. *Surg Neurol* 1980; 13(2):109–113.
6. Maiman DJ, Larson SJ, Luck E, et al: Lateral extracavitary approach to the spine for thoracic disc herniation: Report of 23 cases. *Neurosurgery* 1984; 14(2):178–182.
7. Le Roux PD, Haglund MM, Harris AB: Thoracic disc disease: Experience with the transpedicular approach in twenty consecutive patients. *Neurosurgery* 1993; 33(1):58–66.
8. Fessler RG, Dietze DD, Jr., MacMillan M, et al: Lateral parascapular extrapleural approach to the upper thoracic spine. *J Neurosurg* 1991; 75:349–355.
9. Carson J, Gumpert J, Jefferson A: Diagnosis and treatment of thoracic intervertebral disc protrusions. *J Neurol Neurosurg Psychiatry* 1971; 34:68–77.
10. Hulme A: The surgical approach to thoracic intervertebral disc protrusions. *J Neurol Neurosurg Psychiatry* 1960; 23:133–137.
11. Patterson RH, Jr., Arbit E: A surgical approach through the pedicle to protruded thoracic discs. *J Neurosurg* 1979; 48(5):768–772.
12. Larson SJ, Holst RA, Hemmy DC, et al: Lateral extracavitary approach to traumatic lesions of the thoracic and lumbar spine. *J Neurosurg* 1976; 45(6):628–637.
13. Bohlman HH, Zdeblick TA: Anterior excision of herniated thoracic discs. *J Bone Joint Surg Am* 1988; 70(7):1038–1047.
14. Fidler MW, Goedhart ZD: Excision of prolapse of thoracic intervertebral disc. A transthoracic technique. *J Bone Joint Surg Br* 1984; 66(4):518–522.
15. Perot PL, Jr., Munro DD: Transthoracic removal of midline thoracic disc protrusions causing spinal cord compression. *J Neurosurg* 1969; 31(4):452–458.

16. Lobosky JM, Hitchon PW, McDonnell DE: Transthoracic antero-lateral decompression for thoracic spine lesions. *Neurosurgery* 1984; 14:26–30.

17. Otani K, Yoshida M, Fujii E, et al: Thoracic disc herniation. Surgical treatment in 23 patients. *Spine* 1988; 13(11):1262–1267.

18. Ransohoff J, Spencer F, Siew F, et al: Transthoracic removal of thoracic disc. Report of three cases. *J Neurosurg* 1969; 31(4):459–461.

19. Crafoord C, Hiertonn T, Lindblom K, et al: Spinal cord compression caused by a protruded thoracic disc. Report of a case treated with antero-lateral fenestration of the disc. *Acta Orthop Scand* 1958; 28:103–107.

20. Otani K, Nakai S, Fujimura Y, et al: Surgical treatment of thoracic disc herniation using the anterior approach. *J Bone Joint Surg Br* 1982; 64(3):340–343.

21. Chou SN, Seljeskog EL: Alternative surgical approaches to the thoracic spine. *Clin Neurosurg* 1973; 20:306–321.

22. Sekhar LN, Jannetta PJ: Thoracic disc herniation: Operative approaches and results. *Neurosurgery* 1983; 12:303–305.

23. Ferson PF, Landreneau RJ, Dowling RD, et al: Comparison of open versus thoracoscopic lung biopsy for diffuse infiltrative pulmonary disease. *J Thorac Cardiovasc Surg* 1993; 106:194–199.

24. Dajczman E, Gordon A, Kreisman H, et al: Long-term postthoracotomy pain. *Chest* 1991; 99:270–274.

25. Theodore N, Dickman CA: Current management of thoracic disc herniation. *Contemp Neurosurg* 1996; 18(19):1–7.

26. Broc GG, Crawford NR, Sonntag VKH, et al: Biomechanical effects of transthoracic microdiscectomy. *Spine* 1997; 22(6): 605–612.

27. Horowitz MB, Moossy JJ, Julian T, et al: Thoracic discectomy using video assisted thoracoscopy. *Spine* 1994; 19(9):1082–1086.

28. Rosenthal D, Dickman C, Lorenz R, et al: Thoracic disc herniation: Early results after surgical treatment using microsurgical endoscopy (abstract). *J Neurosurg* 1996; 84:334A

29. Mack MJ, Regan JJ, Bobechko WP, et al: Application of thoracoscopy for diseases of the spine. *Ann Thorac Surg* 1993; 56:736–738.

30. Regan JJ, Mack MJ, Picetti GD, III. A technical report on video-assisted thoracoscopy in thoracic spinal surgery. Preliminary description. *Spine* 1995; 20(7):831–837.

31. Rosenthal D, Rosenthal R, de Simone A: Removal of a protruded thoracic disc using microsurgical endoscopy. A new technique. *Spine* 1994; 19:1087–1091.

32. McAfee PC, Regan JR, Zdeblick T, et al: The incidence of complications in endoscopic anterior thoracolumbar spinal reconstructive surgery. A prospective multicenter study comprising the first 100 consecutive cases. *Spine* 1995; 20(14):1624–1632.

33. Regan JJ, Mack MJ, Picetti GD, III, et al: A comparison of video-assisted thoracoscopic surgery (VATS) with open thoracotomy in thoracic spinal surgery. *Today's Therapeutic Trends* 1994; 11:203–218.

34. Landreneau RJ, Hazelrigg SR, Mack MJ, et al: Postoperative pain-related morbidity: Video-assisted thoracic surgery versus thoracotomy. *Ann Thorac Surg* 1993; 56:1285–1289.

35. Rosenthal D, Dickman CA: Thoracoscopic microsurgical excision of herniated thoracic discs. *J Neurosurg* 1998; 89:224–235.

CHAPTER **19**

Thoracoscopic Resection of Intrathoracic Neurogenic Tumors

Curtis A. Dickman, M.D. and Ronald I. Apfelbaum, M.D.

Transthoracic endoscopic surgery provides an excellent alternative for the resection of thoracic schwannomas, neurofibromas, or other neurogenic tumors with major components that extend into the thoracic cavity. The relatively simple surgical strategies and indications are reviewed in this chapter.

OPERATIVE INDICATIONS

The most ideal tumors for transthoracic endoscopic resection are those located peripherally within the intercostal nerves or those that extend from the neural foramina into the chest cavity. Before the advent of thoracoscopy, these tumors required a thoracotomy for removal (Fig. 19–1).[1–3] Resection of such nerve sheath tumors may be indicated to prevent spinal cord compression from the tumors growing into the spinal canal, to relieve mass effect within the chest when a large tumor has impaired pulmonary function, to prevent malignant transformation of a tumor, or to provide a tissue diagnosis.[1–9]

In the thoracic spine, nerve sheath tumors with a significant component of their mass within the spinal canal compressing the spinal cord (i.e., classic dumbbell tumors) should not be approached endoscopically.[3] These intradural tumors are approached posteriorly or posterolaterally using a laminectomy, transpedicular approach, or costotransversectomy. The dura is opened to allow resection of the intracanalicular tumor and decompression of the spinal cord and is closed in a watertight fashion. If the tumor also extends into the chest, a costotransversectomy approach can be used to resect small to moderate extensions of the tumor (i.e., up to 4 cm). However, if a *large* component of a dumbbell tumor extends into the chest cavity, a thoracotomy or a thoracoscopic approach may be needed to allow adequate visualization and access so that the intrathoracic component of

the tumor (Fig. 19–1) can be resected safely. The risk of a cerebrospinal fluid (CSF) leak can be minimized by resecting the foraminal and intradural tumor *first* and then obtaining a watertight dural closure. Subsequently, thoracoscopy is performed to resect the residual tumor within the thorax.

OPERATIVE TECHNIQUES

Thoracoscopic resection of intrathoracic schwannomas or neurofibromas begins by identifying and protecting the vascular and visceral structures adjacent to the tumor (Figs. 19–2 and 19–3). If the tumor has a cystic component, a long needle can be inserted into the tumor to decompress the lesion internally (Fig. 19–4). The pleura is incised, opened widely, and mobilized from the margins of the tumor (Figs. 19–5 and 19–6). The vascular supply to the tumor is coagulated with bipolar cauterization.

Extradural Tumor

If the tumor is located peripherally on the intercostal nerve and does not enter the neural foramen, the normal segments of the intercostal nerve are identified proximally and distally to the tumor using subperiosteal dissection to mobilize the neurovascular bundle from the rib. The tumor capsule is separated from the surrounding normal tissues using sharp and blunt dissection. The intercostal nerve is sectioned proximally and distally, leaving stumps of normal nerve tissue attached to the tumor that can be used as handles to grasp and manipulate the tumor as it is mobilized circumferentially. The tumor may be resected en bloc as a single specimen. However, to remove a large tumor from the thorax through an endoscopic portal, the tumor may need to be sectioned into pieces or placed within an endoscopic specimen bag (Fig. 19–7).

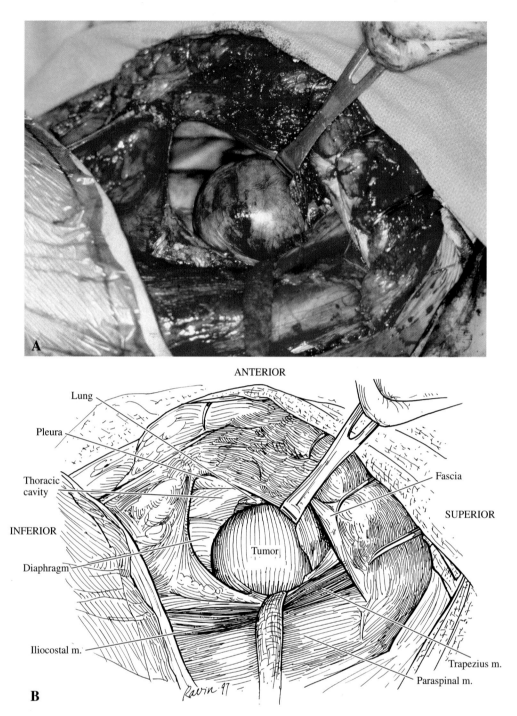

A

ANTERIOR

Lung

Pleura

Thoracic
cavity

Fascia

INFERIOR

SUPERIOR

Diaphragm

Tumor

Iliocostal m.

Trapezius m.

Paraspinal m.

Ravin 97

B

Figure 19–1. Before the advent of thoracoscopy, a thoracotomy was required to resect a large intrathoracic schwannoma. **(A)** Intraoperative photograph and **(B)** corresponding illustration showing an 8-cm, solid tumor arising from the left T10 neural foramen and extending widely into the chest. A 12-inch thoracotomy incision was required for its exposure and resection. The incision extended posteriorly to expose the laminae and spinous processes so that the intradural component of this dumbbell tumor could be resected. The size of this incision contrasts strikingly to the small incisions used for thoracoscopy.

Nerve sheath tumors that extend into the neural foramen are approached using a strategy that avoids extensive manipulation of the tumor, traction on the foraminal component of the tumor, and avulsion of the proximal thoracic nerve root that could cause CSF leakage or spinal cord injury. The intrathoracic tumor is first detached from the distal segment of the intercostal nerve (Fig. 19–25). The distal tumor is mobilized from normal tissues with sharp

and blunt dissection, avoiding traction on the proximal tumor mass within the neural foramen. Once sufficiently mobilized and detached from normal tissues, the tumor is sectioned to detach its main portion from the portion entering the neural foramen (Fig. 19–8). The bulk of the tumor mass can then be removed piecemeal.

The stalk of the proximal tumor that remains within the neural foramen is resected last (Figs. 19–9 to 19–12). To

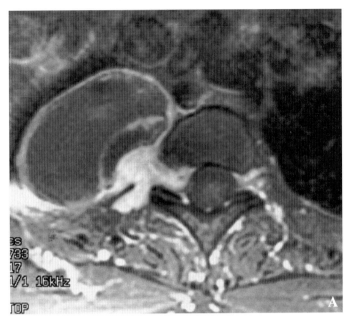 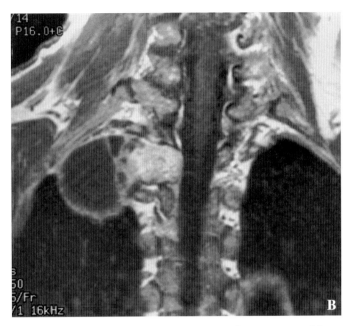

Figure 19–2. **(A)** Axial and **(B)** coronal gadolinium-enhanced magnetic resonance images demonstrating a schwannoma arising from the right T2–T3 neural foramen with a 6-cm, spherical cystic component extending into the apex of the chest. A large portion of the intrathoracic component of the tumor was cystic. The tumor did not extend intradurally. The enhancing tumor had widened the neural foramen. The surgical procedure to remove this tumor is depicted in Figures 19–3 through 19–13.

resect the foraminal component of the tumor completely, the dura and nerve root sleeve must be exposed and identified so that a suture ligature or hemoclip can be placed at the proximal nerve root to prevent CSF leakage. The epidural space is *best* identified by removing the head of the rib and pedicle of the vertebra caudal to the involved foramen (Fig. 19–9). The dorsal edge of the vertebral body may also need to be removed with a drill to provide adequate access to the foramen. Access to the proximal portion of the tumor within the neural foramen can be achieved by reducing the size of the tumor and applying bipolar cauterization to its sheath. The shrunken tumor stalk and proximal nerve root can then be mobilized more easily to identify the epidural space (Fig. 19–10).

Once the dura and normal proximal nerve root are identified, the root sleeve is ligated with an endoscopic suture ligature or a hemoclip (Figs. 19–11 and 19–13). The nerve root is amputated distal to the ligature, and the distal root stump with the attached remaining tumor is removed (Fig. 19–12). The resection bed is inspected to verify that the tumor was totally resected. Hemostasis is completed with bipolar cauterization, and absorbable hemostatic agents are placed over the epidural veins. The dura is inspected, and a Valsalva maneuver is performed to exclude the presence of a CSF leak.

If CSF is leaking from the root sleeve or the dura, the dura should be closed using an endoscopic ligature, endoscopic suturing, dural closure clips, or fibrin glue and a fascial patch graft. The negative pressure within the thorax during normal respiration creates a pressure gradient that could perpetuate a CSF leak postoperatively. Therefore, if

the dura has been opened intraoperatively, the surgeon should obtain a watertight dural closure, place a lumbar drain to divert CSF flow, and avoid placing the chest tube to negative pressure (suction). If a chest tube is needed after surgery to promote reinflation of the lung or drain any fluid collecting within the chest, it should be used briefly, minimizing the amount of suction (i.e., 5 cm H_2O). Alternatively, the chest tube can be placed to water seal, using gravity drainage. If hemostasis is satisfactory, the chest tube can be removed in the operating room or in the recovery room after the lung has fully reinflated.

Intradural Tumor

To remove an intradural extension of a dumbbell tumor using thoracoscopy, a partial corpectomy is required to expose the dura satisfactorily. Endoscopic microscissors are used to incise the dura linearly. The edges of the dural incisions are retracted with dural tack-up sutures. The intradural tumor is resected using microsurgical endoscopic dissection tools. The dural incision is closed using running sutures (4-0 Nurolon or 5-0 Prolene™) that are placed with endoscopic fine-tipped needle holders and fine tissue forceps.

Compared with endoscopy, it is technically much easier to repair the dura and obtain a watertight closure with open techniques. Therefore, if the tumor extends intradurally, we recommend removing the intradural component using an open posterior or a posterolateral approach. Two case examples are illustrated in Figures 19–14 through 19–20 and Figures 19–21 through 19–28.

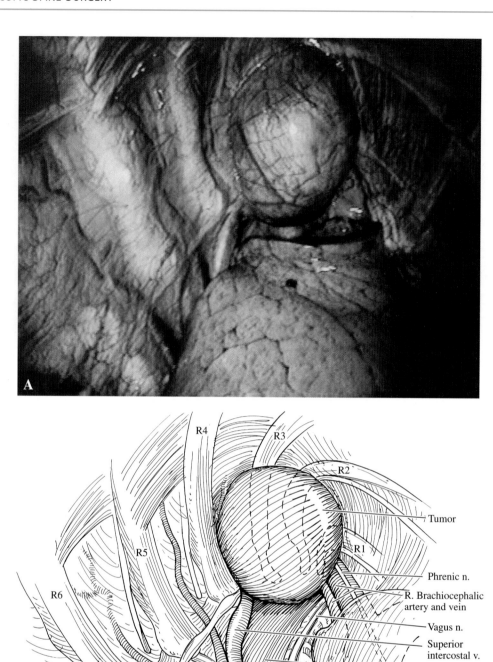

Figure 19–3. **(A)** Thoracoscopic view and **(B)** corresponding illustration of the right-sided apical schwannoma shown in Figure 19–2 and its relationship *(Figure continued next page.)*

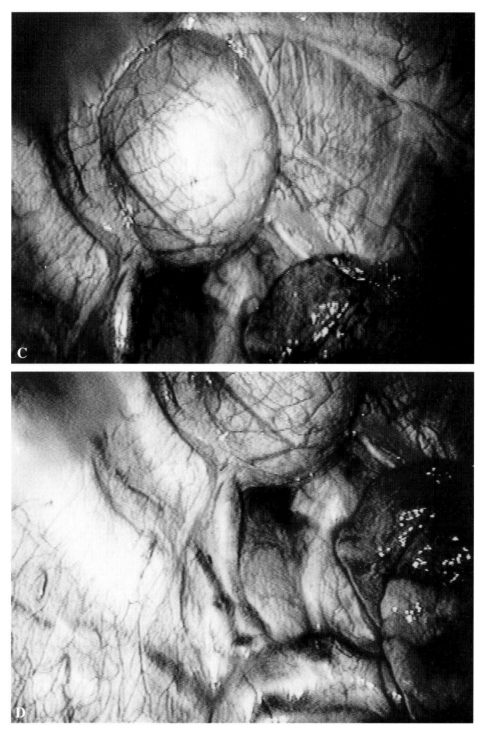

Figure 19–3. *(continued)*   **(C** and **D)** to the surrounding anatomy. The tumor was adjacent to the spine, brachiocephalic vein and artery, phrenic nerve, vagus nerve, trachea, esophagus, and superior intercostal vein.

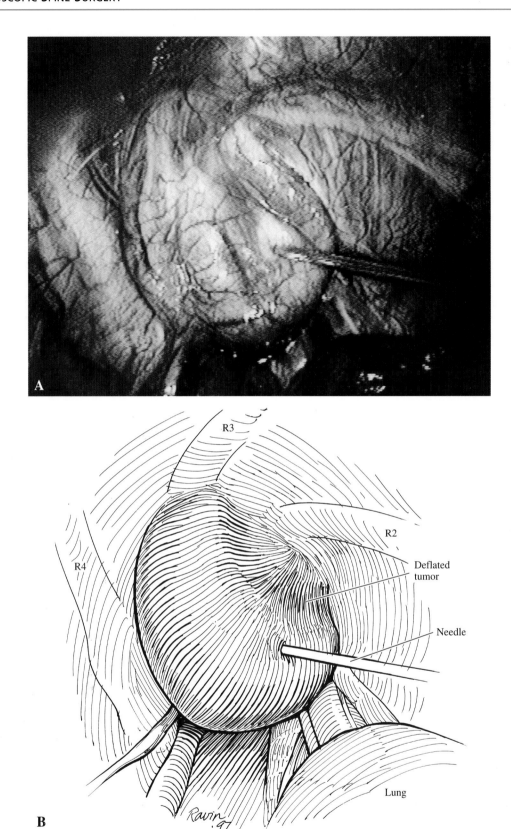

Figure 19–4. **(A)** Intraoperative view and **(B)** corresponding illustration showing a long needle inserted into the tumor cyst. The tumor collapsed after xanthochromic fluid (30 ml) was aspirated from the cyst. Internal decompression of the tumor allowed the tumor to be mobilized more easily and avoided traction on the proximal foraminal tumor and the proximal nerve root. R = rib.

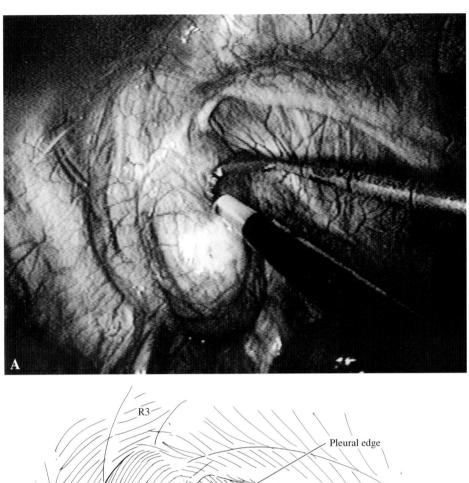

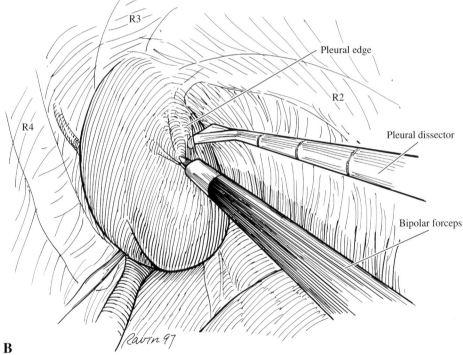

Figure 19–5.   **(A)** Intraoperative view and **(B)** corresponding illustration showing the pleura over the center of the tumor being incised. A pleural dissector was used to separate the pleura from the tumor as well as to open the pleura widely. R = rib.

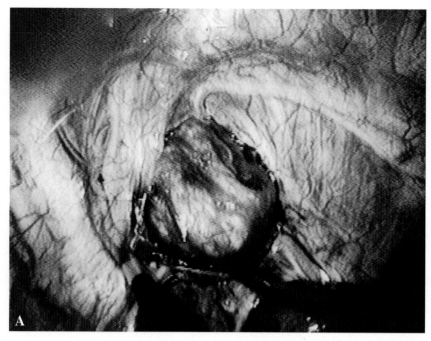

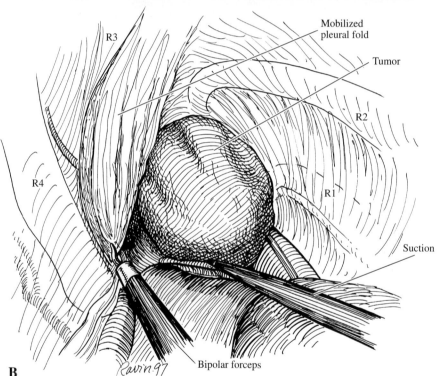

R3

Mobilized
pleural fold

Tumor

R2

R4

R1

Suction

Bipolar forceps

Figure 19–6. In this **(A)** intraoperative view and **(B)** corresponding illustration, the pleura is opened widely to expose and mobilize the margins of the tumor. R = rib.

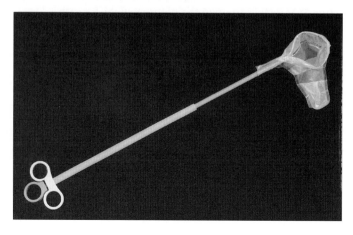

Figure 19–7. This endoscopic specimen pouch can be used to store tumor tissue so that seeding tumor within the thorax or contaminating the portal site can be avoided.

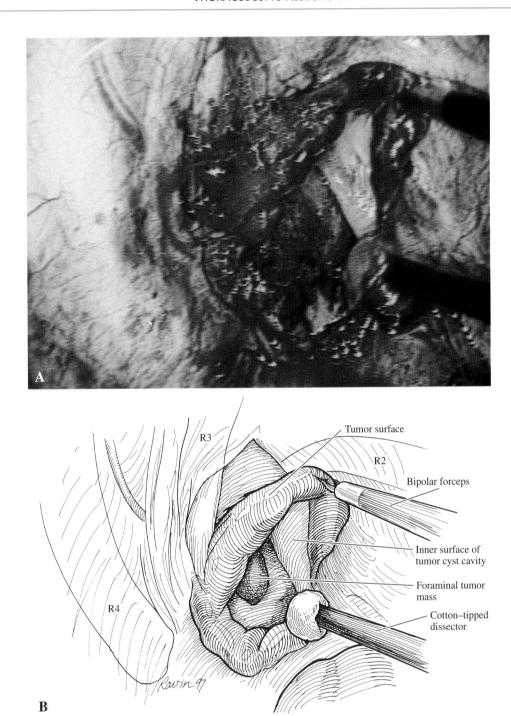

Figure 19–8. The intrathoracic tumor was removed piecemeal. The stalk of tumor, proximally within the neural foramen, was resected after the tumor mass was debulked. The edges of the intrathoracic tumor were grasped and dissected from the adjacent vascular and visceral structures using blunt and sharp dissection. In this **(A)** intraoperative view and **(B)** corresponding illustration, a cotton-tipped endoscopic dissector is being used to mobilize the edges of the tumor. Traction was avoided on the proximal tumor within the neural foramen to avoid avulsing the nerve root, injuring the spinal cord, and causing a cerebrospinal fluid leak. R = rib.

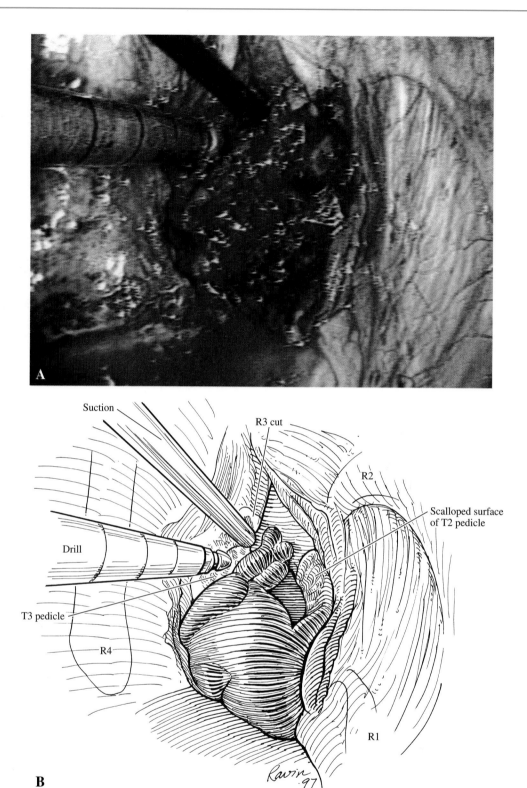

Figure 19–9. In this **(A)** intraoperative view and **(B)** corresponding illustration, the pedicle is thinned with a high-speed drill. It will then be resected with a Kerrison rongeur. The third rib head was removed so the tumor could be followed into the foramen. The epidural space, dura, and proximal nerve root were identified by removing the third rib head and T3 pedicle. R = rib.

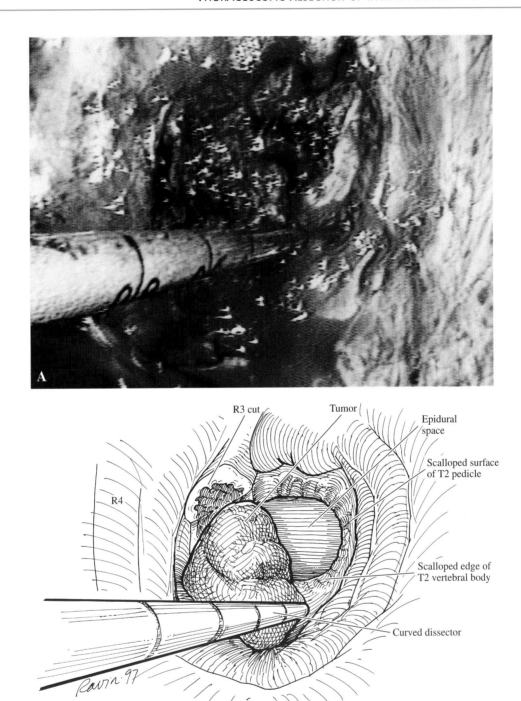

Figure 19–10.   In this **(A)** intraoperative view and **(B)** corresponding illustration, the tumor is mobilized within the neural foramen using an endoscopic microdissector. The tumor capsule was reduced using gentle bipolar cauterization. R = rib.

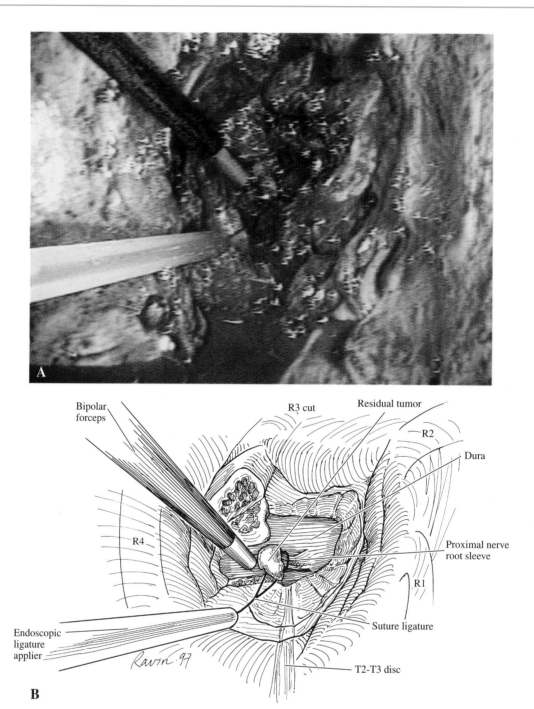

Figure 19–11.   In this **(A)** intraoperative view and **(B)** corresponding illustration, the nerve root sleeve is ligated proximal to the tumor using an endoscopic ligature. The distal root and tumor were then removed. R = rib.

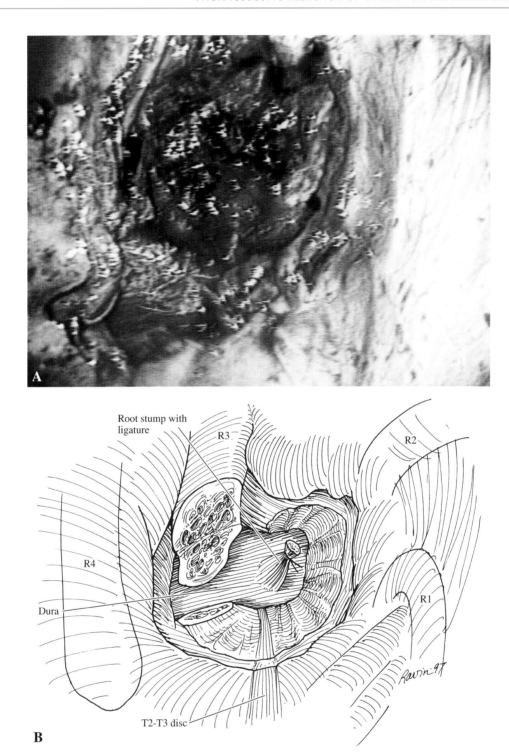

Figure 19–12. **(A)** Intraoperative view and **(B)** corresponding illustration showing complete removal of the tumor. All surrounding anatomical structures were preserved.

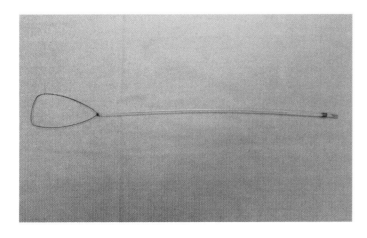

Figure 19–13. Photograph of an endoscopic suture ligature.

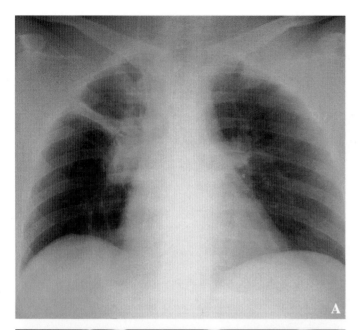

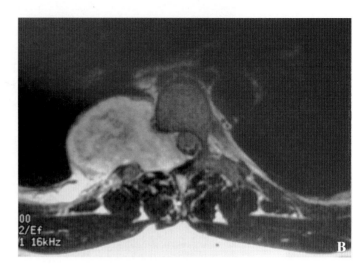

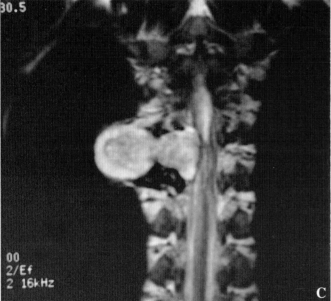

Figure 19–14. **(A)** A 27-year-old man presented with an asymptomatic right-sided posterior mediastinal mass that was discovered on a routine chest x-ray. **(B)** Axial and **(C)** coronal contrast-enhanced magnetic resonance imaging studies demonstrate a large dumbbell-shaped uniformly enhancing tumor at T5–T6 that displaces the spinal cord and has a large extension into the chest. The tumor widens the neural foramen and appears to be extradural with a significant component of tumor within the spinal canal. His operation is depicted in Figures 19–15 through 19–20. [With permission from Barrow Neurological Institute].

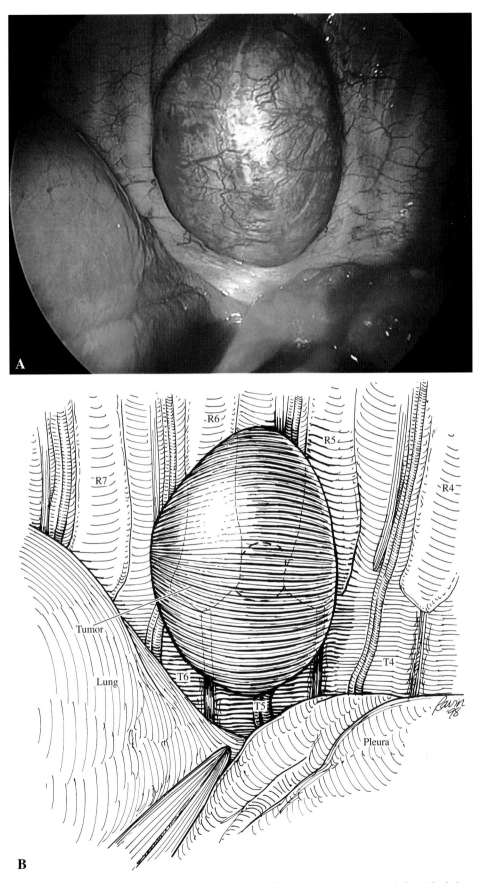

Figure 19–15. **(A)** Intraoperative photograph and **(B)** corresponding illustration showing a right-sided thoracoscopic approach to the thoracic component of this tumor. The tumor was spherical, well demarcated, and not adherent to any thoracic or mediastinal vascular or visceral structures. Histologically, this was a benign ganglioneurofibroma. [With permission from Barrow Neurological Institute].

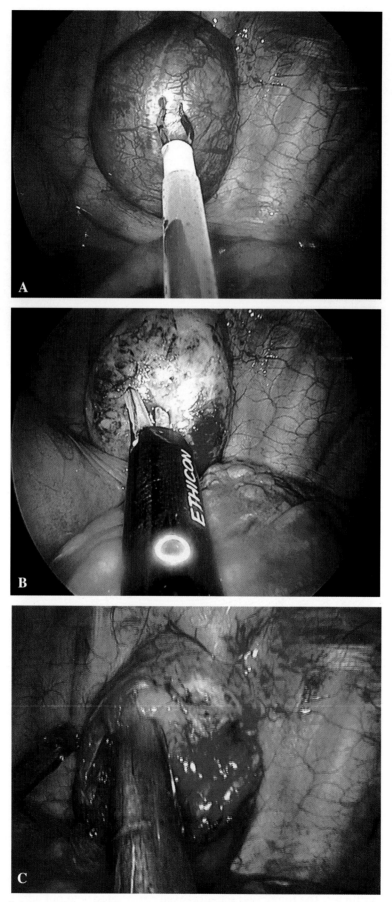

Figure 19–16. **(A)** The superficial vessels on the tumor were sealed with bipolar cauterization. **(B)** The tumor was incised and divided into small sections with a harmonic scalpel. **(C)** The soft tumor was debulked in a piecemeal fashion using biopsy forceps.

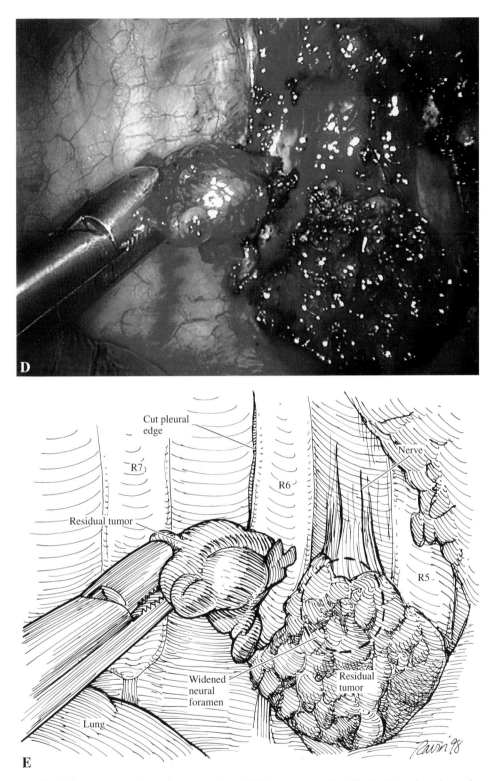

Figure 19–16. *(continued)* **(D)** Intraoperative photograph and **(E)** corresponding illustration showing a large piece of tumor being grasped with a disc rongeur and removed through the endoscopic portal. [With permission from Barrow Neurological Institute.]

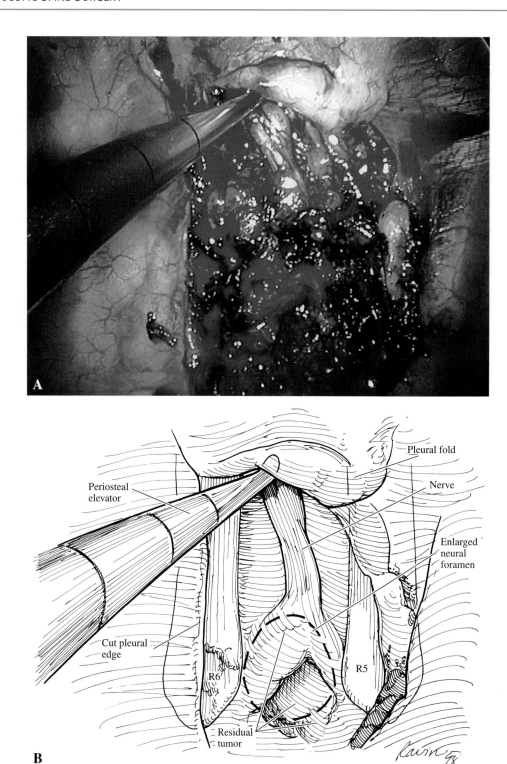

Figure 19–17. **(A)** Intraoperative photograph and **(B)** corresponding illustration demonstrating mobilization of the tumor mass. The normal intercostal nerve was identified and sectioned distal to the tumor to mobilize the neoplasm that completely infiltrated the proximal portion of the nerve. [With permission from Barrow Neurological Institute.]

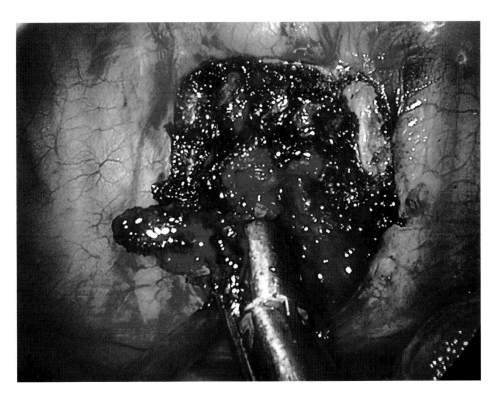

Figure 19–18.   The tumor is removed from the surface of the spine.

Figure 19–19.   (A) The tumor is removed from the neural foramen using microdissection tools and a disc rongeur. **(B)** Intraoperative photograph and **(C)** corresponding illustration showing the residual tumor. The remaining intraspinal portion of the tumor was removed through a posterior approach using a one-level laminectomy. [With permission from Barrow Neurological Institute]

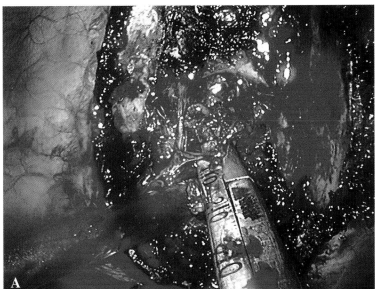

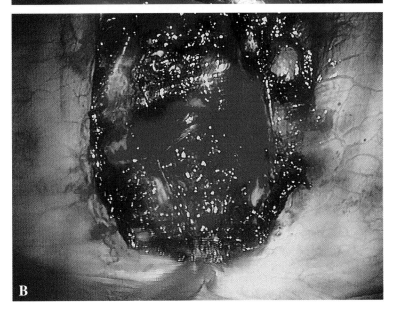

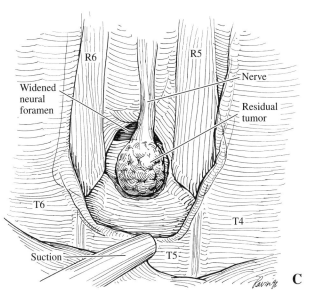

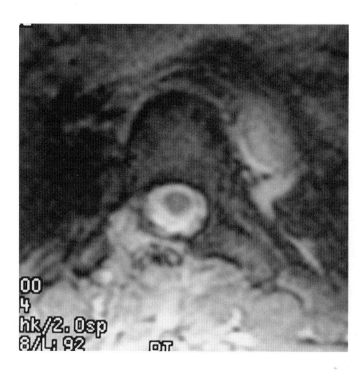

Figure 19–20. Postoperative enhanced magnetic resonance image demonstrating complete resection of the tumor.

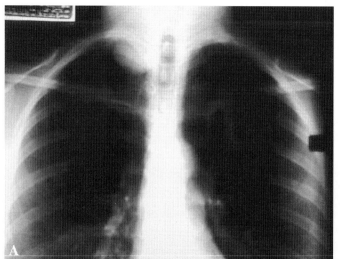

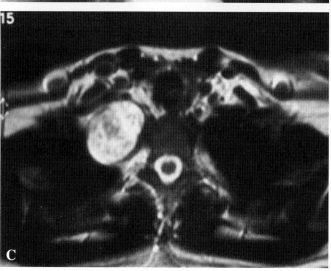

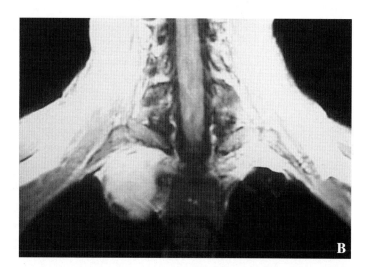

Figure 19–21. A 47-year-old woman presented with a right-sided Horner's syndrome due to a schwannoma arising from the right T2 intercostal nerve. **(A)** The chest x-ray demonstrated an apical soft tissue mass within the right hemithorax. **(B)** Coronal and **(C)** axial magnetic resonance images demonstrated a homogeneously enhancing solid tumor arising from the right T2 foramen. The tumor did not extend intradurally. Her operation is depicted in Figures 19–22 through 19–28.

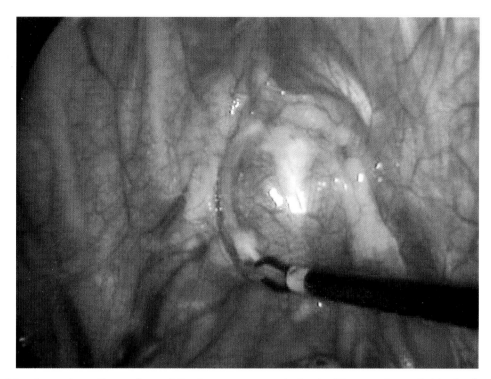

Figure 19–22. The blood vessels on the surface of the tumor were cauterized with an endoscopic bipolar forceps. Note that Figures 19–22 through 19–28 are oriented similar to Figure 19–3.

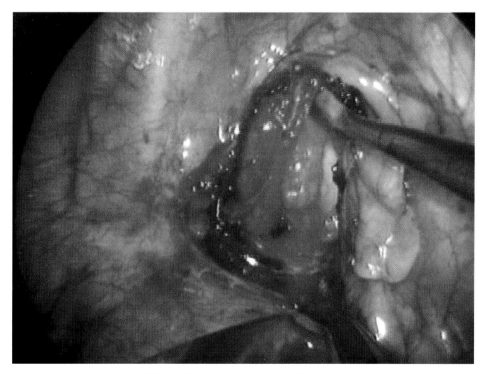

Figure 19–23. The pleura was incised and mobilized from the surface of the tumor.

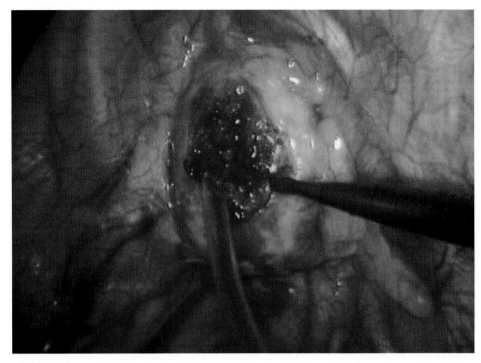

Figure 19–24.   The tumor was incised and internally debulked using soft tissue dissectors. The tumor was soft and relatively avascular.

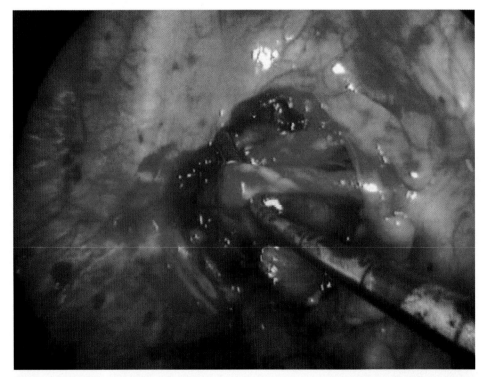

Figure 19–25.   The distal T2 intercostal nerve was identified and sectioned to allow the tumor to be completely mobilized without causing traction on the proximal T2 nerve root.

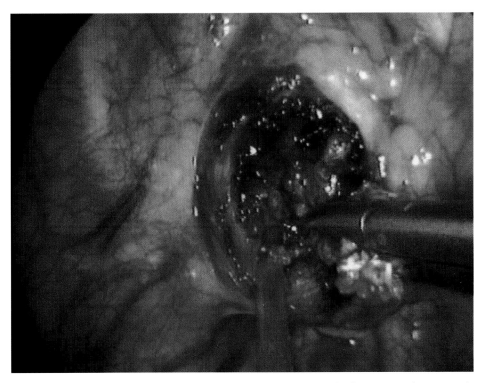

Figure 19–26. The foraminal component of the tumor was mobilized and excised. The proximal T2 root sleeve was ligated with a hemoclip. A complete resection of the tumor was achieved.

DISCUSSION

Various benign and malignant neurogenic tumors can arise from the spinal and paraspinal structures within the posterior mediastinum (Table 19–1).[1-3] Excision is required to diagnose the tissue definitively and remove the tumor. Benign nerve sheath tumors are the most commonly occurring neoplasms (Tables 19–2 and 19–3).[1,2] Schwannomas and neurofibromas are more often round and more than 80% arise outside the spinal canal. They may grow within the segmental thoracic nerves or arise from the phrenic or vagus nerves. The intercostal nerves can be sacrificed without consequences. If, however, tumor arises from the phrenic or vagus nerves, they should be preserved.

Compared to nerve sheath tumors, ganglionic tumors are usually elongated masses with tapered borders. Neurogenic tumors may become symptomatic with neurological symptoms; pain; erosion of the rib, vertebrae, or pedicle; scoliosis; or foraminal enlargement. The most common tumors that become symptomatic with foraminal enlargement are schwannomas and neuroblastomas;[2] those that most often become symptomatic with scoliosis are ganglioneuromas and ganglioneuroblastomas.[2]

Surgery is indicated for the definitive diagnosis and resection of these tumors. Only a few cases using thoracoscopy to excise intrathoracic neurogenic tumors have been reported.[4,6-8] Thoracoscopy, however, can be used successfully and as a preferred method to thoracotomy to resect thoracic neurogenic tumors.

TABLE 19–1   Differentiation of Thoracic Neurogenic Tumors

Origin	Benign	Malignant
Nerve sheath	Schwannoma Neurofibroma	Neurogenic schwannoma (malignant schwannoma)
Autonomic ganglia	Ganglioneuroma	Ganglioneuroblastoma Neuroblastoma
Paraganglionic system	Paraganglioma (pheochromocytoma and chemodectoma)	Malignant pheochromocytoma Malignant paraganglioma
Neuroectoderm	NA	Primitive neuroectodermal tumor

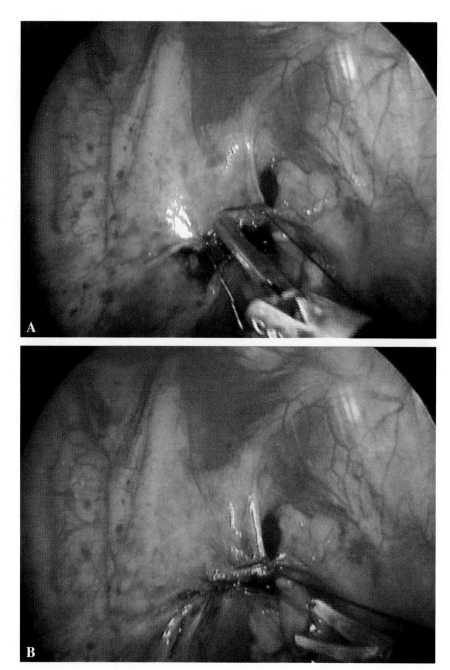

Figure 19–27. **(A)** After totally resecting the tumor, the pleura was closed with an endoscopic suturing device. **(B)** The suture was cut with an endoscopic scissors. A watertight pleural closure was achieved.

TABLE 19–2 Posterior Mediastinal Neural Tumors[1]

Type	No. (%)
Schwannoma	51 (31)
Neurofibroma	16 (10)
Neuroblastoma	24 (15)
Ganglioneuroblastoma	22 (14)
Ganglioneuroma	40 (25)
Paraganglioma	7 (4)
Total	160 (100)

TABLE 19–3 Intrathoracic Neurogenic Tumors[2]

Type	No. (%)
Nerve sheath tumors	
Schwannoma	52 (26)
Neurofibroma	21 (10)
Neurogenic sarcoma	2 (1)
Autonomic ganglion tumors	
Ganglioneuroma	50 (25)
Ganglioneuroblastoma	28 (14)
Neuroblastoma	36 (18)
Paraganglioma	7 (3)
Peripheral neuroectodermal tumor (PNET)	6 (3)
Total	202 (100)

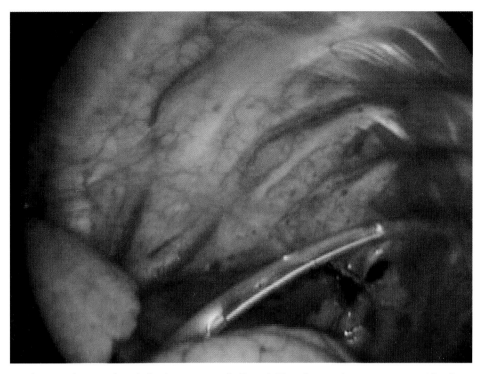

Figure 19–28. A chest tube was inserted and the lung was reinflated. The chest tube was removed in the recovery room. The patient's tumor was completely resected. She had no neurological or clinical complications. The surgical blood loss was 200 ml. The operation took 3.5 hours to complete.

CONCLUSIONS

The operative techniques used for the endoscopic resection of intrathoracic nerve sheath tumors are straightforward and closely resemble the dissection techniques used to resect these tumors with open surgery. Thoracoscopy provides an excellent alternative to thoracotomy for removing tumors from the thorax and thoracic neural foramina. Currently, thoracoscopy is not well suited for treating intradural tumors that compress the spinal cord because achieving a watertight dural closure endoscopically is technically difficult. Large dumbbell tumors that extend intradurally into the spinal canal *and* widely into the thorax can be treated with a staged, open posterolateral resection of the intradural and foraminal portions of the tumor and subsequently with an anterior thoracoscopic approach for the resection of the residual intrathoracic component.

REFERENCES

1. Shields TW, Reynolds M: Neurogenic tumors of the thorax. *Surg Clin North Am* 1988; 68(3):645–668.
2. Reed JC, Hallet KK, Feigin DS: Neural tumors of the thorax: Subject review from the AFIP. *Radiology* 1978; 126(1):9–17.
3. Grillo HC, Ojemann RG, Scannell JG, et al: Combined approach to "dumbbell" intrathoracic and intraspinal neurogenic tumors. *Ann Thorac Surg* 1983; 36(4):402–407.
4. Landreneau RJ, Dowling RD, Ferson PF: Thoracoscopic resection of a posterior mediastinal neurogenic tumor. *Chest* 1992; 102(4): 1288–1290.
5. Landreneau RJ, Dowling RD, Castillo WM, et al: Thoracoscopic resection of an anterior mediastinal tumor. *Ann Thorac Surg* 1992; 54(1):142–144.
6. McNulty PS, McAfee PC, Regan JJ: Biopsy of discs, vertebrae, and paraspinal masses. In Regan JJ, McAfee PC, Mack MJ, eds: *Atlas of Endoscopic Spine Surgery*. St. Louis: Quality Medical Publishing; 1995:151–164.
7. Lyons MK, Gharagozloo F: Video assisted thoracoscopic resection of intercostal neurofibroma. *Surg Neurol* 1995; 43(6):542–545.
8. Weder W, Schlumpf R, Schimmer R, et al: Thoracoscopic resection of benign schwannoma. *Thorac Cardiovasc Surg* 1992; 40(4):192–194.
9. Dickman CA, Apfelbaum RI: Thoracoscopic microsurgical excision of a thoracic schwannoma. Case report. *J Neurosurg* 1998; 88:898–902.

CHAPTER 20

Thoracoscopic Corpectomy

Curtis A. Dickman, M.D. and Daniel J. Rosenthal, M.D.

Patients with pathology affecting the spine may become symptomatic with myelopathy, myelo-radiculopathy, radiculopathy, or mechanical back pain. Overt structural instability of the thoracic spine tends to be associated with spinal cord dysfunction. The goals of surgical treatment are to reduce spinal deformity, to decompress the spinal cord and nerves, to reconstruct the anterior column, to provide axial load-bearing, to restore anatomic alignment, to immobilize unstable vertebrae, and to eliminate destructive processes.[1-9] This chapter focuses on the most salient features of thoracoscopic corpectomy. The specific issues pertaining to surgical preparation and exposure are discussed in Chapters 10, 11, and 12.

INDICATIONS

As an alternative approach to thoracotomy, thoracoscopy can be used to perform thoracic corpectomies; to decompress the spinal cord and nerve roots; or to resect, reconstruct, and fixate a portion of the spinal column affected by destructive processes. Thoracoscopic corpectomy can be used to treat unstable thoracic fractures, to resect thoracic spinal tumors, to debride vertebrae infected with osteomyelitis, to drain epidural abscesses, to resect congenital hemivertebrae, and remove large herniated thoracic discs.[1,5,9]

PREOPERATIVE PLANNING

Computed tomography and magnetic resonance imaging are both used to delineate the soft tissue and osseous anatomy. An anterior approach is indicated when the surgeon must access and visualize the anterior spinal cord and the anterior vertebral bodies.[1-10] Posterior or posterolateral approaches to the thoracic spine only provide a view of the lateral and posterior dura, *not* the ventral dura.[11-17] Although posterolateral approaches can be used for partial corpectomy and reconstruction, the surgeon can never see the ventral surface of the dura. The surgeon must therefore select the approach that best fits the patient's pathology and the surgeon's individual skills. The same issues involved in planning a discectomy are present in planning a corpectomy (see Chapter 16).

TECHNIQUE OF THORACOSCOPIC CORPECTOMY

The patient is positioned in a standard lateral decubitis position with the back exactly perpendicular to the operating table. The patient is then secured to the table with cloth tape. Maintaining this exact orientation becomes important if the spine is to be fixated with screw plates.

Fluoroscopy is used to localize the pathology and orient the trajectory of the hardware. The skin is marked to identify the portal sites and the pathologic vertebrae. The portals may be positioned like those used for a discectomy. If, however, a screw plate is planned, coaxial portals are needed.

After a standard exposure has been performed, the lung is mobilized from the surface of the spine and the spinal level is localized visually and radiographically. The pleura is incised and mobilized over the proximal ribs of the involved vertebrae (Fig. 20–1). The segmental vessels are ligated with hemoclips and transected. The initial steps for vertebral body resection and spinal cord decompression resemble the basic steps initially used for discectomy. However, a wider surface area of the spine is exposed.

The neurovascular bundles, intercostal muscles, and ligaments are detached from the proximal 2 cm of each rib. The proximal 2 cm of each rib and the pedicles are removed

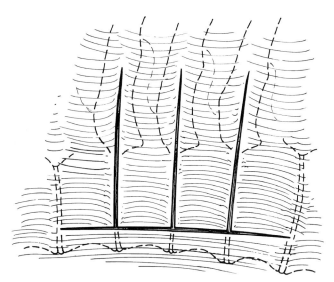

Figure 20–1. Pleural incision for thoracic corpectomy exposes multiple ribs, discs, and vertebral bodies for the decompression of the spinal cord and reconstruction of the spine.

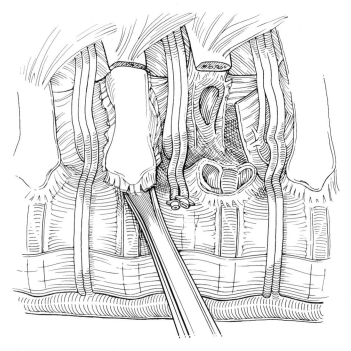

Figure 20–2. The first step in performing a corpectomy is to ligate the segmental vessels and remove the proximal ribs over the involved vertebrae. The bone is saved for graft material. The ribs are removed to expose the pedicles. [With permission from Barrow Neurological Institute.]

at the level(s) to be resected (Fig. 20–2). The ribs are saved and used as bone graft material for the reconstruction.

The pedicles are removed so the surgeon can identify the dura and avoid injuring the spinal cord by observing its position during the dissection (Fig. 20–3). Next, the discs are incised adjacent to the pathology to delineate the cephalad and caudal boundaries of the bone resection. The disc spaces can be opened and incised with an osteotome, Cobb elevator, or curettes (Fig. 20–4).

A large cavity is made in the center of the vertebral body, preserving the anterior and posterior cortices and the contralateral side of the vertebrae (Fig. 20-5). A rectangular

central corpectomy cavity is created using high-speed drills, osteotomes, oscillating saws, rongeurs, and curettes. The cavity creates a working space to decompress the spinal cord and reconstruct the spine with bone grafts. Posteriorly, the remaining thin shell of cortical bone, posterior longitudinal ligament, and any pathology compressing the spinal cord are removed by curetting the material into the cavity in the bodies. The spinal cord can thus be safely decompressed under direct visualization (Fig. 20–6).

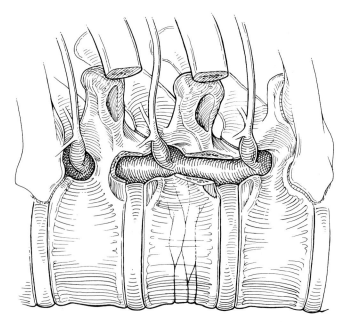

Figure 20–3. The pedicles are removed so the dura can be clearly visualized. The remainder of the procedure can then be performed while all maneuvers in relationship to the spinal cord are observed directly. [With permission from Barrow Neurological Institute.]

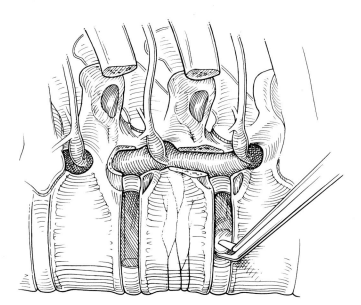

Figure 20–4. The discs at the rostral and caudal margins of the corpectomy site are removed to delineate the boundaries of the bone resection. [With permission from Barrow Neurological Institute.]

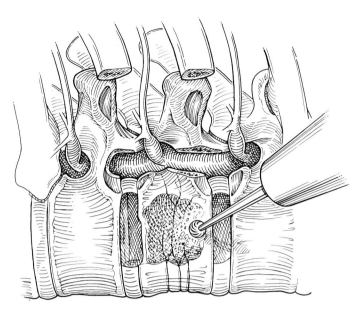

Figure 20–5.   A large cavity is created in the vertebral bodies. The bone is resected with drills, curettes, rongeurs, and osteotomes. [With permission from Barrow Neurological Institute.]

Next, the corpectomy site is prepared for the reconstruction (Fig. 20–7). The corpectomy should be extended until normal, healthy, viable, vascularized bone surface is exposed to facilitate incorporation of the reconstructive grafts. All disc material, soft tissue, and the cartilaginous end plates are removed from the corpectomy bed.

Precise carpentry techniques are used to prepare a rectangular-shaped mortise within the corpectomy bed. The

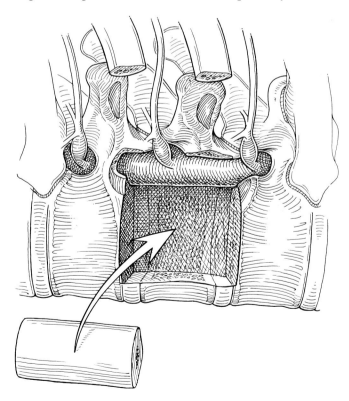

Figure 20–7.   The corpectomy bed is prepared to fit the bone graft. The end plates are decorticated and the bone graft is inserted into the fusion bed. [With permission from Barrow Neurological Institute.]

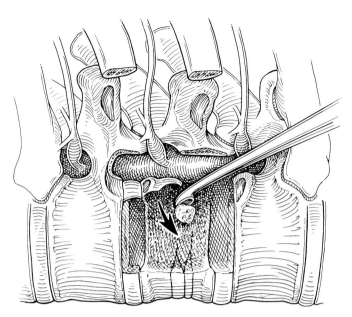

Figure 20–6.   The posterior cortex of the vertebrae, the posterior longitudinal ligament, and the pathology compressing the spinal cord are resected. The bone and ligament are dissected away from the spinal cord into the cavity in the vertebral body. [With permission from Barrow Neurological Institute.]

bone surfaces must be flush and contact the surfaces of the reconstructive grafts evenly. The dimensions of the corpectomy bed are precisely measured with a plastic ruler cut to match the size of the bone defect. A long suture is tied to the ruler so that it will be anchored externally and easy to extract from the chest. Using suture to anchor any loose items (i.e., graft, screws, bolts, plates, rulers, etc.) is a useful technique that saves the surgeon from trying to locate a disengaged item within the thorax.

The surgeon then proceeds with the vertebral reconstruction and, if needed, internal fixation. These topics are discussed in the next few chapters. The techniques for closing the chest after corpectomy are identical to the closure techniques used after discectomy.

ILLUSTRATIVE CASE

During an unsuccessful attempt at removing a herniated disc at T8–T9 through a costotransversectomy and transpedicular approach at another hospital facility, a 48-year-old women developed thoracic myelopathy and became severely paraparetic. The disc was not resected, and the patient's neurological deficits worsened during the subsequent year.

A left-sided thoracoscopic approach was used to perform T8 and T9 corpectomies to expose the spinal canal fully (Figs. 20–8 to 20–26). The base of the pedunculated disc was transected with a drill and grasped. The disc attachments were removed from the dura and from the arachnoid and pial surface of the spinal cord with microdissection tools. The disc fragments were removed to decompress the dura completely. The patient underwent a staged posterior

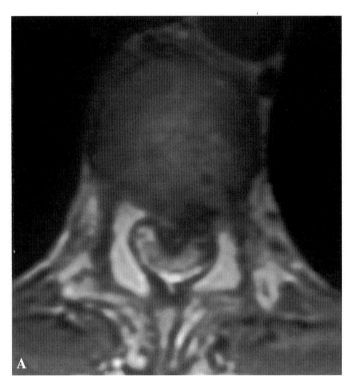
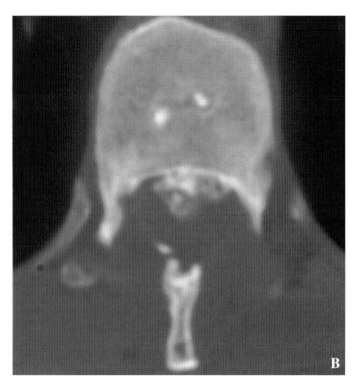

Figure 20–8. **(A)** Axial magnetic resonance image demonstrates severe compression and deformity of the spinal cord. **(B)** Computed tomographic scan demonstrates the broad-based, ossified, lobulated herniated thoracic disc at T8–T9. The left pedicle and rib and part of the right pedicle had been removed during a prior posterolateral approach that failed to resect this calcified disc.

fixation of the thoracic spine using hooks and rods to stabilize the spine. Within 2 years of surgery, her neurological condition had gradually improved to normal.

CLINICAL RESULTS OF THORACOSCOPIC CORPECTOMY

In 1996, we published the clinical outcomes of our first 17 patients treated with thoracoscopic corpectomy and reconstruction.[1] Thirteen patients presented with myelopathy and four with radiculopathy. The abnormalities causing thoracic vertebral body destruction and neural compression included tumors ($n = 7$), fractures ($n = 6$), infection ($n = 3$), or multilevel calcified herniated discs ($n = 1$). The location of the abnormalities ranged from T3 to T10 and involved either a single vertebra ($n = 11$) or two adjacent vertebrae ($n = 6$).

All operative decompressive procedures were performed satisfactorily by thoracoscopy alone. *No* patient required conversion to a thoracotomy. Most procedures were approached from the right side ($n = 15$); a left-sided approach was reserved for left-sided eccentric abnormalities ($n = 2$). The number of portals averaged 4.3 per patient (range: 3–6). Vertebral bodies were reconstructed with methylmethacrylate ($n = 5$) or bone grafts ($n = 9$). The reconstruction grafts included autogenous iliac crest bone struts ($n = 5$), allograft humerus shafts filled with autologous rib grafts ($n = 2$), or titanium mesh cages filled with

autologous bone ($n = 2$). No reconstructive grafts were placed in the three patients who required subtotal vertebrectomies for focal abnormalities.

Internal fixation was performed in 14 patients with a thoracoscopically placed ventral screw plate ($n = 11$) or posterior hook-rod instrumentation ($n = 3$). Hook-rod instrumentation was reserved for patients with kyphotic deformities or involvement of the posterior spinal elements that required posterior reduction and stabilization. Anterior thoracic screw plates were used to treat spinal instability, compress the grafts or methacrylate against the adjacent vertebrae, to prevent displacement of the reconstructive grafts, and to maintain spinal immobilization until the fusion healed.

There were no nonunions, and no patient developed loss of fixation, progression of spinal deformity, loosening of hardware, or displacement of reconstructive grafts. No patients had persistent pain from spinal instability or compression of the spinal cord or nerve root.

The neurological outcome primarily depended on the patient's status at presentation. All nine patients with mild or moderate spinal cord injuries (Frankel Grades C and D) improved. Six were neurologically normal, and three had mild residual motor deficits. None of the patients who presented with severe spinal cord dysfunction improved neurologically (Frankel Grades A and B). The pain of all four patients who initially presented with radiculopathy completely resolved.

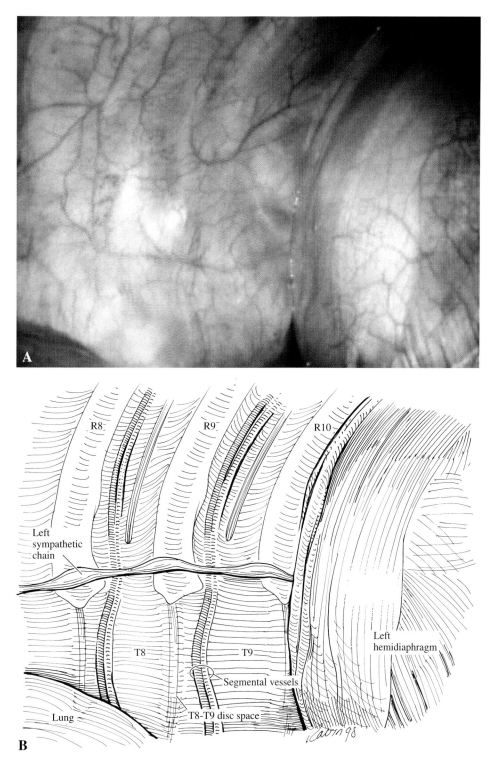

Figure 20–9. The patient underwent a left-sided thoracoscopic approach. **(A)** Intraoperative photograph and **(B)** corresponding illustration showing the diaphragm, ribs, rib heads, and vertebral bodies before the beginning of the spine dissection. R = rib.

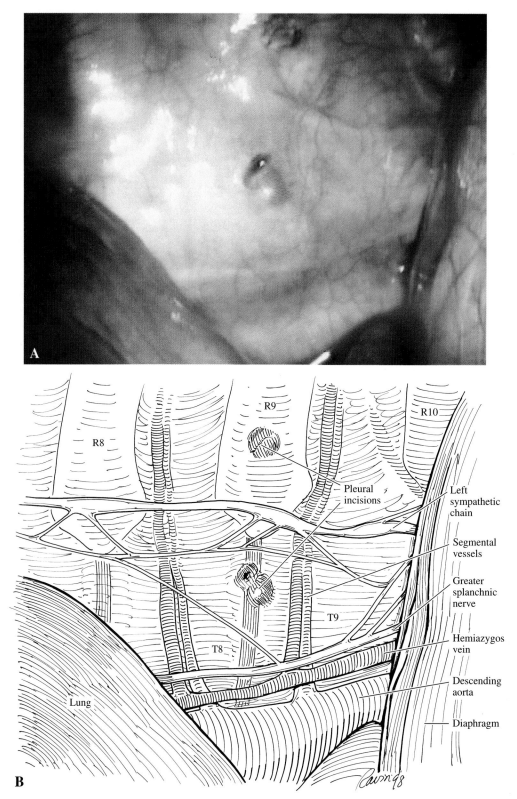

Figure 20–10.   **(A)** Intraoperative photograph and **(B)** corresponding illustration showing the pleural incision over the T9 rib head and the T8–T9 disc space that marks the level after the location is verified radiographically. The aorta, hemiazygos vein, segmental vessels, and the greater splanchnic nerves are visible at the operative site. R = rib.

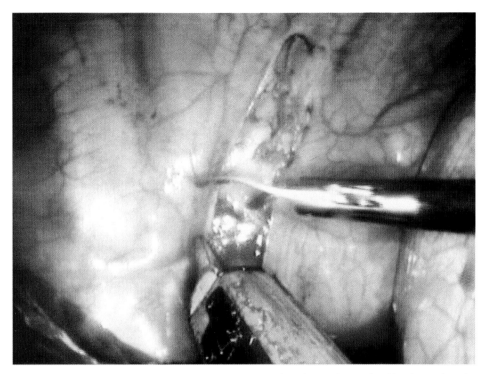

Figure 20–11. The parietal pleura is incised and mobilized to expose the ribs and vertebral bodies. The pleural edges are grasped with a forceps, everted, and incised with a scissors.

COMPARISON OF THORACOSCOPY AND THORACOTOMY FOR CORPECTOMY

Table 20–1 compares the clinical data associated with thoracoscopy and thoracotomy for a concurrent cohort of patients undergoing anterior corpectomy and reconstruction. These data were derived from a combined series of 17 thoracoscopic corpectomies performed at Johann Wolfgang Goethe University, Frankfurt, Germany, and the Barrow Neurological Institute.[1] The two groups of patients did not differ in terms of age, male-to-female ratio, type of pathol-

ogy, severity of neurological defects, or the extent of decompression and stabilization procedures performed.

No differences in the extent of decompression, reconstruction, and fixation were achieved between the two groups. No patients had residual compressive pathology. There were no significant differences between the lengths of the procedures. Thoracoscopic procedures were associated with less blood loss, less chest tube drainage, less usage of pain medication, and shorter stays in the intensive care unit and hospital compared to thoracotomy patients.

Complications in the thoracotomy group included pneumonia ($n = 2$), pleural effusion ($n = 1$), tension pneumothorax ($n = 1$), deep venous thrombosis ($n = 1$), and

TABLE 20–1   Clinical Data Comparing Vertebrectomies Performed by Thoracoscopy and Thoracotomy

Clinical Variable	Thoracoscopic Vertebrectomy Mean (Range) $n = 17$	Thoracotomy for Vertebrectomy Mean (Range) $n = 7$
Operative time (min)	347 (133–712)	393 (235–510)
Estimated blood loss (ml)	1117 (250–2000)	1557 (300–2500)
Duration of chest tube (days)	2.8 (1–8)	3.9 (1–10)
Chest tube drainage (ml)	1309 (120–3500)	1741 (128–4800)
Narcotic pain medications* (days)	4.1 (0.5–24)	8.9 (1–20)
ICU stay (days)	2.6 (1–17)	6.4 (1–22)
Hospital stay (days)	8.7 (4–31)	15.8 (5–60)

* Duration of intravenous, intramuscular, or epidural narcotic analgesic adminstration; ICU = intensive care unit.

[From Dickman CA, Rosenthal D, Karahalios DG, et al: Thoracic vertebrectomy and reconstruction using a microsurgical thoracoscopic approach. *Neurosurgery* 1996; 38(2):279–293. Reprinted with permission from Williams & Wilkins.]

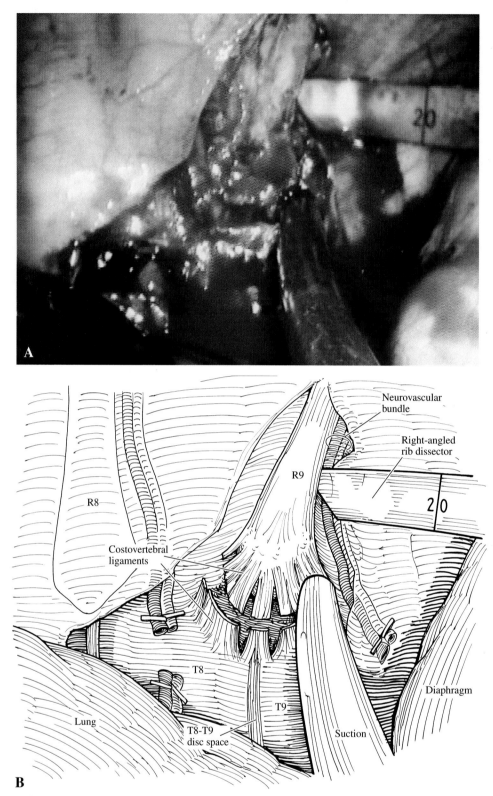

Figure 20–12. **(A)** Intraoperative photograph and **(B)** corresponding illustration showing a right–angle rib dissector being used to cut the costotransverse ligaments from the ninth rib after the neurovascular bundle has been detached from the caudal rib edge. R = rib.

intercostal neuralgia ($n = 3$). Complications in the thoracoscopy group included myocardial infarction leading to one postoperative death, transient intercostal neuralgia ($n = 2$), pleural effusion ($n = 1$), and pneumonia ($n = 1$). Intercostal neuralgia and pain syndromes were more common and more severe after thoracotomy. Two patients who underwent thoracotomy had prolonged, moderately severe pain syndromes. In contrast, the symptoms of both patients who experienced intercostal neuralgia after thoracoscopy were mild and transient.

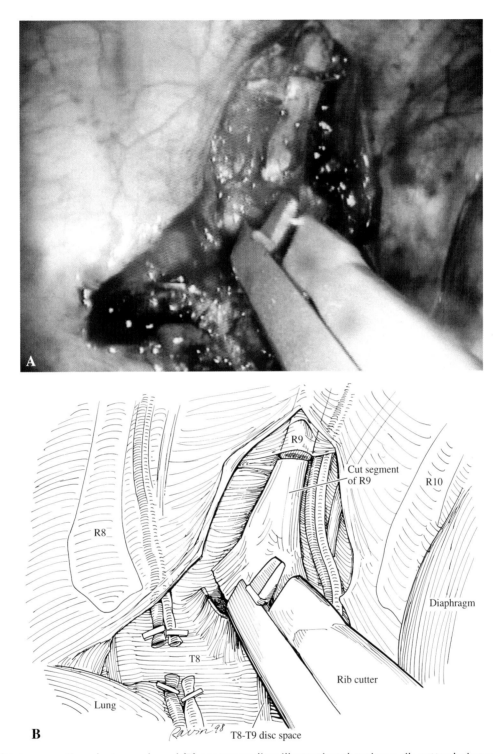

Figure 20–13. **(A)** Intraoperative photograph and **(B)** corresponding illustration showing a rib cutter being used to transect the rib. R = rib.

CONCLUSIONS

Thoracoscopy is an excellent method for performing a single-level or multiple–level corpectomy. The technique is very similar to the techniques used for microdiscectomy. However, more bone is resected and a more extensive reconstruction is required. Technically, corpectomy can be easier to perform than a thoracoscopic microdiscectomy because the larger operative field provides more mobility and visibility for the surgeon.

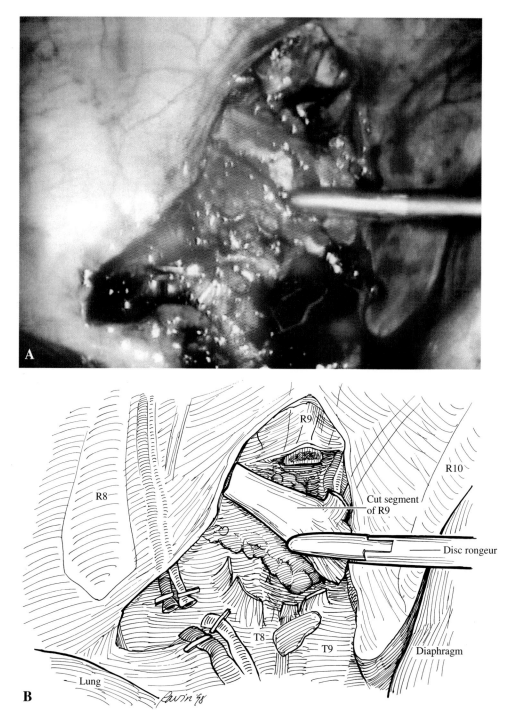

Figure 20–14. **(A)** Intraoperative photograph and **(B)** corresponding illustration showing the proximal rib and rib head being removed en bloc. The bone is saved for graft material. R = rib.

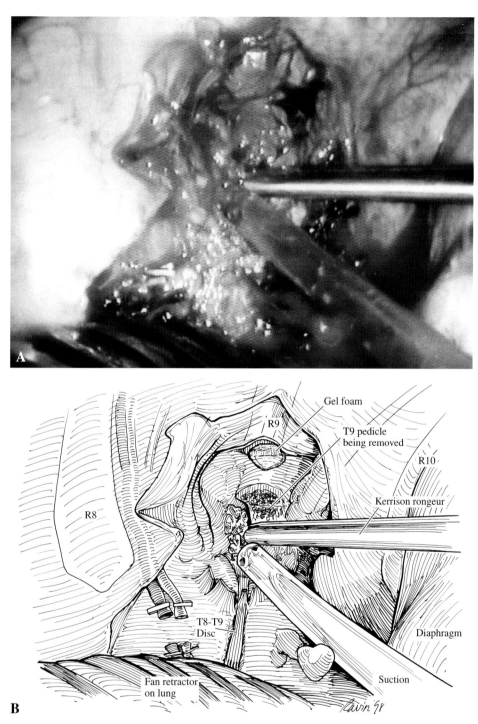

Figure 20–15. **(A)** Intraoperative photograph and **(B)** corresponding illustration showing a Kerrison rongeur being used to remove the pedicle of T9 so the epidural space can be identified before the vertebral body is resected. R = rib.

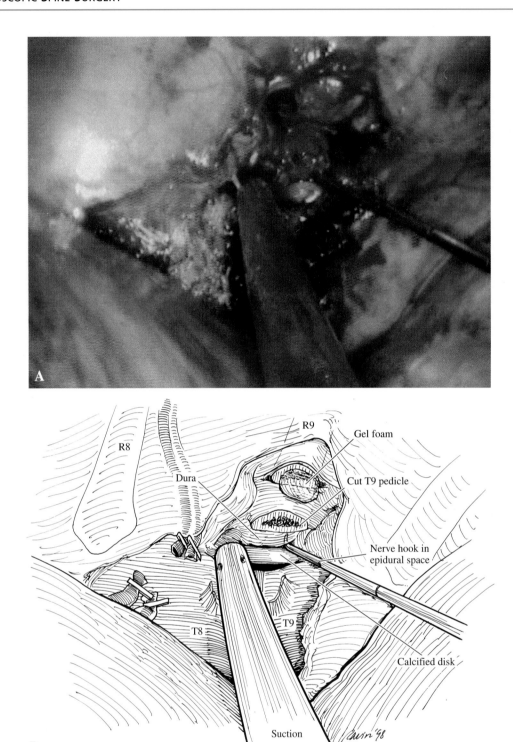

Figure 20–16.   **(A)** Intraoperative photograph and **(B)** corresponding illustration showing a nerve hook being placed into the epidural space to feel the calcified disc fragment. R = rib.

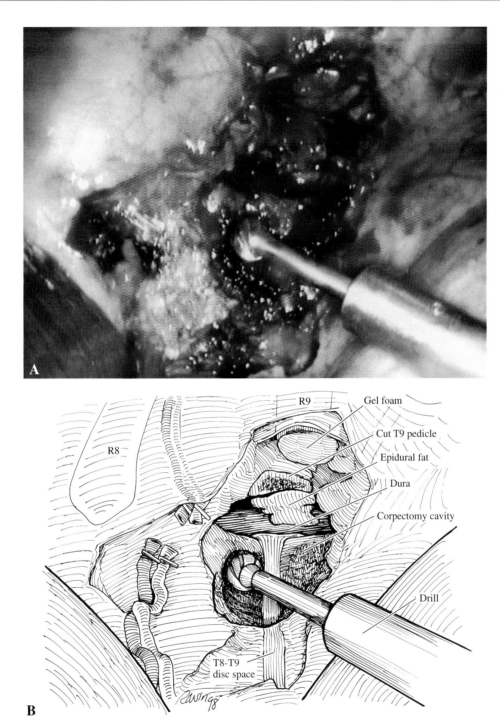

Figure 20–17. **(A)** Intraoperative photograph and **(B)** corresponding illustration showing a cutting burr being used to resect the vertebral bodies. R = rib.

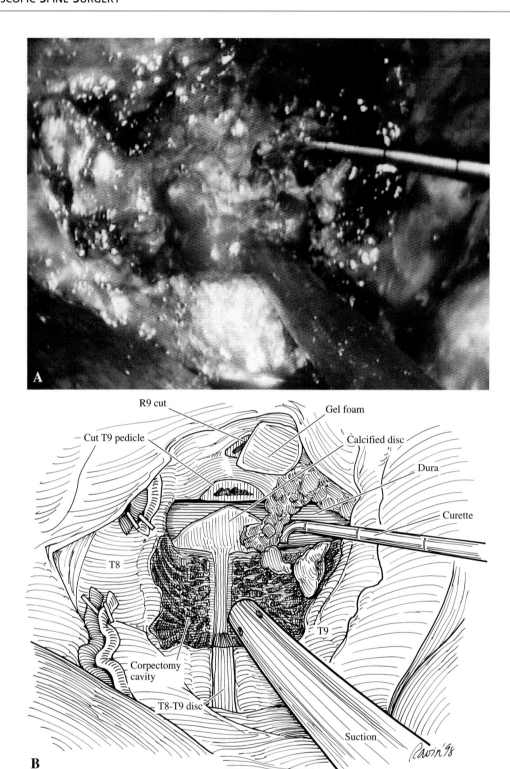

Figure 20–18. **(A)** Intraoperative photograph and **(B)** corresponding illustration showing a large rectangular cavity being created in the T8 and T9 vertebral bodies. The posterior longitudinal ligament is removed with a curved curette, and normal dura is exposed above and below the large intradural disc. The cavity is then deepened across the spinal canal. R = rib.

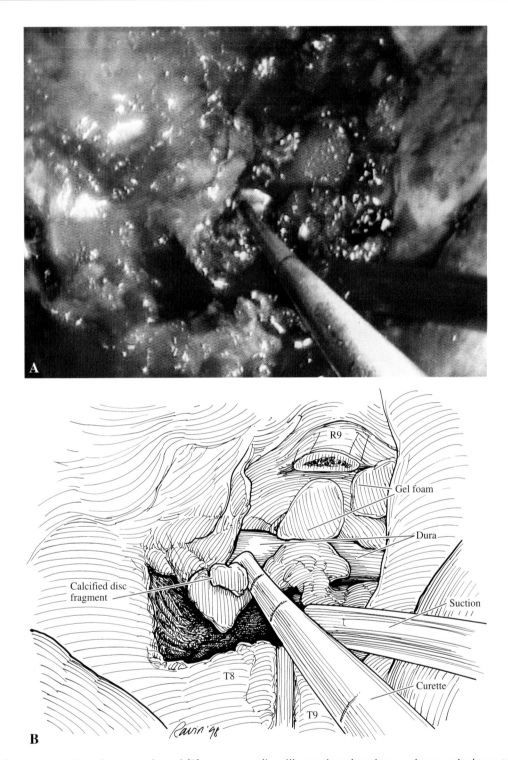

Figure 20–19. **(A)** Intraoperative photograph and **(B)** corresponding illustration showing a microsurgical curette being used to remove a large lobular piece of calcified disc. The disc is being pulled away from the spinal cord into the corpectomy cavity. R = rib.

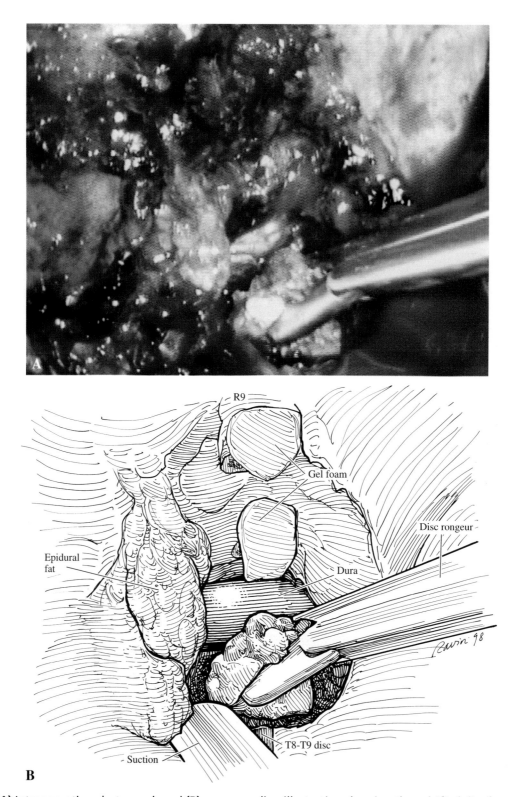

Figure 20–20.   **(A)** Intraoperative photograph and **(B)** corresponding illustration showing the calcified disc fragment being removed with a disc rongeur. R = rib.

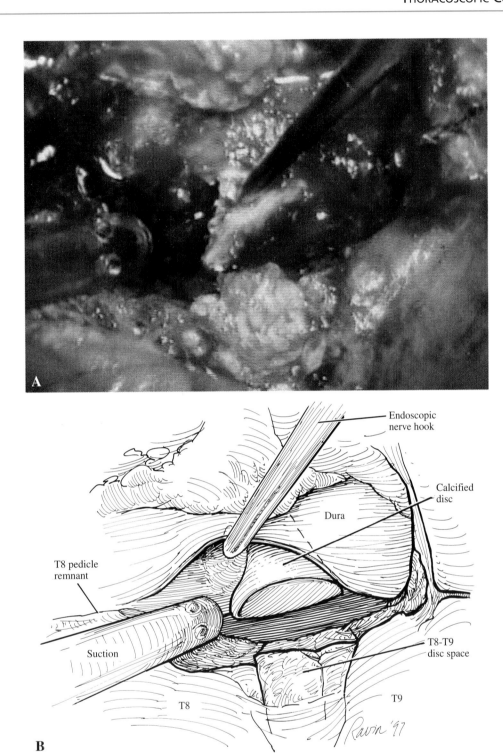

Figure 20–21. **(A)** Intraoperative photograph and **(B)** corresponding illustration showing a remaining fragment of peduncular disc that extended intradurally. The disc is separated from its dural attachments. [From Rosenthal D and Dickman CA: Thoracoscopic microsurgical excision of herniated thoracic discs. J Neurosurg 1998; 89:224–235. With permission from the Journal of Neurosurgery.]

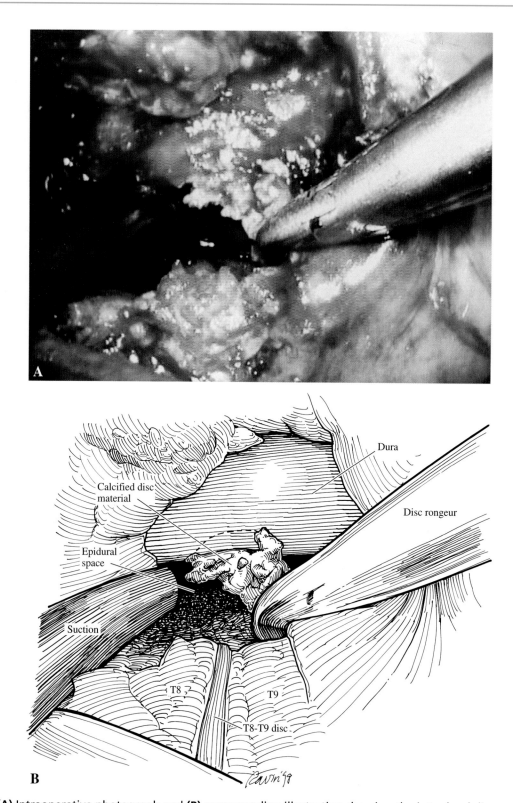

Figure 20–22. **(A)** Intraoperative photograph and **(B)** corresponding illustration showing the intradural disc material being gently removed with a disc rongeur.

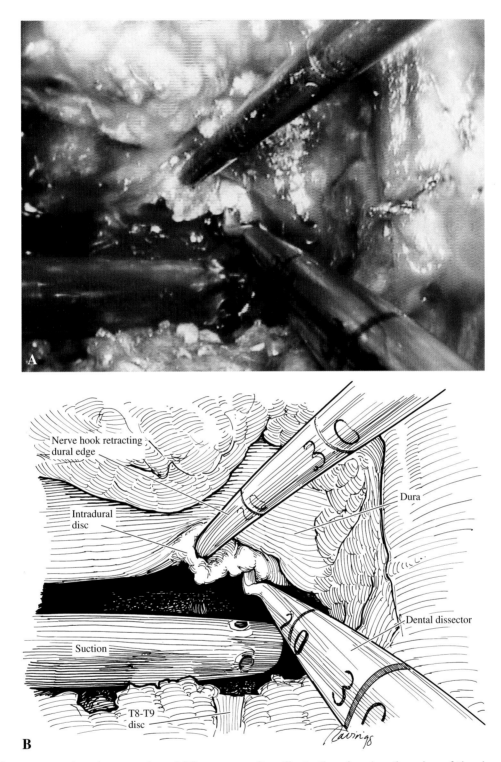

Figure 20–23. **(A)** Intraoperative photograph and **(B)** corresponding illustration showing the edge of the dura being retracted with an endoscopic nerve hook, while an endoscopic dental dissector is used to gently dissect the intradural disc material from the pial surface of the spinal cord.

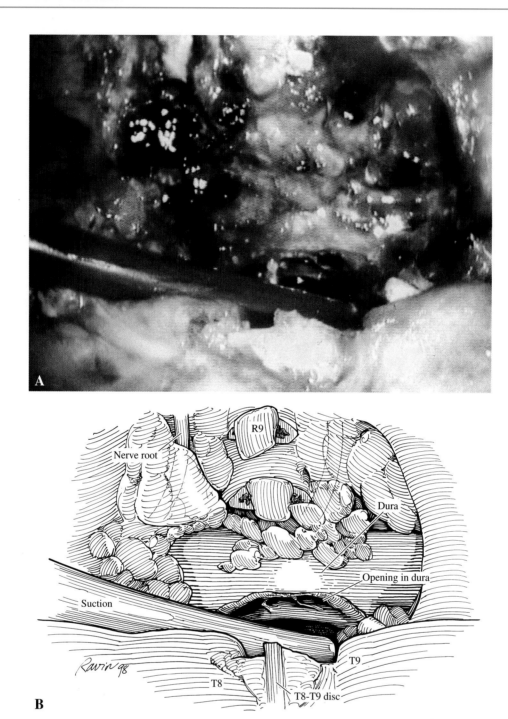

Figure 20–24. **(A)** Intraoperative photograph and **(B)** corresponding illustration showing the spinal cord after it was completely decompressed. All the intradural disc material has been removed. The linear dural defect is sealed with fibrin glue, and a lumbar drain is placed prophylactically to prevent a subarachnoid-pleural cerebrospinal fluid fistula from developing. R = rib.

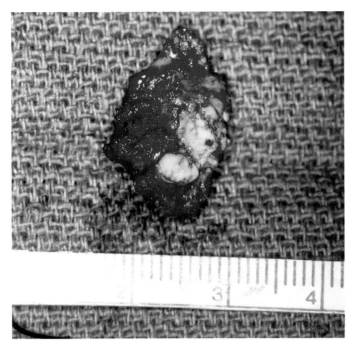

Figure 20–25. Photograph of the calcified intradural disc fragment.

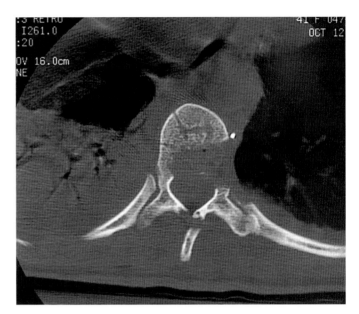

Figure 20–26. Postoperative computed tomographic scan demonstrates complete resection of the calcified disc and the rectangular corpectomy cavity.

REFERENCES

1. Dickman CA, Rosenthal D, Karahalios DG, et al: Thoracic vertebrectomy and reconstruction using a microsurgical thoracoscopic approach. *Neurosurgery* 1996; 38(2):279–293.

2. Sundaresan N, Galicich JH, Lane JM, et al: Treatment of neoplastic epidural cord compression by vertebral body resection and stabilization. *J Neurosurg* 1985; 63:676–684.

3. Sundaresan N, Galicich JH, Bains MS, et al: Vertebral body resection in the treatment of cancer involving the spine. *Cancer* 1984; 53:1393–1396.

4. McAfee PC, Zdeblick TA: Tumors of the thoracic and lumbar spine: Surgical treatment via the anterior approach. *J Spinal Disord* 1989; 2(3):145–154.

5. Rosenthal D, Marquardt G, Lorenz R, et al: Anterior decompression and stabilization using a microsurgical endoscopic technique for metastatic tumors of the thoracic spine. *J Neurosurg* 1996; 84:565–572.

6. Sundaresan N, Shah J, Foley KM, et al: An anterior surgical approach to the upper thoracic vertebrae. *J Neurosurg* 1984; 61:686–690.

7. Otani K, Yoshida M, Fujii E, et al: Thoracic disc herniation. Surgical treatment in 23 patients. *Spine* 1988; 13(11):1262–1267.

8. Lobosky JM, Hitchon PW, McDonnell DE: Transthoracic anterolateral decompression for thoracic spine lesions. *Neurosurgery* 1984; 14:26–30.

9. McAfee PC, Regan JR, Zdeblick TA, et al: The incidence of complications in endoscopic anterior thoracolumbar spinal reconstructive surgery. A prospective multicenter study comprising the first 100 consecutive cases. *Spine* 1995; 20(14):1624–1632.

10. Harrington KD: Anterior cord decompression and spinal stabilization for patients with metastatic lesions of the spine. *J Neurosurg* 1984; 61:107–117.

11. Larson SJ, Holst RA, Hemmy DC, et al: Lateral extracavitary approach to traumatic lesions of the thoracic and lumbar spine. *J Neurosurg* 1976; 45(6):628–637.

12. Patterson RH, Jr., Arbit E: A surgical approach through the pedicle to protruded thoracic discs. *J Neurosurg* 1978; 48(5):768–772.

13. Fessler RG, Dietze DD, Jr., Mac Millan M, et al: Lateral parascapular extrapleural approach to the upper thoracic spine. *J Neurosurg* 1991; 75:349–355.

14. Le Roux PD, Haglund MM, Harris AB: Thoracic disc disease: Experience with the transpedicular approach in twenty consecutive patients. *Neurosurgery* 1993; 33:58–66.

15. Maiman DJ, Larson SJ, Luck E, et al: Lateral extracavitary approach to the spine for thoracic disc herniation: Report of 23 cases. *Neurosurgery* 1984; 14(2):178–182.

16. Garrido E: Modified costotransversectomy: A surgical approach to ventrally placed lesions in the thoracic spinal canal. *Surg Neurol* 1980; 13(2):109–113.

17. Stillerman CB, Chen TC, Day JD, et al: The transfacet pedicle–sparing approach for thoracic disc removal: Cadaveric morphometric analysis and preliminary clinical experience. *J Neurosurg* 1995; 83:971–976.

CHAPTER 21

Thoracoscopic Spinal Reconstruction Techniques

Curtis A. Dickman, M.D. and Daniel J. Rosenthal, M.D.

Thoracoscopy provides several alternatives for interbody fusion and vertebral body reconstruction. The goals of these techniques are to fill in structural defects, to achieve mechanical stability, to restore axial load-bearing, to prevent spinal deformity from developing, and to achieve arthrodesis of the involved spine segments.

DISC SPACE ARTHRODESIS

Fusion across single disc spaces or across multiple disc levels may be desired after osteotomies or anterior releases to treat scoliosis or kyphotic deformities or for epiphysiodesis to prevent the crankshaft phenomenon in skeletally immature patients with scoliosis (i.e., continued progression of the deformity due to mismatched growth across the unfused ventral spinal segments and no growth across the fused posterolateral segments). Fusion across the disc space can also be elected after a thoracic microdiscectomy is performed for a herniated intervertebral disc.

The options for grafting or reconstructive material across a thoracic disc space include autograft rib or iliac crest (solid blocks or a morcellized slurry), allograft, or demineralized bone matrix. In the future, bone morphogenic protein and interbody threaded fusion cages may also become available clinically for use in the thoracic spine.

THORACOSCOPIC ANTERIOR RELEASE OF SPINAL DEFORMITY

Anterior release refers to the transection of anterior attachment of spinal soft tissue (i.e., annulus, anterior longitudinal ligament, and scar tissue) required to correct chronic progressive kyphotic or scoliotic curvatures.[1-3] This technique consists of modified multilevel discectomies and has been used extensively in orthopedic surgery for spinal deformities. This topic is discussed in more depth in Chapters 15 and 16.

The pleura is incised over the disc spaces of interest; however, the dura need not be exposed. The rib heads are not removed unless a thoracoplasty is being performed in association with the correction of the curvature. At each disc space, the annulus is incised; disc material is removed with curettes and rongeurs; and the end plates are decorticated with curettes, osteotomes, or drills. After the vertebral end plates are decorticated, the bone grafts (solid struts or a slurry of bone) are inserted to serve as the substrate for fusion. We prefer solid bone grafts because they can be impacted into the disc spaces under compression to facilitate interbody fusion (Fig. 21–1). After the anterior release is performed, the curvature is reduced and fixated, typically with a posteriorly applied universal hook-rod system.

INTERBODY FUSION AFTER THORACIC DISCECTOMY

If a moderate-sized cavity is made in the vertebrae to perform a discectomy, a fusion may be considered, especially if the patient has osteoporosis or has undergone a prior posterior approach to the spine at that level. The patients' own rib graft, harvested during the exposure, can be used as a strut to bridge the bone defect. A recessed mortise should be created to anchor the graft into position and prevent it from migrating (Fig. 21–2). The thoracic BAK™ threaded interbody fusion cage (SpineTech, Inc., Minneapolis, MN) is another device that may be useful for thoracic interbody fusion (Fig. 21–3). Their use in the thoracic spine, however, is experimental. Currently, these cages have only been approved for use for posterior and anterior interbody fusion in the lumbar spine. When used for thoracic interbody

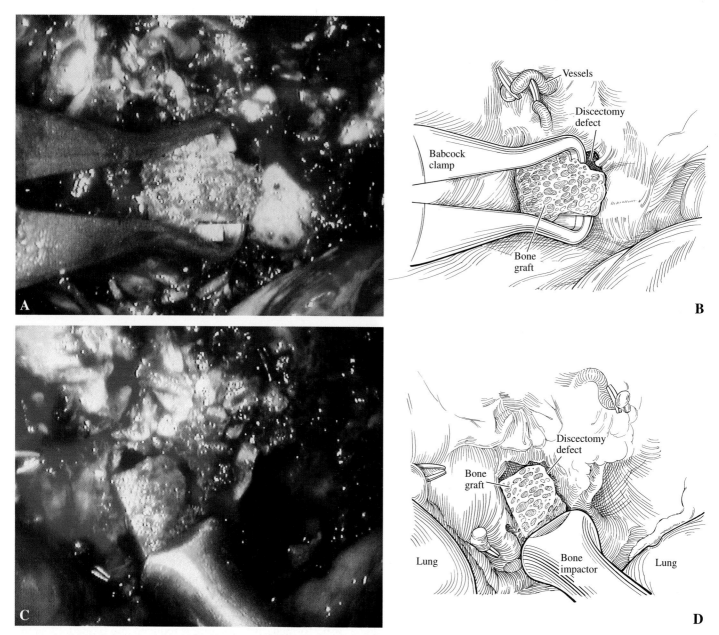

Figure 21–1. **(A)** Intraoperative photograph and **(B)** corresponding illustration show corticocancellous autografts being inserted onto the surface of the spine with an endoscopic Babcock clamp. **(C)** Intraoperative photograph and **(D)** corresponding illustration show the solid bone grafts being compressed into the decorticated disc space with a graft impactor after a multilevel anterior release and discectomy have been performed. The vertebral end plates have been removed to facilitate graft incorporation. [From Dickman CA and Mican CA. Multilevel anterior thoracic discectomies and anterior interbody fusion using a microsurgical thoracoscopic approach. Case report. *J Neurosurg* 1996;84:104–109. With permission from the Journal of Neurosurgery.]

fusion, a single cage is inserted from a lateral approach, with a coronal orientation across the disc space.

VERTEBRAL BODY RECONSTRUCTION

A vertebral body defect may be reconstructed after a corpectomy with autogenous tricortical iliac crest bone struts, whole shaft humerus allograft struts, titanium mesh cages, or methylmethacrylate. The grafts or reconstruction material must be strong enough to withstand the large forces transmitted to the thoracic spine. The grafts must be narrow enough to fit within the corpectomy, yet preserve space for the spinal cord.

Before a corpectomy site is reconstructed, the defect must be precisely mortised with level, smooth, decorticated bone surfaces that are free of soft tissue. This step provides flush contact with the graft and maximizes the incorporation of the graft. The upper or lower edge of the bone graft may be beveled slightly to facilitate insertion of the graft. The length, width, and depth of the corpectomy defect are measured precisely with a ruler.

Reconstruction with Bone Grafts

If a thoracic kyphotic deformity is present, the surgeon reduces it by applying direct manual compression against the apex of the kyphosis, pushing ventrally on the patient's

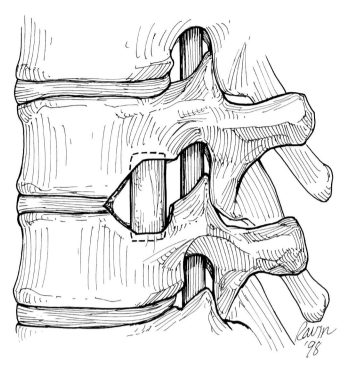

Figure 21–2. An autologous rib graft can be used to fuse the disc space after a thoracoscopic microdiscectomy.

back against the spinous process (Fig. 21–4). Reducing the kyphosis enlarges the corpectomy defect and aligns the end plates in parallel positions. While the reduction is held, the graft is sized to fit precisely within the defect (Fig. 21–5). After the external reductive force is released, the spine recoils, compressing the graft against the end plates.

Reconstructive grafts are placed into the chest end-on through a 20-mm portal through a tissue dilator or an enlarged intercostal incision (i.e., mini-utility thoracotomy; Fig. 21–6). The grafts are grasped securely with an endoscopic clamp within the chest and precisely delivered into the corpectomy bed. The movement of the graft must be completely controlled and visualized to ensure that the graft does not become displaced or compress the spinal cord. The

grafts are wedged into position in the corpectomy bed using a bone graft impactor. By manually reducing the kyphosis, sizing the grafts precisely, and beveling the corners of the graft, the grafts can be compressed into the surrounding bone (Figs. 21–5 to 21–22).

Vertebral body defects can also be reconstructed with titanium mesh cages. A titanium mesh cages can be filled with the patient's own bone graft (rib or other bone) and used as a strut. The cage provides a structural spacer between the vertebral bodies. The fenestrations in the cage allow bone ingrowth (Figs. 21–23 to 21–31). Humerus allograft struts can also be used like a "biological" cage. The center of the graft can be filled with the patient's own bone to promote its incorporation and fusion. Dense cortical allograft provides structural support and remodels and incorporates much more slowly than cancellous autograft bone.

Reconstruction with Methylmethacrylate

If a tumor has been resected, reconstruction can be performed relatively easily with methylmethacrylate.[4–9] The dimensions of the vertebrectomy defect are measured. The adjacent normal vertebrae are used to anchor the methylmethacrylate. A sterile, flexible, silastic tube is cut so that it is 5 or 6 mm longer than the end plates at the margin of the vertebrectomy defect. The end plates of the adjacent normal vertebrae are penetrated, and large holes are made into the adjacent vertebrae with drills and curettes to fit the diameter of the tube. The silastic tube, which serves as a template for the methylmethacrylate until it sets, is telescoped into the bodies of the adjacent vertebrae. A hole is cut in the middle of the tube to allow the injection of the methylmethacrylate. A long, wide-bore needle with a pressure syringe is used to inject the methylmethacrylate. Slow-setting cranioplasty methylmethacrylate is preferred to rapid-setting methylmethacrylate because it allows the polymer to be injected. It also produces much less heat as it

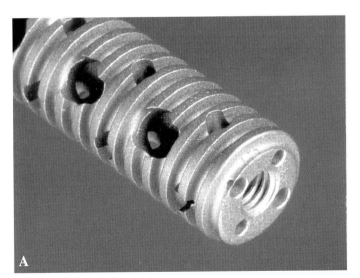
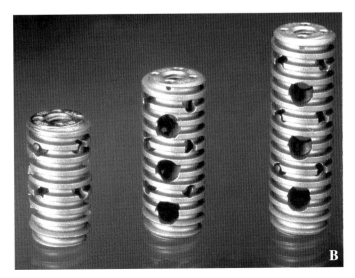

Figure 21–3. **(A)** The BAK™ (SpineTech, Minneapolis, MN) threaded thoracic interbody fusion cage is made of titanium. The hollow fenestrated cage is packed with bone graft. **(B)** The thoracic cages are available in several sizes.

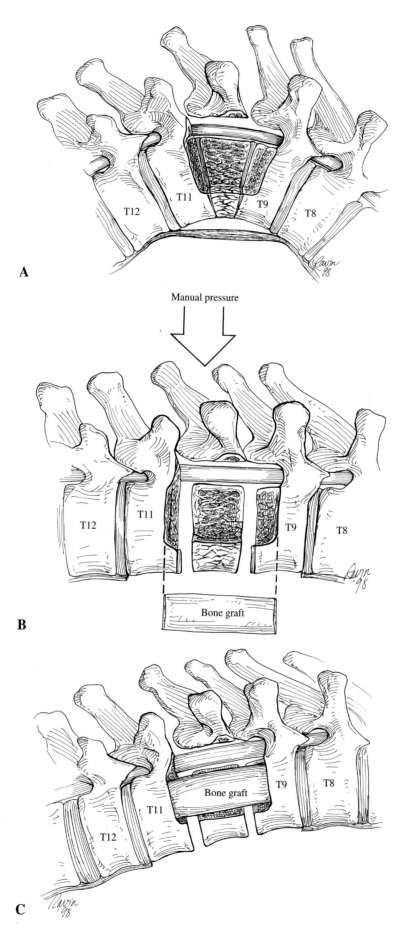

Figure 21–4. **(A)** A thoracic kyphotic deformity is most easily reduced directly by the surgeon pushing ventrally with his or her hand against the spinous processes externally at the apex of the kyphosis. **(B)** The force manually reduces the kyphosis, expands the corpectomy defect, and brings the end plates parallel. **(C)** The graft is precisely sized and inserted into the defect. The manual force is then released. The spine recoils back toward the kyphosed position, locking the strut under compression. The compressed strut is anchored, preventing further deformity.

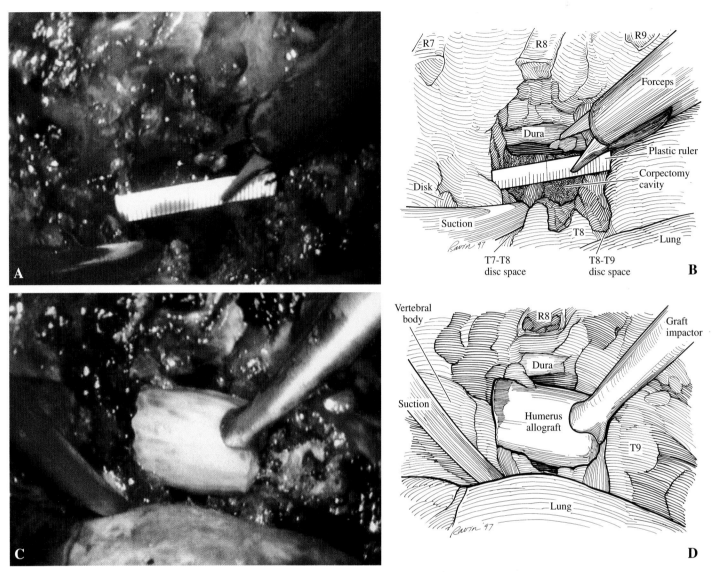

Figure 21–5. **(A)** Intraoperative photograph and **(B)** corresponding illustration of a left-sided corpectomy performed to decompress a compression fracture at T8. A plastic ruler is inserted into the cavity to measure the dimensions of the bone graft. **(C)** Intraoperative photograph and **(D)** corresponding illustration show a humerus allograft filled with autograft bone being inserted into the corpectomy defect. The space for the spinal cord is preserved.

sets, thereby minimizing the risk of thermal injury to the spinal cord. The methylmethacrylate is injected until it completely fills the silastic tubing and "toothpastes" through the ends into the adjacent vertebrae. The silastic tube acts like a mold while the methylmethacrylate hardens. The methylmethacrylate must be extruded into the adjacent bone to provide an anchor that prevents the polymer from loosening or becoming displaced. Additional methylmethacrylate can be added ventral and lateral to the tube; however, care should be taken to ensure that the dura and spinal cord are not compressed by any of the acrylic material (Figs. 21–32 to 21–34).

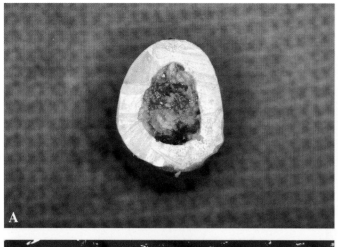

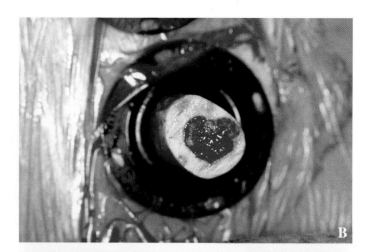

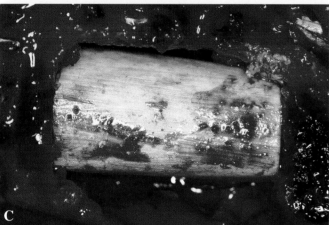

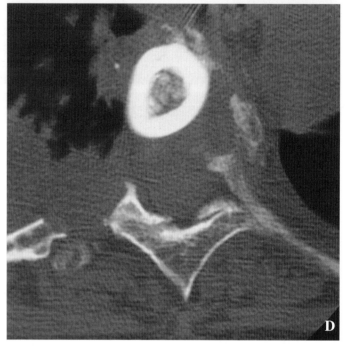

Figure 21–6. **(A)** A 16-mm diameter humerus allograft is filled with the patient's rib. **(B)** The graft is inserted into the chest through a 20-mm diameter portal. **(C)** The graft is positioned precisely into the corpectomy site, preserving the space for the spinal cord. **(D)** Postoperative computed tomographic scan demonstrates the graft in position in the T5 vertebral body. [B used with permission from Barrow Neurological Institute.]

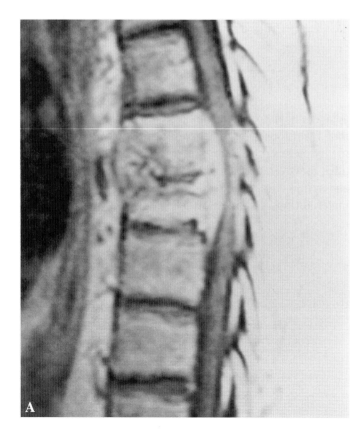

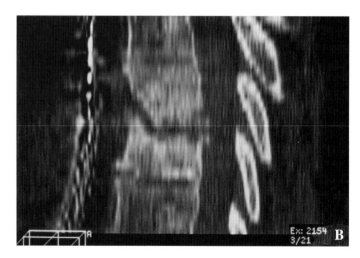

Figure 21–7. A 50-year-old man presented with acute paraparesis from an epidural abscess and vertebral osteomyelitis at T6–T7. **(A)** A sagittal magnetic resonance image demonstrates the epidural abscess and infected bone. The spinal cord is compressed by the abscess. **(B)** The vertebrae show lytic erosion from the infection. The patient was treated with a right-sided approach for thoracoscopic corpectomy and reconstruction. This surgical procedure is presented in Figures 21–8 to 21–22.

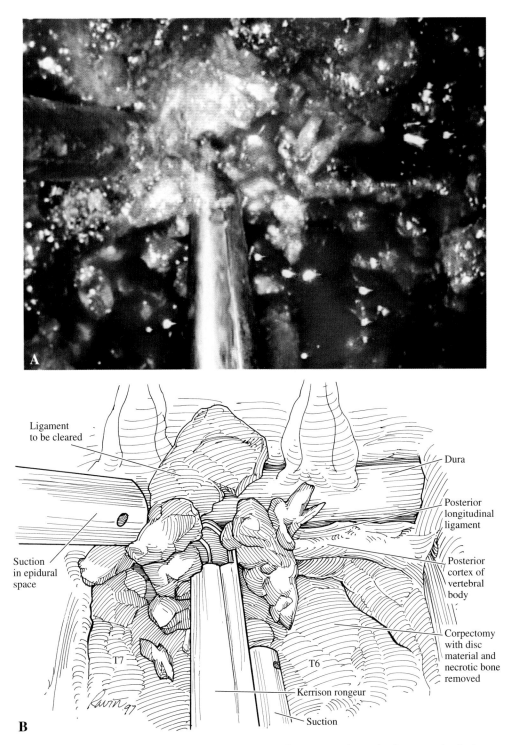

Figure 21–8. **(A)** Intraoperative photograph and **(B)** corresponding illustration show the large cavity being created in the T6 and T7 vertebral bodies. The posterior longitudinal ligament is removed with a Kerrison rongeur. The spinal cord is completely decompressed, and all necrotic and devitalized bone is debrided.

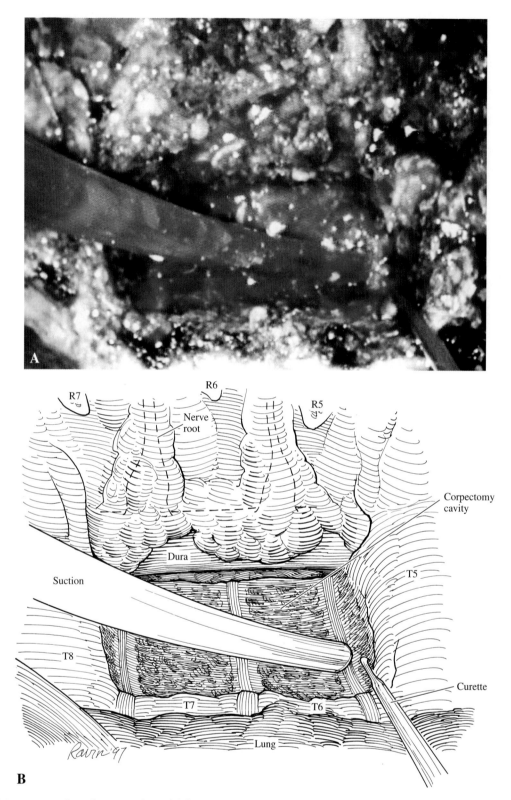

Figure 21–9. **(A)** Intraoperative photograph and **(B)** corresponding illustration show the corpectomy being mortised into a smooth rectangular bed. The disc material and end plates are removed to facilitate incorporation of the graft. The entire ventral surface of the spinal cord is visible. R = rib.

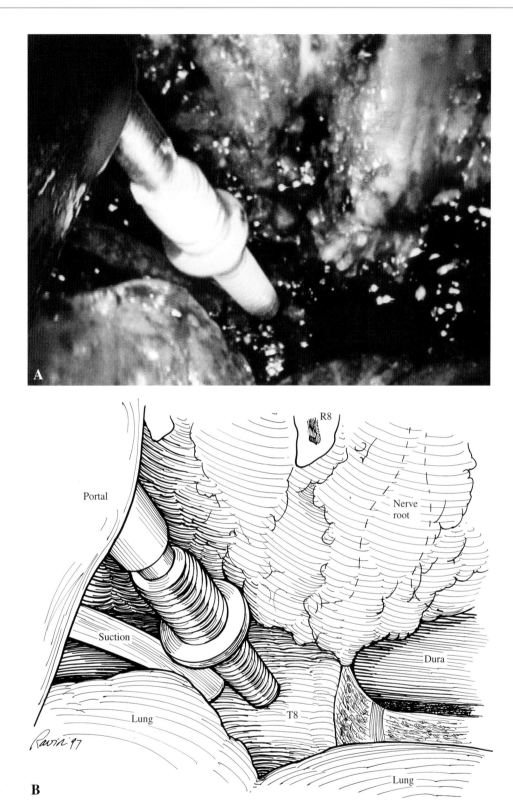

Figure 21–10. **(A)** Intraoperative photograph and **(B)** corresponding illustration show a bolt being placed in the vertebral body caudal to the corpectomy. The trajectory of the bolt is monitored under direct endoscopic vision and fluoroscopically. The bolt is angled 10° *away* from the spinal cord. R = rib.

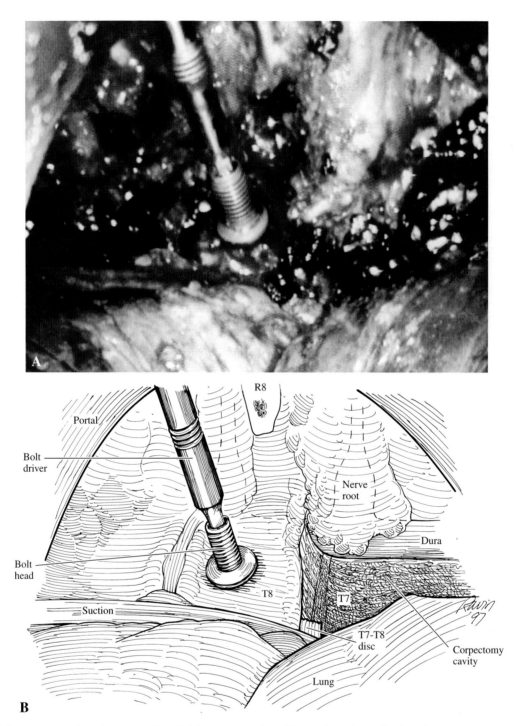

Figure 21–11. **(A)** Intraoperative photograph and **(B)** corresponding illustration show the bolt being positioned flush against the bone surface. R = rib.

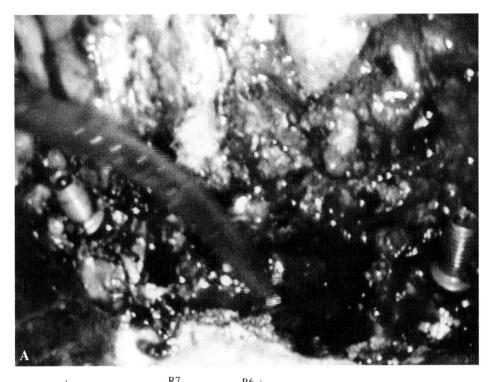

A

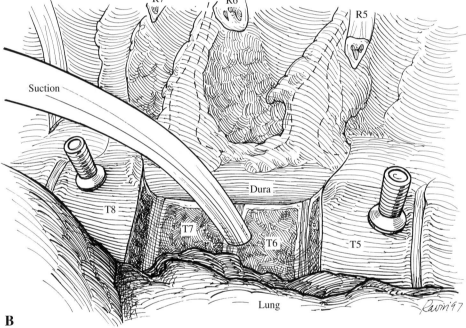

B

Figure 21–12. (A) Intraoperative photograph and (B) corresponding illustration show bolts being placed into the vertebrae rostral and caudal to the corpectomy site before the bone graft is inserted so that the trajectory of the bolts can be observed in relationship to the spinal cord. R = rib.

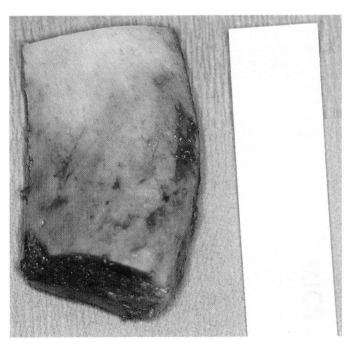

Figure 21–13. A large, tricortical, iliac crest autograft is harvested to reconstruct the vertebral bodies. The graft is cut to fit the dimensions of the corpectomy site precisely.

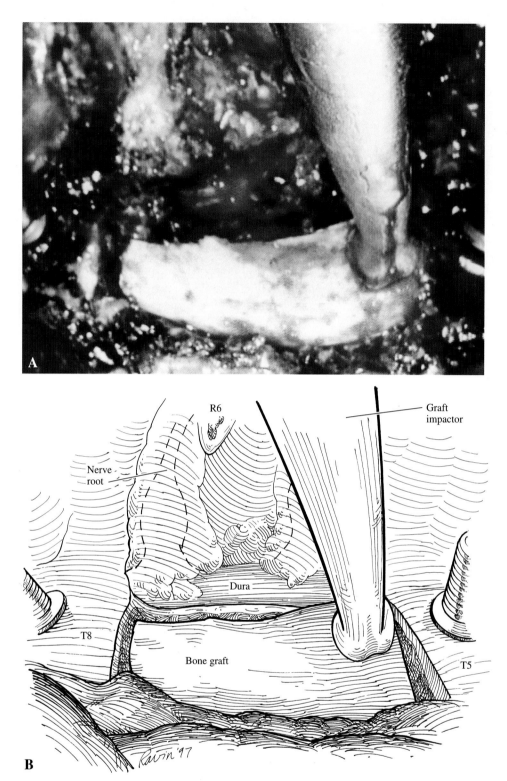

Figure 21–14. **(A)** Intraoperative photograph and **(B)** corresponding illustration show the graft being inserted precisely into the corpectomy site. The space for the spinal cord is clearly visualized and preserved. R = rib.

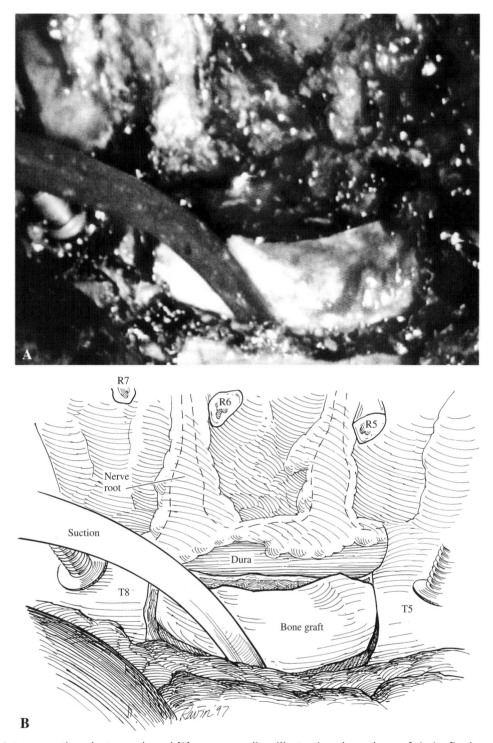

Figure 21–15. **(A)** Intraoperative photograph and **(B)** corresponding illustration show the graft in its final position compressed against the end plates of the adjacent vertebrae. The spinal cord decompression is fully preserved. R = rib.

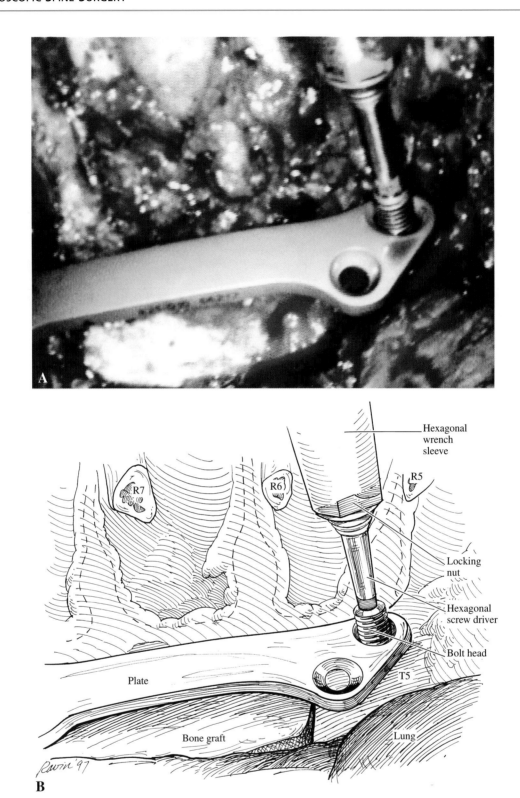

Figure 21–16. **(A)** Intraoperative photograph and **(B)** corresponding illustration show a Z-plate being inserted on top of the bolts. Locking nuts are inserted onto the bolts to lock the plate and bolts together. R = rib.

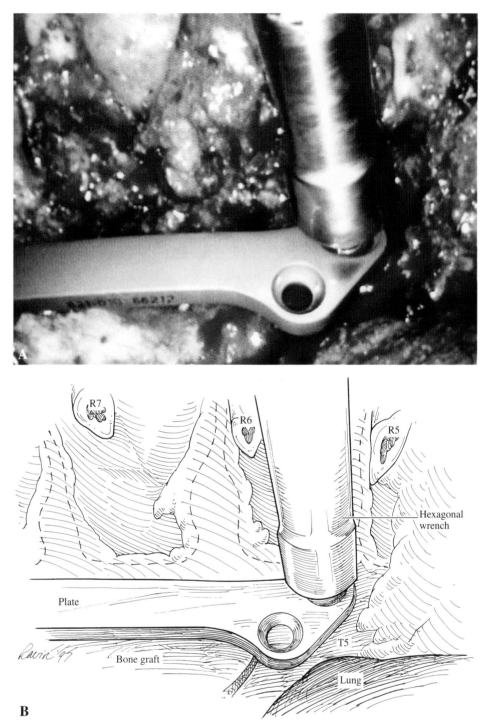

Figure 21–17. **(A)** Intraoperative photograph and **(B)** corresponding illustration show the nuts being secured with a hexagonal wrench that is integrated onto the shaft of the screwdrivers. R = rib.

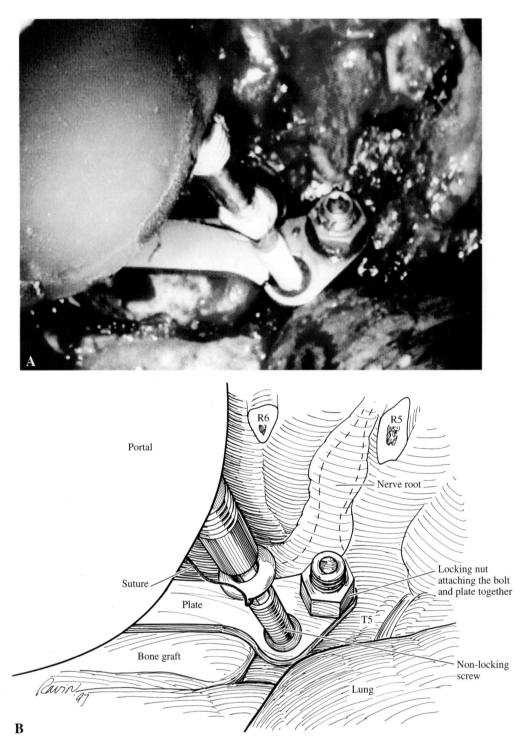

Figure 21–18. **(A)** Intraoperative photograph and **(B)** corresponding illustration show a nonlocking screw being inserted into the T5 vertebrae. The screw converges 10° toward the midline. A suture is tied to the screw in case the screw needs to be retrieved from the chest. R = rib.

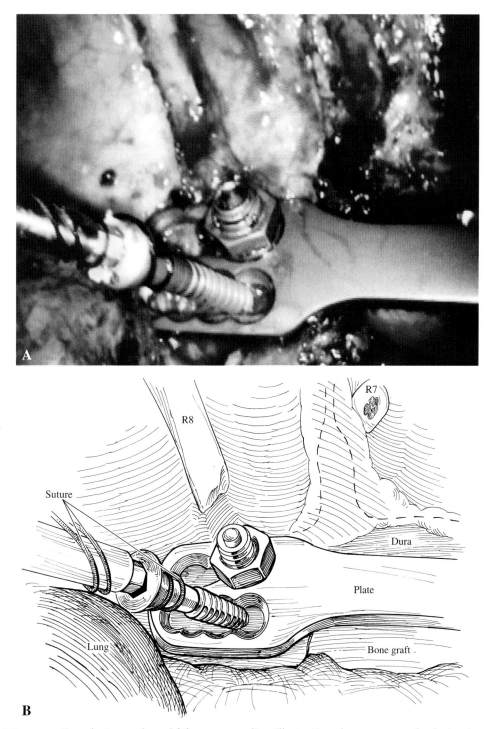

Figure 21–19. **(A)** Intraoperative photograph and **(B)** corresponding illustration show a screw also being inserted into the T8 vertebral body to anchor the plate. R = rib.

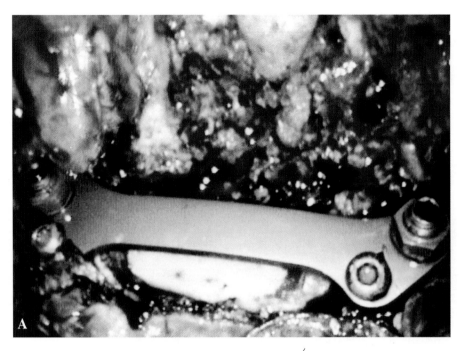

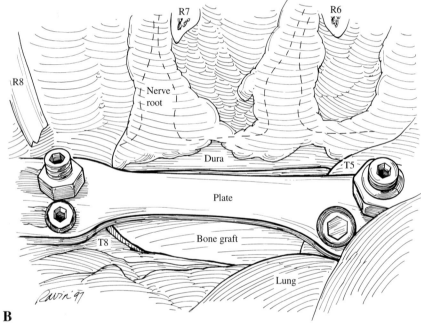

Figure 21–20. **(A)** Intraoperative photograph and **(B)** corresponding illustration show the screws, plate, and graft in their final position. R = rib.

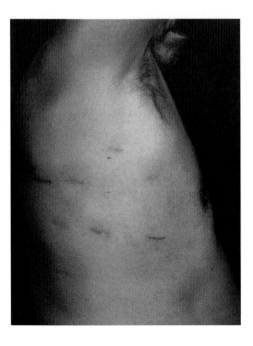

Figure 21–21. Postoperative photograph showing the patient's chest incisions.

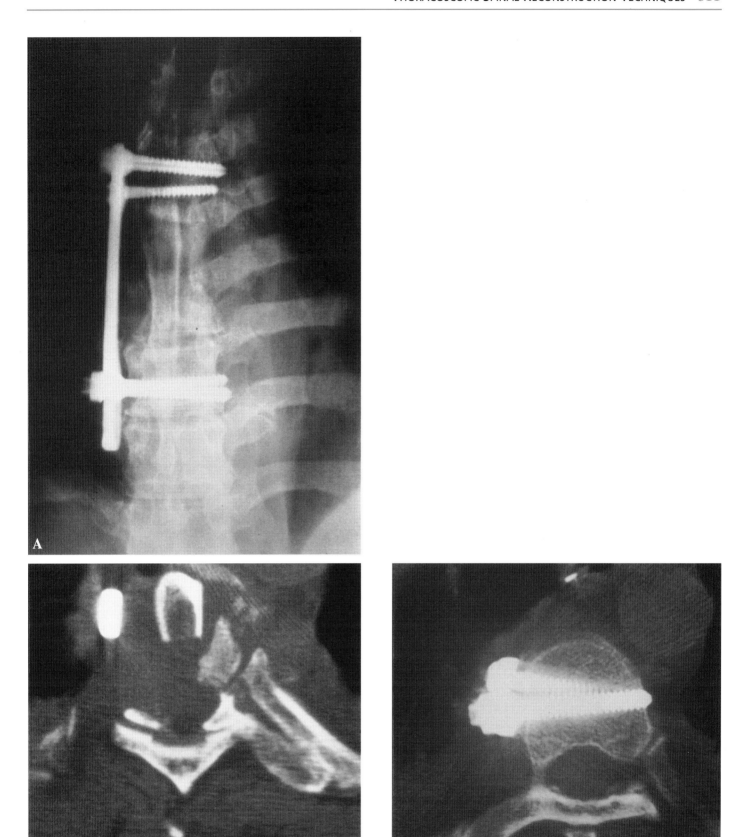

Figure 21–22. **(A)** Postoperative anteroposterior radiograph and **(B)** axial computed tomographic (CT) scan showing the corpectomy site. **(C)** Axial CT through the level of the screws and bolts. Postoperatively, the patient had minimal pain and was discharged to a spinal rehabilitation unit on the fifth postoperative day. He had no postoperative complications; his infection cleared with antibiotic treatment; and he completely recovered normal neurological function. At a follow-up examination 3 years after surgery, he had an osseous union. His hardware was intact and his neurological function was normal.

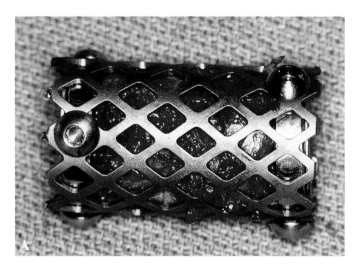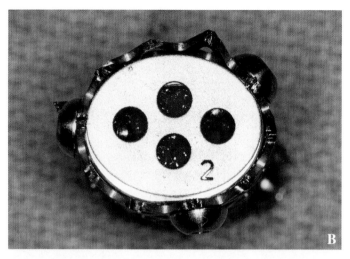

Figure 21–23. A titanium mesh cage can be filled with autograft bone and used to reconstruct a corpectomy defect. **(A)** The cage has wide fenestrations to allow bone ingrowth. **(B)** The cages can be reinforced with end caps to prevent subsidence or telescoping of the cages into the adjacent vertebrae. The caps, too, are fenestrated to allow bone ingrowth.

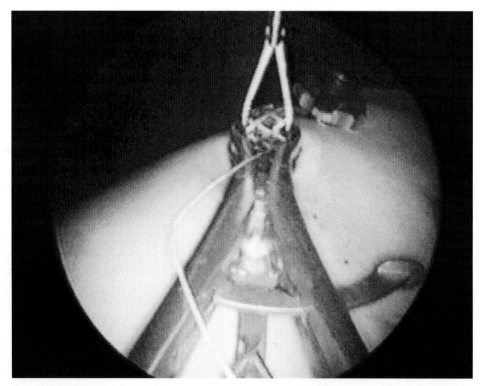

Figure 21–24. A tissue dilator is used to widen a portal incision to insert a titanium mesh cage into the chest. A suture is tied to the cage to retrieve it if necessary.

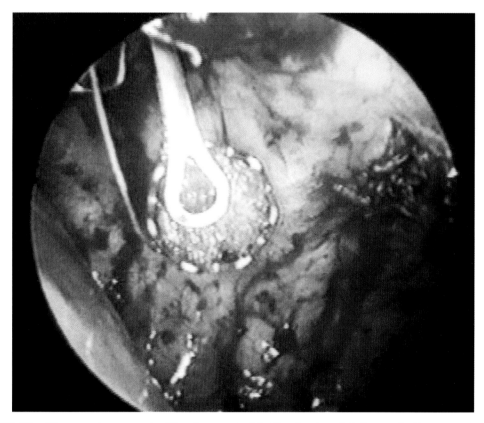

Figure 21–25.   The cage is grasped with a forceps inside the chest and delivered to the corpectomy site.

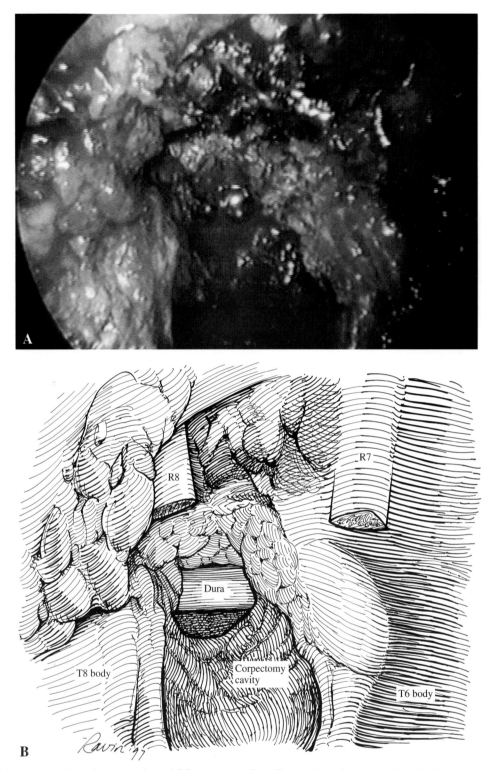

Figure 21–26. **(A)** Intraoperative photograph and **(B)** corresponding illustration show a right-sided T7 corpectomy being performed to decompress a metastatic tumor. A wide corpectomy is created to decompress the spinal cord. R = rib.

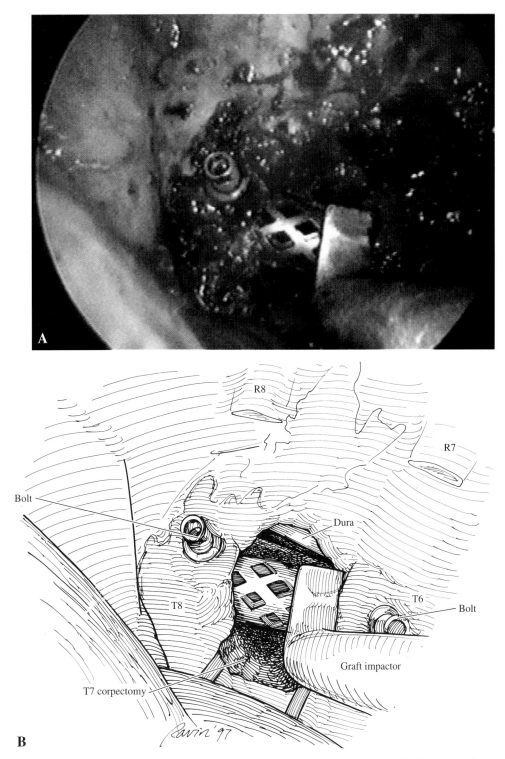

Figure 21–27. **(A)** Intraoperative photograph and **(B)** corresponding illustration show bolts that were being placed into the vertebrae adjacent to the corpectomy before the vertebral body was reconstructed. A titanium mesh cage is inserted to span the bone defect. The cage is inserted with a graft impactor.

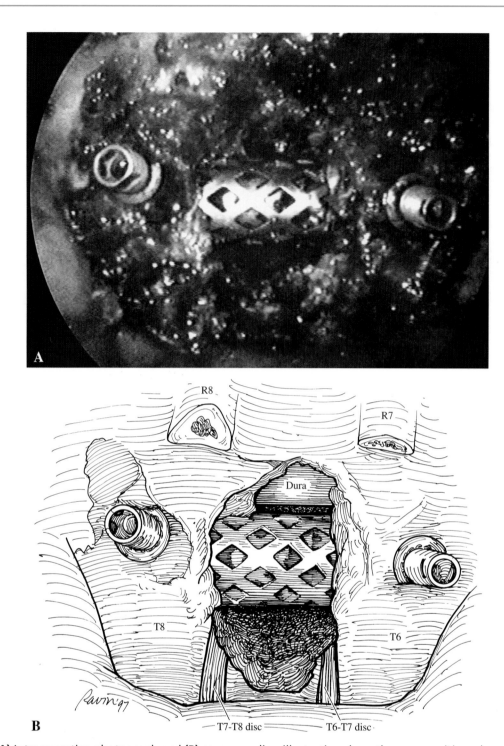

Figure 21–28. **(A)** Intraoperative photograph and **(B)** corresponding illustration show the cage positioned precisely to preserve space for the spinal cord. The ends of the cage are compressed against the adjacent end plates. R = rib.

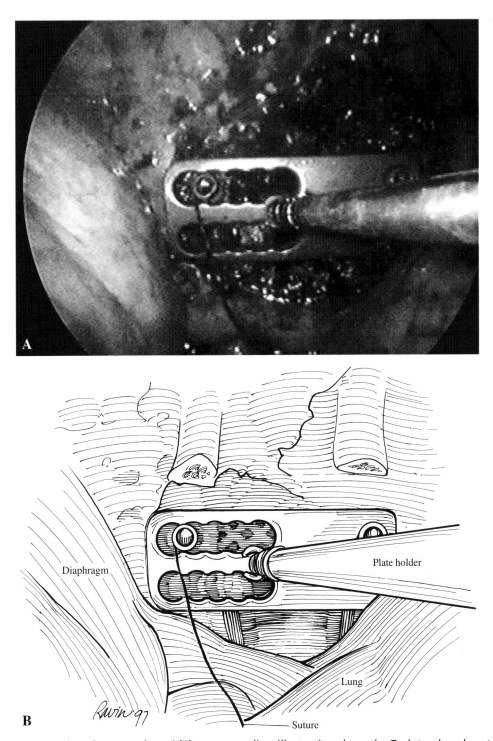

Diaphragm

Plate holder

Lung

Suture

Ravin '97

B

Figure 21–29. **(A)** Intraoperative photograph and **(B)** corresponding illustration show the Z-plate placed on top of the bolts. A suture is tied to the plate in case it needs to be retrieved.

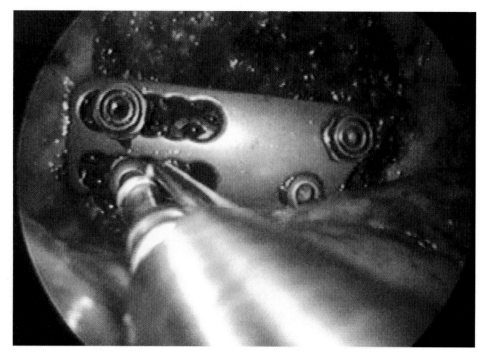

Figure 21–30.   The plate is locked to the bolts with nuts. A self-retaining screwdriver is used to insert the nonlocking screws into the bone.

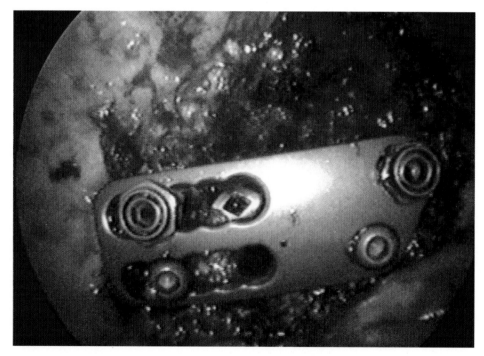

Figure 21–31.   The final intraoperative appearance of the screws, plate, and cage.

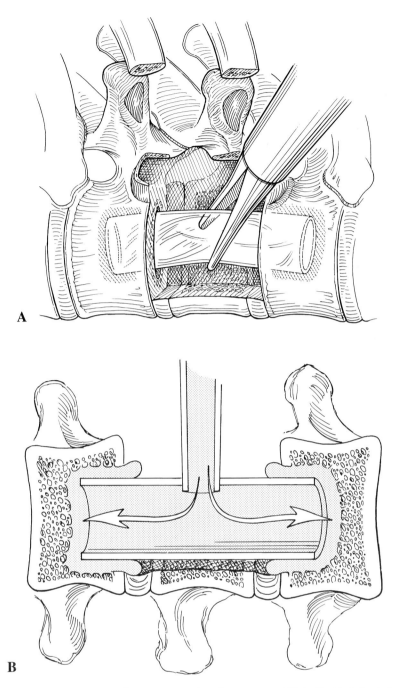

Figure 21–32. Methylmethacrylate vertebral body reconstruction for tumors. **(A)** A silastic tube is inserted into holes in the adjacent vertebral bodies. **(B)** Methylmethacrylate injected into the tube extrudes beyond the ends of the tube into the surrounding bone. After the acrylic hardens, it becomes anchored within the surrounding bone. [With permission from Barrow Neurological Institute.]

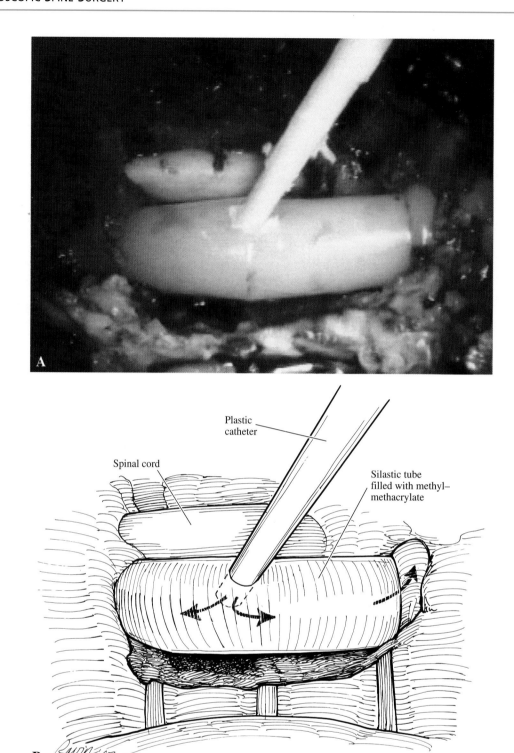

Figure 21–33. **(A)** Intraoperative photograph and **(B)** corresponding illustration show a vertebral body reconstruction performed with methylmethacrylate. The silastic tube is filled with the liquefied polymer.

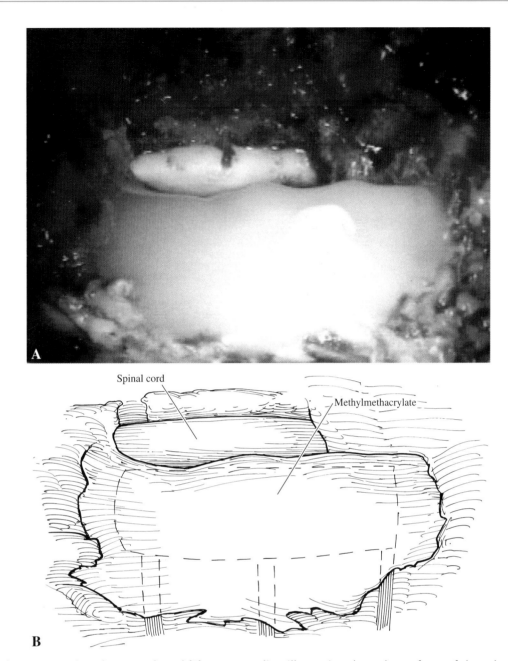

Spinal cord

Methylmethacrylate

Figure 21–34. **(A)** Intraoperative photograph and **(B)** corresponding illustration show the surfaces of the tube covered with methylmethacrylate and space preserved for the spinal cord.

REFERENCES

1. Dwyer AF, Schafer MF: Anterior approach to scoliosis. Results of treatment in fifty-one cases. *J Bone Joint Surg Br* 1974; 56(2):218–224.
2. Simmons ED, Jr., Kowalski JM, Simmons EH: The results of surgical treatment for adult scoliosis. *Spine* 1993; 18(6):718–724.
3. Dickman CA, Mican CA: Multilevel anterior thoracic discectomies and anterior interbody fusion using a microsurgical thoracoscopic approach. *J Neurosurg* 1996; 84:104–109.
4. Errico TJ, Cooper PR: A new method of thoracic and lumbar body replacement for spinal tumors: Technical note. *Neurosurgery* 1993; 32:678–681.
5. Cooper PR, Errico TJ, Martin R, et al: A systematic approach to spinal reconstruction after anterior decompression for neoplastic disease of the thoracic and lumbar spine. *Neurosurgery* 1993; 32:1–8.

6. Kostuik JP, Errico TJ, Gleason TF, et al: Spinal stabilization of vertebral column tumors. *Spine* 1988; 13(3):250–256.
7. Harrington KD: Anterior cord decompression and spinal stabilization for patients with metastatic lesions of the spine. *J Neurosurg* 1984; 61:107–117.
8. Dickman CA, Rosenthal D, Karahalios DG, et al: Thoracic vertebrectomy and reconstruction using a microsurgical thoracoscopic approach. *Neurosurgery* 1996; 38(2):279–293.
9. McAfee PC, Regan JR, Zdeblick T, et al: The incidence of complications in endoscopic anterior thoracolumbar spinal reconstructive surgery. A prospective multicenter study comprising the first 100 consecutive cases. *Spine* 1995; 20:1624–1632.

CHAPTER 22

Thoracoscopic Internal Fixation Techniques

Daniel J. Rosenthal, M.D. and Curtis A. Dickman, M.D.

*I*nternal fixation of the unstable thoracic spine can be performed with thoracoscopy using spinal instrumentation with screws that are inserted into the vertebral bodies. The screws can be anchored together with plates or rods to restore spinal stability. The tools for inserting the hardware must be long enough for percutaneous use. The fixation devices restrict spinal motion, keep the bone grafts compressed, and prevent displacement of the spine and the bone grafts. Fluoroscopy and direct inspection with endoscopy are used to accurately guide the trajectory of the hardware into the bone. Frameless stereotactic navigation techniques may also facilitate the insertion of endoscopic hardware.

SCREW PLATES FOR INTERNAL FIXATION OF THE THORACIC SPINE

Screw plates can be readily applied using a thoracoscopic operative approach. A low-profile titanium screw plate is available with long tools that can be used to insert fixation devices percutaneously (Z-plate, Sofamor-Danek, Memphis, TN). The components of this locking screw plate make it relatively easy to insert thoracoscopically (Fig. 22–1). The screws and plate are applied to the lateral surfaces of the vertebral bodies positioned away from the spinal cord, great vessels, heart, and mediastinum.

Before surgery begins, the portals for insertion of the bolts and screws are determined by using fluoroscopy, which minimizes the need for additional portal incisions (Fig. 22–2). Intraoperative fluoroscopy and direct visualization with the thoracoscope are required to guide the trajectory of the screws and bolts precisely into the bones.

Plate application is relatively simple (Fig. 22–3). After the corpectomy and decompression of the spinal cord are completed, the dura is visualized directly. The surfaces of the adjacent vertebrae are prepared so that osteophytes and irregular contours of the bone surfaces can be removed to allow the plate to sit flush against the bone surface. The rib heads adjacent to the plate must be removed to permit the plate to fit flush.

Preoperative magnetic resonance imaging or computed tomography studies are used to measure the width of the vertebrae. The bolts and screws are selected so that they achieve bicortical purchase but penetrate no more than 1 to 2 mm beyond the opposite cortical surface of the vertebral body.

The vertebrae rostral and caudal to the corpectomy are measured individually. Bolts and screws of the appropriate length are selected. The screws should be 5 mm longer than the bolts to compensate for the height of the plate.

Intraoperative fluoroscopy and direct endoscopic observation are essential for determining the appropriate trajectory for the bolts and screws. *Direct* visualization of the dura with the endoscope and *precise* positioning of the patient in a true lateral position allow the surgeon to confirm the exact trajectory of the screws. The bolts and screws are placed parallel to the vertebral end plates on anteroposterior fluoroscopic imaging. In relation to the transverse plane, the bolts are directed 10° anteriorly and the screws are angled 10° posteriorly. The bolts are inserted 1 cm from the posterior edge of the vertebral body and 1 cm from the edge of the distal end plates. A bone awl or drill is used to create a proximal pilot hole 10 to 15 mm deep in the bone.

The self-tapping bolts are placed parallel to the vertebral end plates and are angled 10° away from the spinal canal. The bolts are placed on a bolt driver and inserted so that the shoulders of the bolts are positioned flush with the surface of the vertebrae.

Before the plate is inserted onto the bolts, the reconstruction graft is inserted into the corpectomy defect. The plate is inserted, grasped with a plate holder inside the

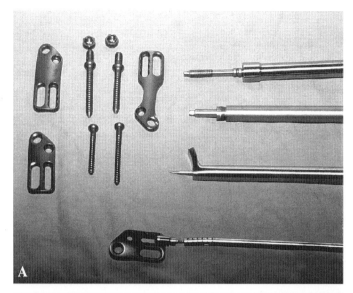

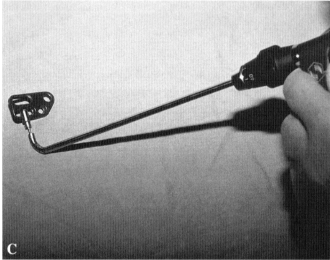

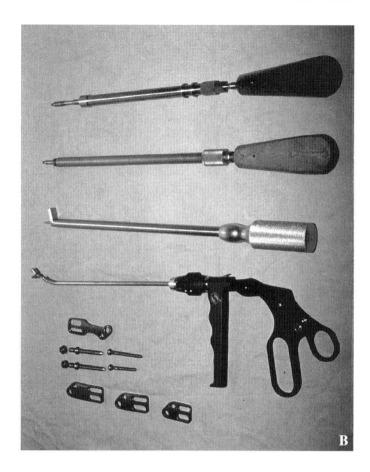

Figure 22–1. Thoracoscopic screw-plate application is performed using a locking thoracic screw plate and long tools to apply the plates endoscopically (Z-plate, Sofamor Danek, Memphis, TN). **(A)** Endoscopic plate tools include (right, top to bottom) a bolt and nut driver with a threaded shaft and an integrated hexagonal wrench, a self-retaining screwdriver, a bone awl and plate guide, and a variable angle plate holder. The plates are available in a variety of sizes. **(B)** The long tools permit percutaneous plate and screw insertion through the portals. **(C)** The adjustable plate holder can be bent and maneuvered inside the thorax to facilitate positioning the plate onto the bolts.

thoracic cavity, and positioned onto the two bolts. A compression tool can be applied to the bolt drivers/wrenches outside the surface of the chest to compress the graft against the end plates (Fig. 22–4). Locking nuts are applied to secure the plate to the bolts. The nuts are applied with a hexagonal wrench that is integrated into a sleeve on the shaft of the bolt driver. After the nuts are applied to lock the plate to the bolts, screws are placed in the ventral slot and the ventral hole on the plate. Screws that are 5 mm longer than the bolts are selected to accommodate the height of the plate. Compared to the bolts, the screws are angled 10° toward the spinal canal and are positioned more ventrally and proximally to the vertebrectomy defect. Unlike the bolts, the screws do not lock to the plate. The screws have a bicortical purchase to anchor them into position. Other types of screw plates can be used so long as the tools are long enough to be inserted endoscopically.

Illustrative Case: Right Thoracoscopic T9 Corpectomy and Screw-Plate Fixation

A 72-year-old woman presented with a progressive myelopathy. At another hospital she had previously undergone a posterolateral approach to treat a large calcified midline T9–T10 disc. The disc was incompletely removed, and the procedure was terminated because the patient's somatosensory evoked potentials disappeared with attempted manipulation of the calcified disc fragment. Her postoperative course was complicated by the development of a *Staphylococcal* deep wound infection, which was treated with 3 months of intravenous antibiotics. She presented 6 months later with an acute myelopathy due to collapse of the T9 vertebral body, a kyphotic deformity, and compression of the spinal cord (Fig. 22–5).

A thoracoscopic approach was performed with microsurgical removal of the ossified disc fragment (Figs. 22–6

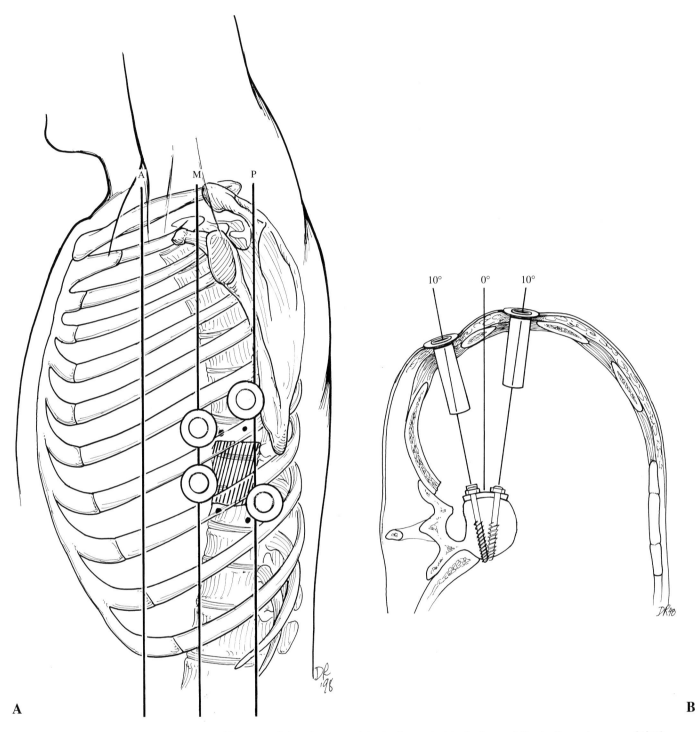

Figure 22–2. The portals are positioned in a coaxial trajectory with the intended trajectory of the bolts and screws. **(A)** The portals are positioned on the chest wall in a trapezoidal shape. The location is evaluated fluoroscopically. **(B)** Cross section of the thorax demonstrating the trajectory of the hardware.

through 22–19). Corpectomy of T9 was required to expose and excise the disc. The vertebral bodies were reconstructed with a humerus allograft filled with the patient's rib. Anterior instrumentation was performed with a locking screw plate. A staged posterior spinal fixation was performed 2 days later because the patient had a prior laminectomy with posterior element instability and moderately severe kyphosis. Postoperatively, her myelopathy slowly improved. Six months later, she was ambulating independently and had recovered almost full motor function (Fig. 22–20).

SCREW RODS AND OTHER FIXATION DEVICES

Chapter 16 details the application of the Blackman-Luque anterior spinal fixation system for anterior endoscopic correction of scoliotic deformities. This top-loading screw rod system can be completely inserted thoracoscopically.

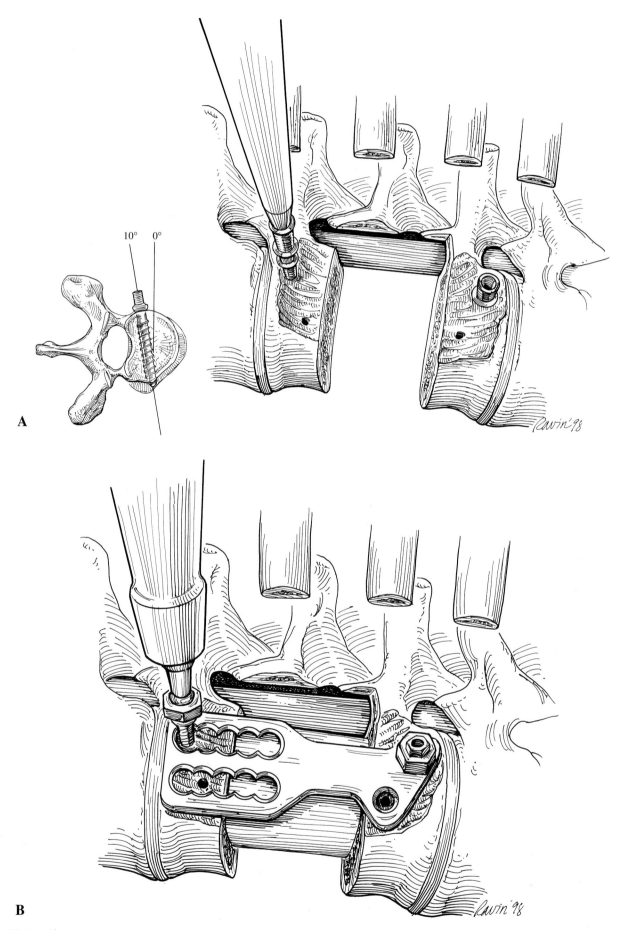

Figure 22–3. Thoracoscopic Z-plate application. The sequence of bolt, plate, and screw insertion is identical to the open technique. The nuts are castellated and create a friction fit with the bolt head. **(A)** The bolts are inserted 1 cm from the distal end plates and 1 cm from the posterior edges of the vertebral bodies. The shoulder of the bolts are positioned flush with the bone surface. *(Inset)* The bolts are angled 10° *away* from the spinal canal. **(B)** The plate is placed over the bolts. Nuts are applied to lock the plate to the bolts.

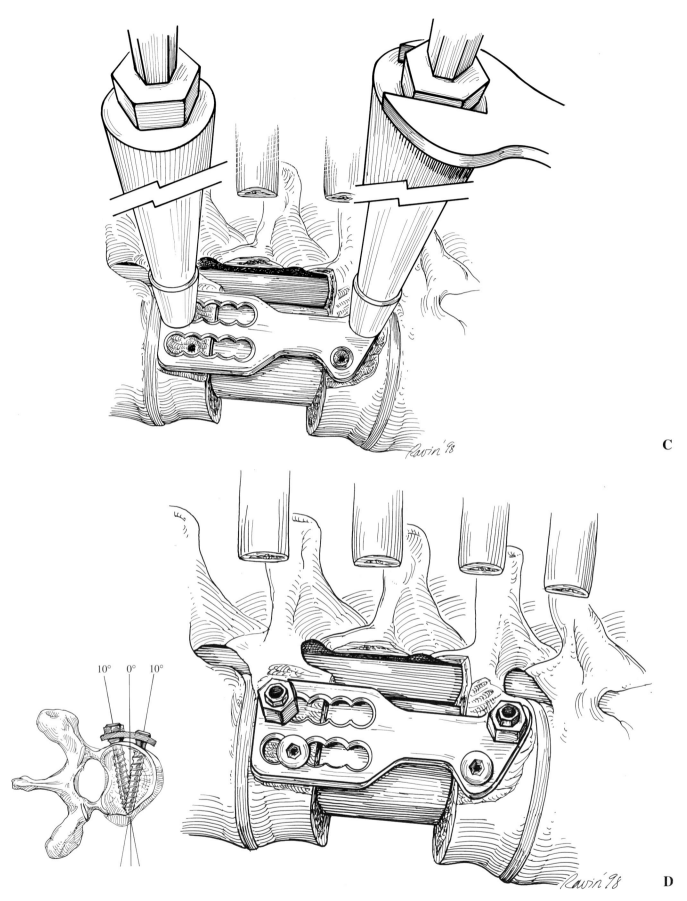

C

D

Figure 22–3.   *(continued)*   **(C)** The nuts are tightened using a wrench that is applied to a hex-wrench sleeve. **(D)** Screws, 5 mm longer than the bolts, are placed in the anterior slot and hole in the plate and angled 10° toward the spinal canal. *(Inset)* The tips of the screws converge toward the tips of the bolts to resist plate pullout.

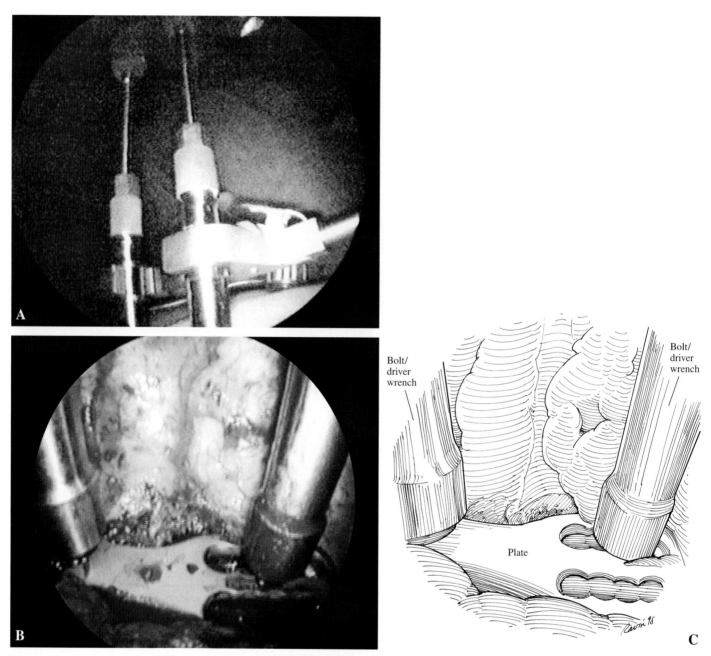

Figure 22–4. **(A)** A compressor is applied to the bolt drivers/wrenches outside the surface of the chest. This device can be used to compress the vertebral bodies against the graft in the corpectomy site. **(B)** Intraoperative photograph and **(C)** corresponding illustration showing an endoscopic view of the bolt drivers/wrenches attached onto the bolts during compression of the construct.

Another system, the HMA rod system (Aesculap, Tuttlingen, Germany) uses wide fenestrated vertebral body screws that can be locked together with a rod (Figs. 22–21 through 22–33). The system provides a tension band and buttress effect. Primarily, it resists flexion, extension, and lateral bending. Its resistance to axial rotation and transla-tion of the spine is potentially limited because only single screws are used to fixate each vertebral body. The design for these devices, which are currently unavailable for clinical use in the United States, is being modified to improve their mechanical strength.

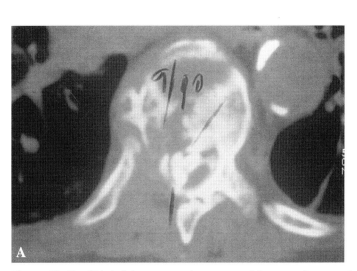

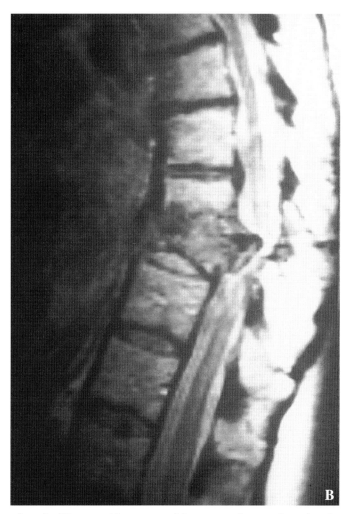

Figure 22–5. **(A)** Axial computed tomographic scan after myelography of a 72-year-old woman with progressive myelopathy. A calcified disc fragment on the right side of the spinal cord compressed and deformed the spinal cord. A prior transpedicular approach had been attempted, but was unsuccessful in removing the disc. **(B)** Sagittal magnetic resonance image demonstrates collapse of the T9 vertebral body and the residual calcified disc fragment compressing the spinal cord. The surgical removal of this pathology is shown in Figures 22–6 through 22–20.

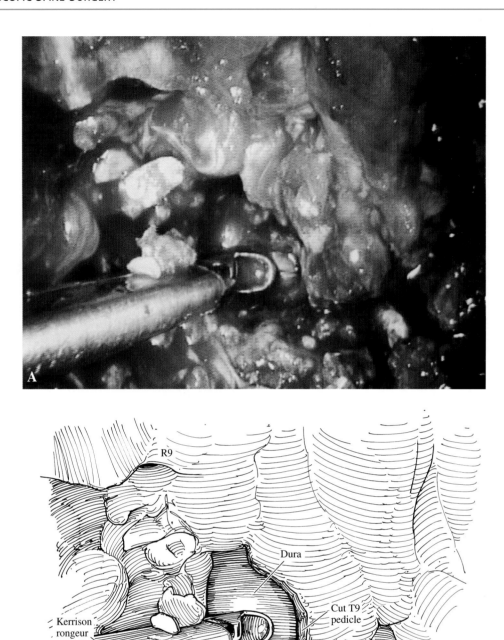

Figure 22–6. **(A)** Intraoperative photograph and **(B)** corresponding illustration showing the removal of T9 and T10 pedicles with a Kerrison rongeur to clearly identify the epidural space before proceeding with the corpectomy. A right-sided thoracoscopic approach was used.

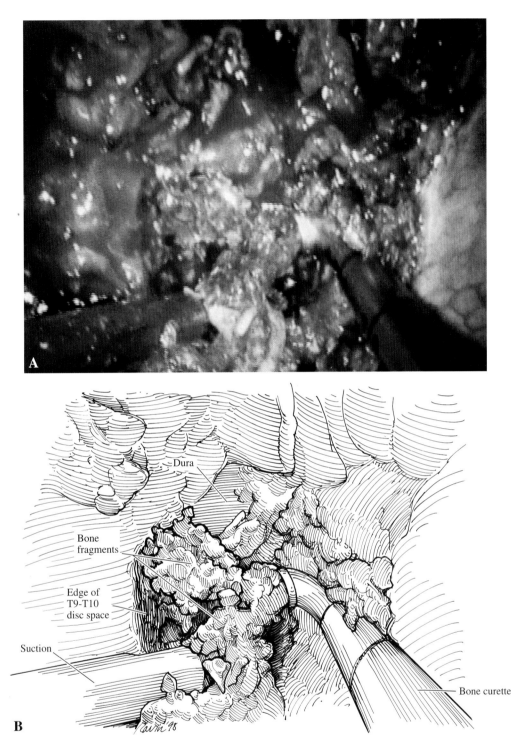

Figure 22–7. **(A)** Intraoperative photograph and **(B)** corresponding illustration showing the removal of the osteoporotic bone from the collapsed, pathological T9 vertebral body with a large endoscopic bone curette.

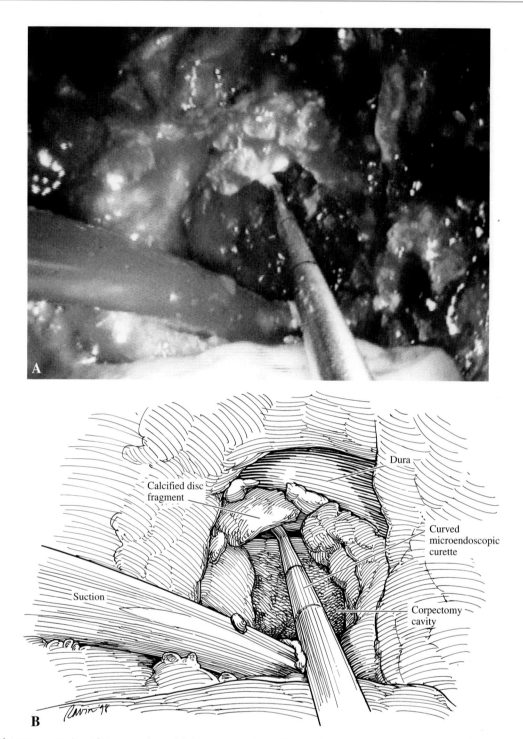

Figure 22–8. **(A)** Intraoperative photograph and **(B)** corresponding illustration showing the creation of a large corpectomy cavity to provide sufficient room to work with tools to extract the disc fragment without placing any tools in the compromised epidural space. The large calcified disc, which was compressing and distorting the spinal cord, was removed with a curved microendoscopic curette.

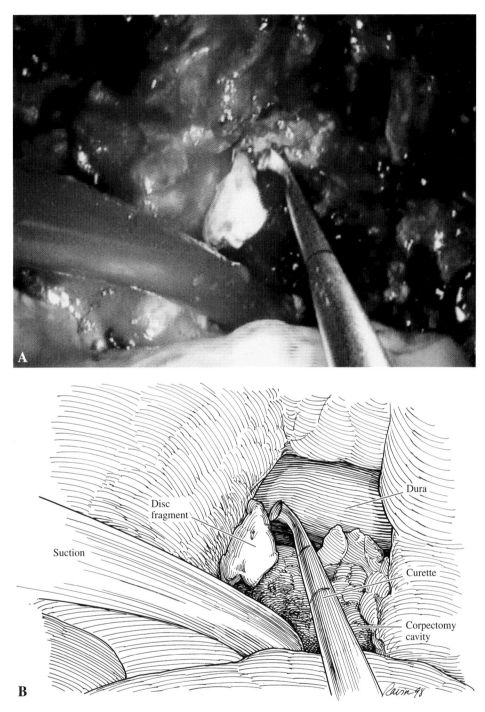

Figure 22–9. **(A)** Intraoperative photograph and **(B)** corresponding illustration showing the large disc fragment being pulled away from the dura and spinal cord using sharp microdissection with a small curved curette.

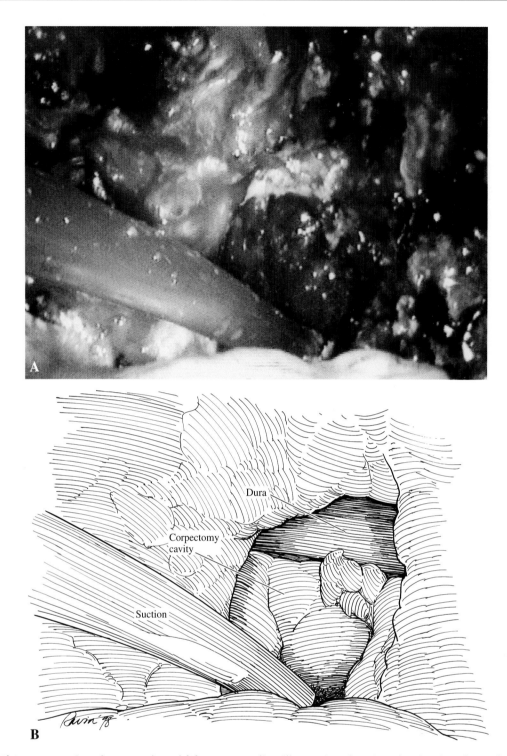

Figure 22–10. **(A)** Intraoperative photograph and **(B)** corresponding illustration showing the dural surface after it was completely decompressed. The entire ventral surface of the dura was visible.

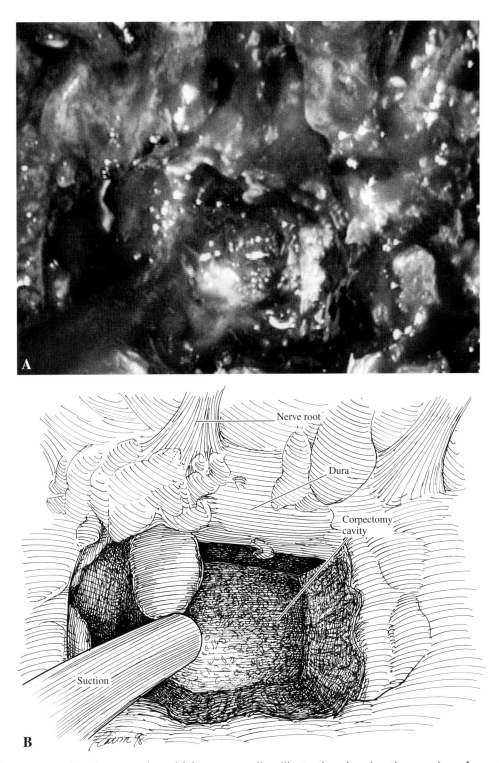

Figure 22–11. **(A)** Intraoperative photograph and **(B)** corresponding illustration showing the creation of a rectangular corpectomy defect. All soft tissue, disc material, and the vertebral end plates were removed to facilitate incorporation of the bone graft.

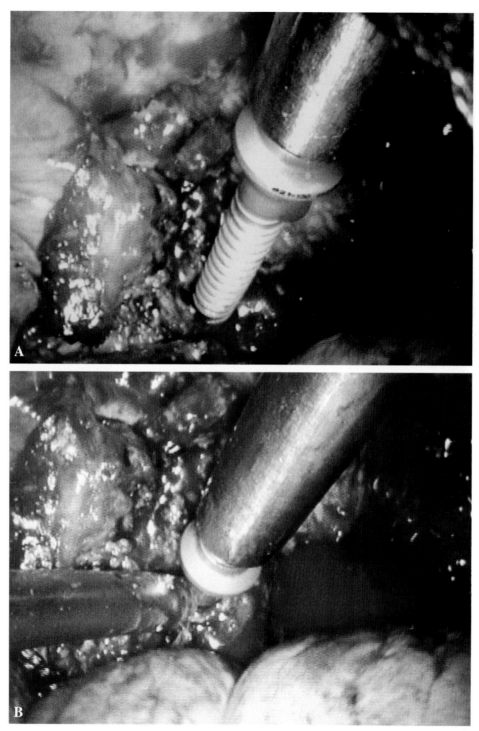

Figure 22–12. **(A)** The insertion of the bolt into the vertebra caudal to the decompression site was observed endoscopically. The bolt was angled 10° away from the spinal canal. **(B)** The bolt was inserted so that its shoulder was flush with the surface of the vertebral body.

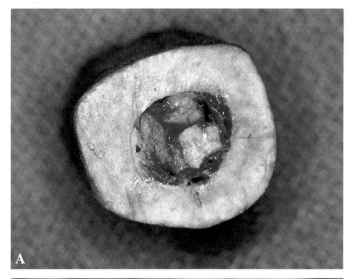

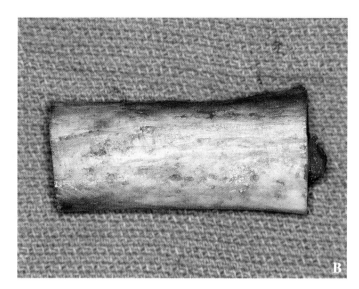

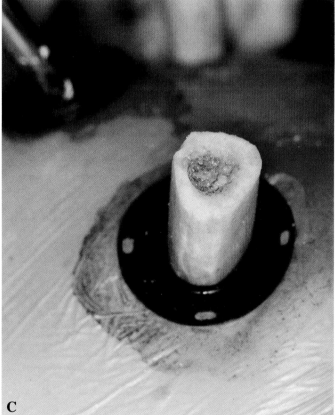

Figure 22–13. **(A)** A 17-mm diameter humerus allograft was filled with the patient's bone (from the ribs and vertebral body). **(B)** Lateral view of the bone graft. **(C)** The graft was inserted end on into the endoscopic portal.

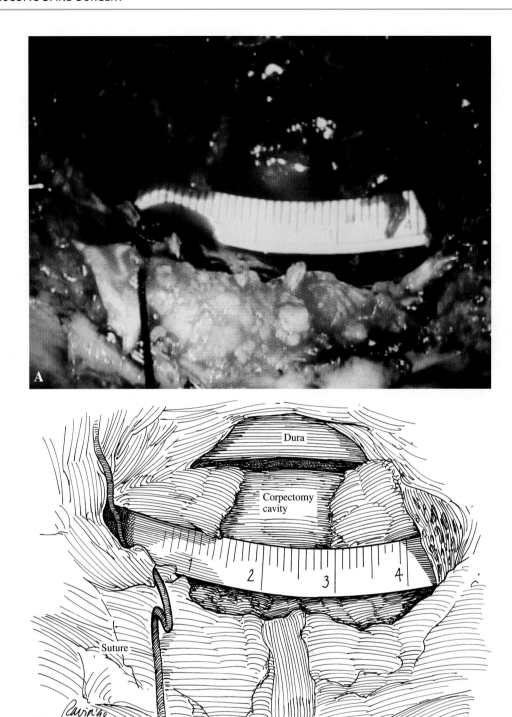

Figure 22–14. **(A)** Intraoperative photograph and **(B)** corresponding illustration showing a plastic ruler being used to measure the dimensions of the corpectomy site. A suture was tied to the ruler for its retrieval.

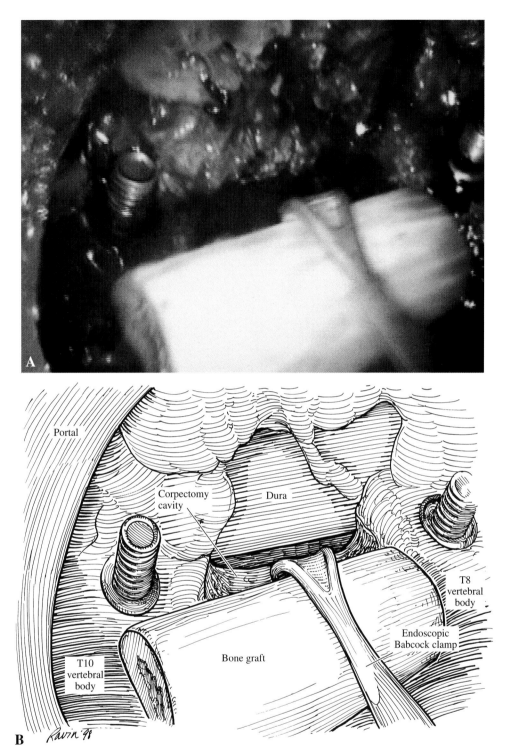

Figure 22–15. **(A)** Intraoperative photograph and **(B)** corresponding illustration showing the bone graft being grasped with an endoscopic Babcock clamp and positioned into the corpectomy site.

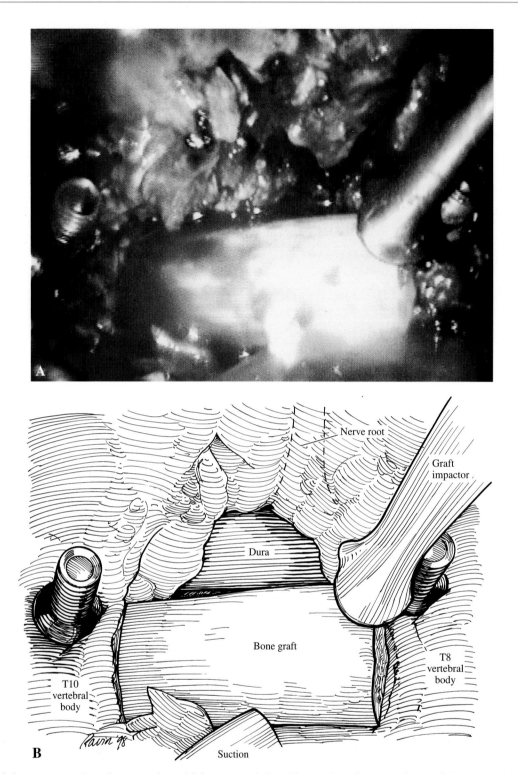

Figure 22–16.   **(A)** Intraoperative photograph and **(B)** corresponding illustration showing the graft being carefully impacted into the corpectomy bed, preserving the space for the spinal cord.

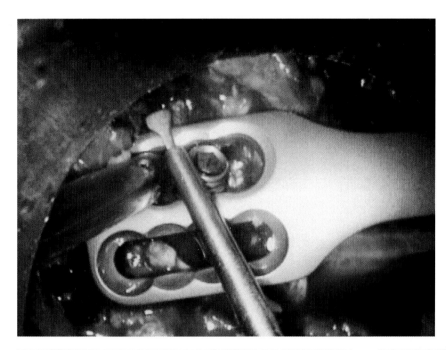

Figure 22–17. The plate was positioned on top of the bolts. The plate was locked to the bolts with nuts.

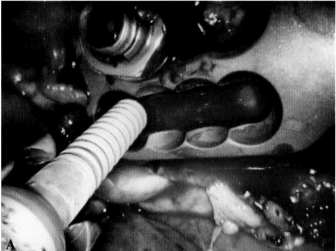

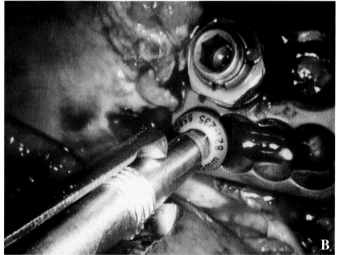

Figure 22–18. **(A)** Nonlocking screws were inserted into the vertebral bodies. The screws converged toward the bolts and were angled 10° toward the spinal canal. **(B)** The screws were held with a self-retaining screwdriver. The heads were positioned flushly against the plate.

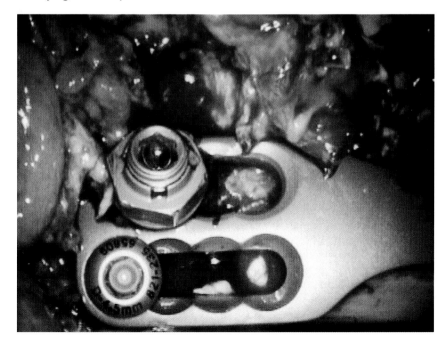

Figure 22–19. Final view of the lower end of the plate, demonstrating the appearance of the bolt, screw, and graft in relationship to the plate.

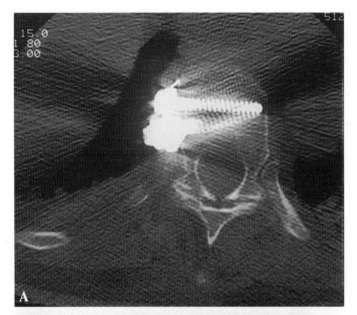

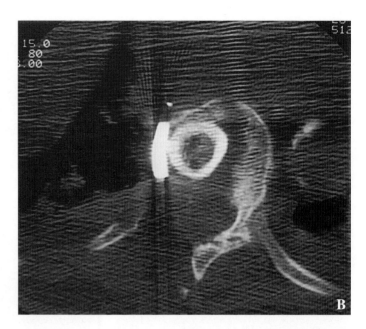

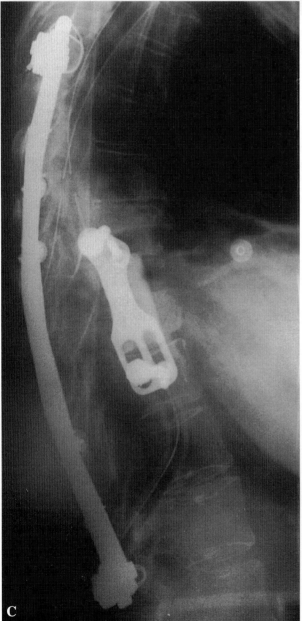

Figure 22–20. Postoperative computed tomography (CT) scans **(A)** demonstrate the position of the screws in the vertebral body. **(B)** The graft and plate are positioned satisfactorily. The space for the spinal cord is completely preserved. **(C)** Postoperative lateral radiograph. A posterior thoracolumbar spinal fixation was performed to supplement the screw plate because of the patients' severe osteoporosis and her prior posterior spinal surgery. [With permission from Williams and Wilkins.]

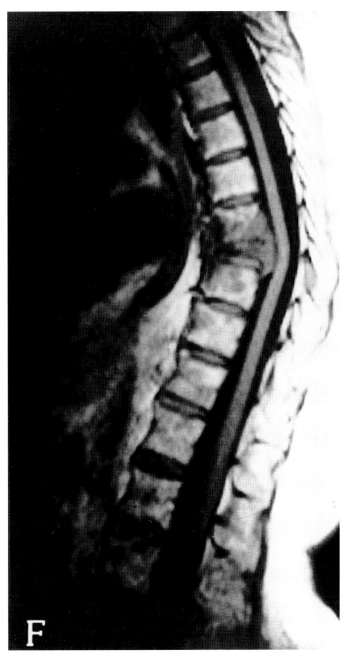

Figure 22–21.   Preoperative magnetic resonance imaging demonstrating collapse and tumor infiltration of the T5 vertebral body with a kyphotic deformity. A metastatic breast cancer also compressed the ventral surface of the spinal cord causing paraparesis in this patient.

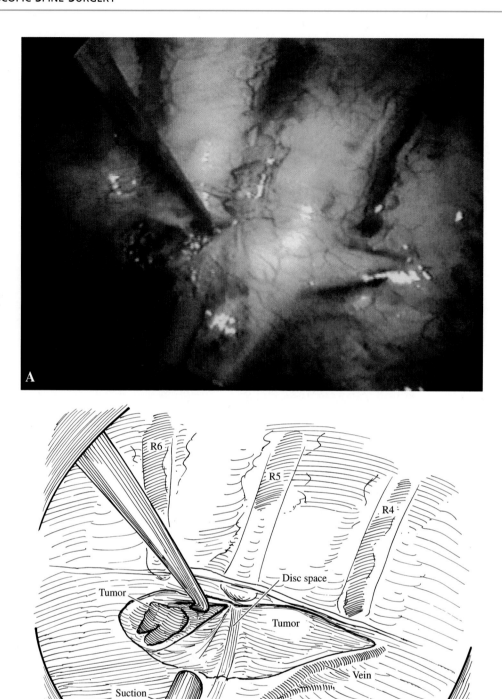

Figure 22–22.   (A) Intraoperative photograph and **(B)** corresponding illustration showing a right-sided thoracoscopic approach being used to resect the metastatic breast carcinoma, which had destroyed the T5 vertebral body and caused severe paraparesis. The pleura was dissected from the surface of the tumor, which was exophytic on the surface of the spine.

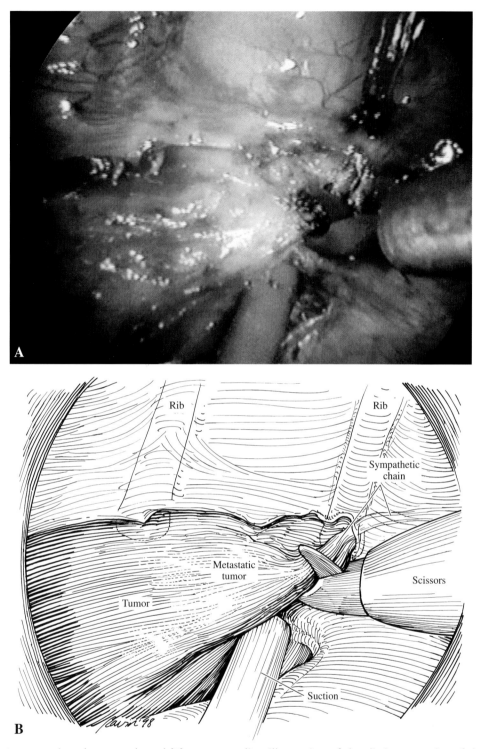

Figure 22–23. **(A)** Intraoperative photograph and **(B)** corresponding illustration of the distinct margins of the tumor. The margins were defined to isolate the tumor.

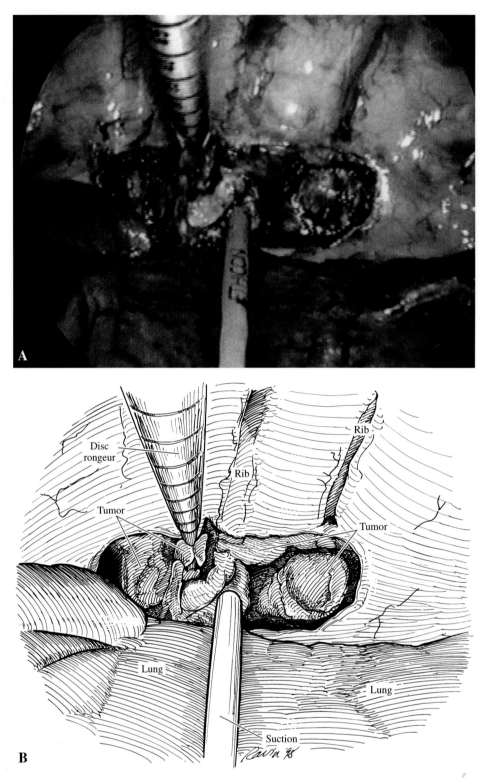

Figure 22–24. **(A)** Intraoperative photograph and **(B)** corresponding illustration showing the removal of the avascular soft, fleshy tumor from the surface of the spine with disc rongeurs.

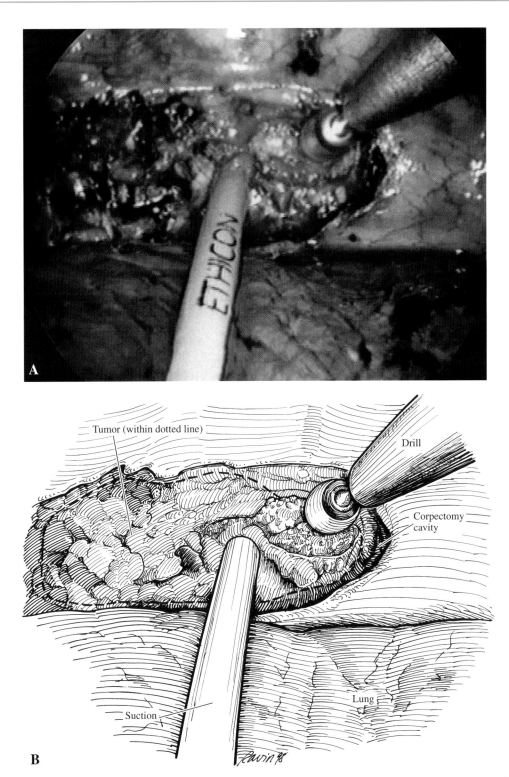

Figure 22–25. **(A)** Intraoperative photograph and **(B)** corresponding illustration showing a corpectomy cavity being drilled into the T5 vertebral body using a cylindrical-shaped drill bit.

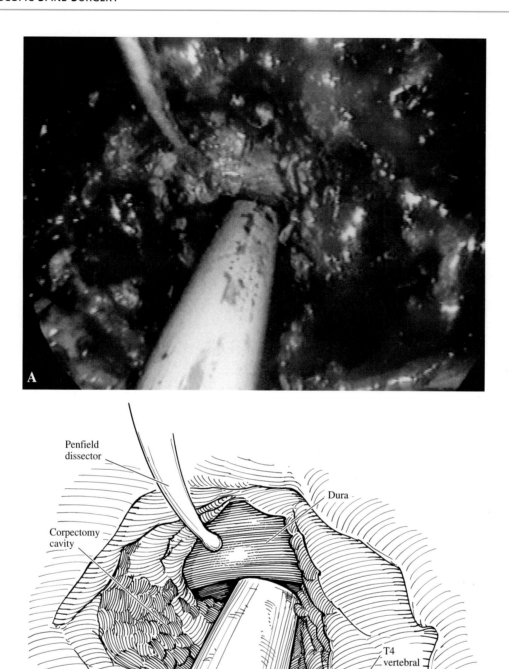

Figure 22–26. **(A)** Intraoperative photograph and **(B)** corresponding illustration showing the decompression of the entire ventral surface of the spinal cord. Gross total resection of the tumor was achieved.

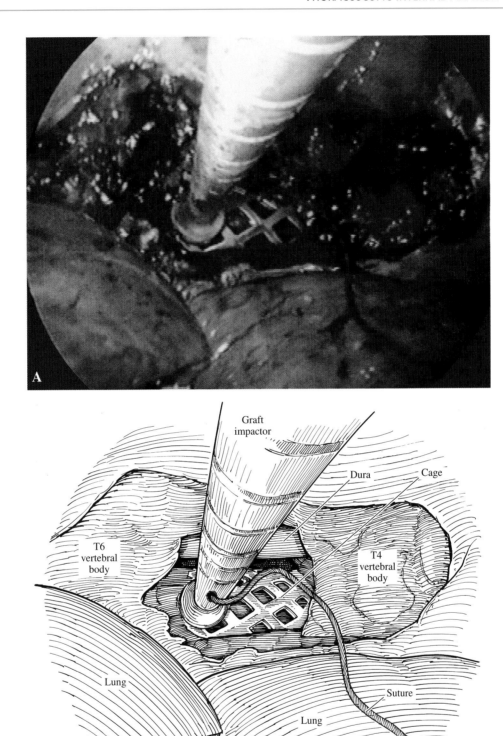

Figure 22–27. **(A)** Intraoperative photograph and **(B)** corresponding illustration showing the insertion of a titanium mesh cage to reconstruct the defect within the vertebral body.

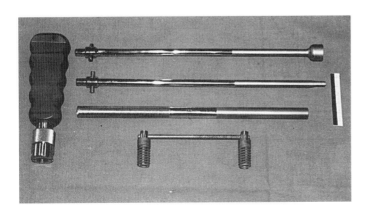

Figure 22–28. Photograph of the HMA screw rod system and its insertion tools.

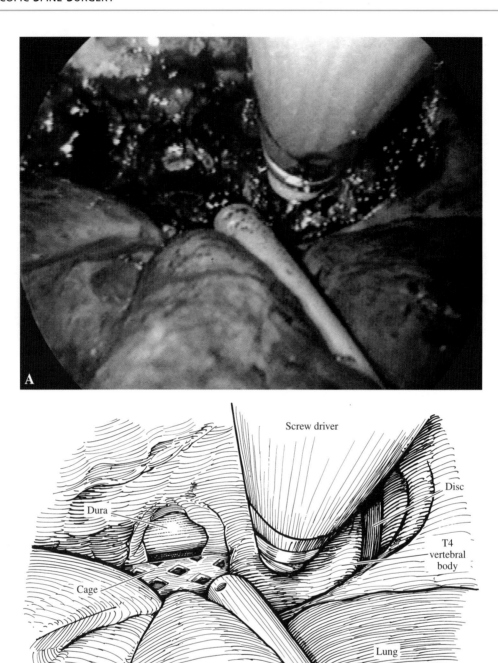

Figure 22–29. **(A)** Intraoperative photograph and **(B)** corresponding illustration showing the insertion of large anchor screws into the vertebrae adjacent to the corpectomy.

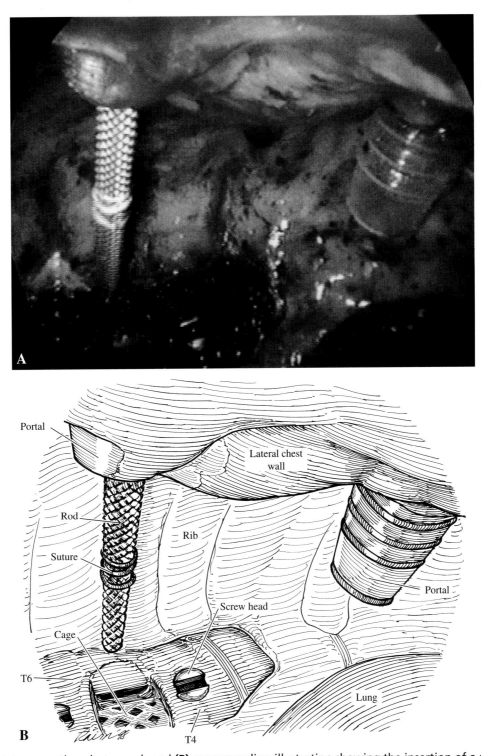

Figure 22–30. **(A)** Intraoperative photograph and **(B)** corresponding illustration showing the insertion of a rod through the portal into the chest. A suture was tied to the rod for its retrieval.

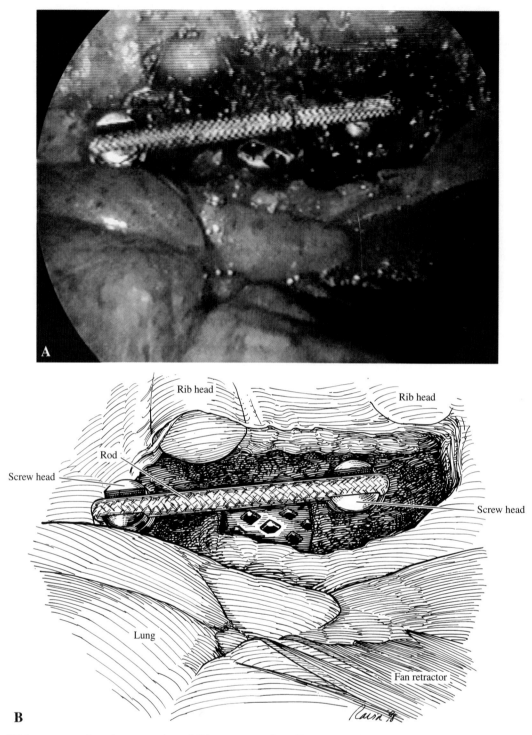

Figure 22–31. **(A)** Intraoperative photograph and **(B)** corresponding illustration showing the rod being positioned onto slots in the heads of the anchor screws.

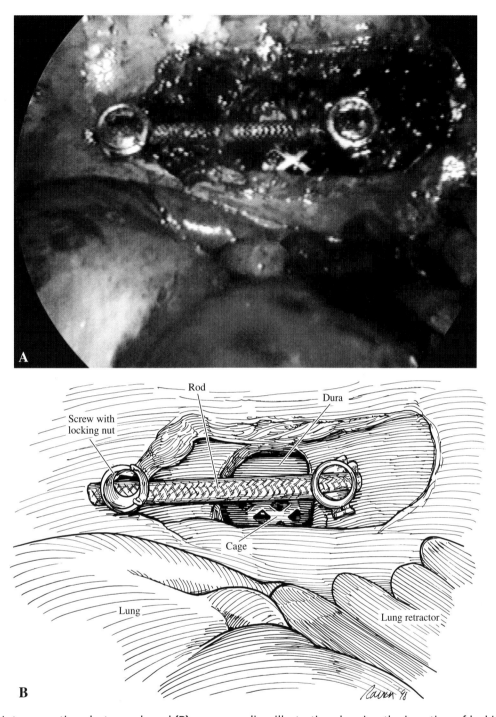

Figure 22–32. **(A)** Intraoperative photograph and **(B)** corresponding illustration showing the insertion of locking nuts on top of the screw heads to lock the rod to the screws.

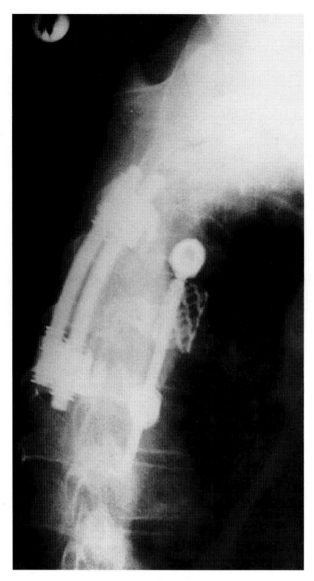

Figure 22–33. Postoperative lateral radiograph of the thoracic spine demonstrating the position of the screw rod system and the titanium mesh cage. The kyphotic deformity was corrected during the anterior endoscopic procedure. The fixation was reinforced with posterior short segment hook-rod instrumentation.

CONCLUSIONS

Anterior spinal fixation devices can be applied endoscopically to restore spinal stability and to correct spinal deformities. The hardware is inserted with techniques that are similar to those used for open surgery. The tools to insert the hardware endoscopically must be long enough for percutaneous use. The clinical experience with endoscopic spine stabilization has been excellent, achieving the same extent of stabilization as open techniques to anteriorly fixate the thoracic spine.

RECOMMENDED READINGS

1. Dickman CA, Rosenthal D, Karahalios DG, et al: Thoracic vertebrectomy and reconstruction using a microsurgical thoracoscopic approach. *Neurosurgery* 1996; 38(2):279–293.
2. McAfee PC, Regan JR, Zdeblick T, et al: The incidence of complications in endoscopic anterior thoracolumbar spinal reconstructive surgery. A prospective multicenter study comprising the first 100 consecutive cases. *Spine* 1995; 20:1624–1632.
3. Regan JJ, Mack MJ, Picetti GD III, et al: A comparison of video–assisted thoracoscopic surgery (VATS) with open thoracotomy in thoracic spinal surgery. *Today's Therapeutic Trends* 1994; 11:203–218.
4. Kaneda K, Abumi K, Fujiya M: Burst fractures with neurologic deficits of the thoraco–lumbar spine. Results of anterior decompression and stabilization with anterior instrumentation. *Spine* 1984; 9:788–795.
5. Kostuik JP: Anterior fixation for fractures of the thoracic and lumbar spine with or without neurologic involvement. *Clin Orthop* 1984; 189:103–115.
6. Dickman CA, Mican C: Thoracoscopic approaches for the treatment of anterior thoracic spinal pathology. *BNI Quarterly* 1996; 12(1):4–19.
7. Dwyer AF, Schafer MF: Anterior approach to scoliosis. Results of treatment in fifty–one cases. *J Bone Joint Surg Br* 1974; 56: 218–224.
8. Zdeblick TA: Z–plate anterior thoracolumbar instrumentation. In Hitchon PW, Traynelis VC, Rengachary SS, eds: *Techniques in Spinal Fusion and Stabilization.* New York: Thieme; 1995: 279–289.
9. Cooper PR, Errico TJ, Martin R, et al: A systematic approach to spinal reconstruction after anterior decompression for neoplastic disease of the thoracic and lumbar spine. *Neurosurgery* 1993; 32(1):1–8.
10. Rosenthal D, Marquardt G, Lorenz R, et al: Anterior decompression and stabilization using a microsurgical endoscopic technique for metastatic tumors of the thoracic spine. *J Neurosurg* 1996; 84:565–572.
11. Harrington KD: Anterior cord decompression and spinal stabilization for patients with metastatic lesions of the spine. *J Neurosurg* 1984; 61:107–117.
12. Kostuik JP, Errico TJ, Gleason TF, et al: Spinal stabilization of vertebral column tumors. *Spine* 1988; 13(3):250–256.
13. Dickman CA, Mican CA: Multilevel anterior thoracic discectomies and anterior interbody fusion using a microsurgical thoracoscopic approach. *J Neurosurg* 1996; 84:104–109.

CHAPTER 23

Future Directions for Spinal Thoracoscopy

Curtis A. Dickman, M.D., Daniel J. Rosenthal, M.D., and Noel I. Perin, M.D.

An outdated concept in surgery is "to make the largest incision possible for exposure, and you will only need to enlarge it more to provide enough room for adequate access." Complications and pain, however, can be reduced when the surgeon avoids cutting through or retracting *normal* anatomical structures to remove a pathological lesion. Thoracoscopy reduces the approach-related complications of surgery while preserving or improving the effectiveness of dissection. This field is a fertile area for development and further improvements to benefit patients. The development of thoracoscopic surgery has evolved in parallel with other specialties that also use minimally incisional surgery.

Compared to a thoracotomy for an anterior transthoracic exposure, thoracoscopic surgery reduces approach-related morbidity. Unlike costotransversectomy, however, it does not compromise the extent of exposure and visualization or the ability to perform extensive surgical dissections on the ventral thoracic spine and around the ventral surfaces of the spinal cord and nerve roots. Thoracoscopy permits pathology to be manipulated identical to that possible during open surgical approaches.

Current experience with thoracoscopic spinal surgery has demonstrated that a wide spectrum of surgical procedures and techniques is feasible. These techniques are safe and associated with reduced complications, better cosmetic results, less pain, and faster recovery times than open surgical techniques. Clinical outcomes completely depend on the surgeon's training, practice, skill, and experience. Our teaching experiences have indicated that vigorous, dedicated laboratory training and clinical preceptorships are mandatory prerequisites for performing these techniques safely. The continued growth and development of thoracoscopic spinal surgery depend on four major issues: (1) educating and credentialing of surgeons; (2) collecting prospective data, analyzing outcomes, and performing rigorously controlled scientific studies; (3) developing and implementing new technology; and (4) expanding clinical and surgical applications.

EDUCATION

The education and credentialing processes are fully discussed in Chapter 3. Surgeons need both a comprehensive didactic and practical background to perform thoracoscopic surgery safely. Surgeons cannot rely on their own initiative and existing skill level. Having performed a large number of open thoracic spinal surgeries does not adequately prepare surgeons to undertake thoracoscopic spinal surgery.

Endoscopy requires new and unfamiliar dissection skills, new psychomotor skills, new perceptions of anatomy, and extensive practice to master the techniques. Only by following a progressive, graduated training and preceptorship experience will surgeons be satisfactorily prepared to perform thoracoscopic surgery. Failure to adhere to these recommendations could result in serious technical complications that otherwise would have been avoidable.

The future of spinal thoracoscopy depends on the implementation of rigorous standards and credentialing processes for spine applications to ensure safe and effective practice. This process is best implemented by professional medical societies, while credentialing requirements can be verified and established by individual hospital facilities. The information superhighway will facilitate teaching by allowing telementoring and teleproctoring from remote sites.

SCIENTIFIC ASSESSMENT

The available data on the clinical utility of spinal thoracoscopy show that the technique has been associated with excellent results in tertiary referral centers. More data are needed to assess the technology further, including cost and outcome analyses and prospective clinical trials. Data collection studies have been organized and are in progress in many centers. In the future, collaborative, multicenter studies will provide the most comprehensive assessments.

TECHNOLOGICAL DEVELOPMENTS

Technological developments will continue to improve the performance of thoracoscopic spinal surgery. Improvements in imaging technology that can be anticipated include better resolution of optical images, zoom capabilities (adjustable magnification), adjustable focus, narrower diameter endoscopes, improved flexible steerable endoscopes, greater use of working channels, improved three-dimensional endoscopic imaging, virtual reality endoscopy (Fig. 23–1), and holographic imaging. Thoracoscopy of the future will be performed with better visualization and better tools and through fewer incisions. Operative planning, surgical navigation, and the precision of dissection will be enhanced by frameless stereotactic navigation devices, computer interfacing, intraoperative imaging, virtual reality systems, and robotic devices.

Some robotic devices are already available for use in thoracoscopic surgery (Fig. 23–2). A voice-controlled robotic arm (Automated Endoscopic System for Optimal Positioning, AESOP) has been approved by the Food and Drug Administration (FDA) as a holder for endoscopes (Computer Motion, Golita, CA). The surgeon wears a microphone headset and verbally commands the robotic arm to reposition the endoscope within the operative field. Intraoperatively, the robot can memorize several anatomical positions and immediately return to the designated positions. AESOP provides the surgeon with direct control of the endoscope, resulting in a more stable and sustainable endoscopic image. This device reduces operating time by immediately adjusting and repositioning the endoscope, thereby freeing the surgeons' hands for the dissection. It greatly facilitates surgery.

A robotic surgical system is under development (Zeus, Computer Motion, Golita, CA). Viewing the surgery with computer-enhanced video images, the surgeon sits at a control panel and manipulates surgical robotic instruments (Figs. 23–3, 23–4, and 23–5). Using robotic arms to perform the dissection enhances surgical dexterity, eliminates hand tremor, and scales motion (reduces or amplifies movements). The result is greater precision and the ability to perform microdissections that are not possible today (e.g., microvascular anastomoses, dural closure). Zeus also improves ergonomics: the surgeon will be able to sit while operating instead of standing for hours. Using this robotics control system will also allow surgical procedures to be performed from a remote site if desired—for example, to treat wounded soldiers in military combat zones. Potentially, surgeons could use Zeus or a similar system to perform a sur-

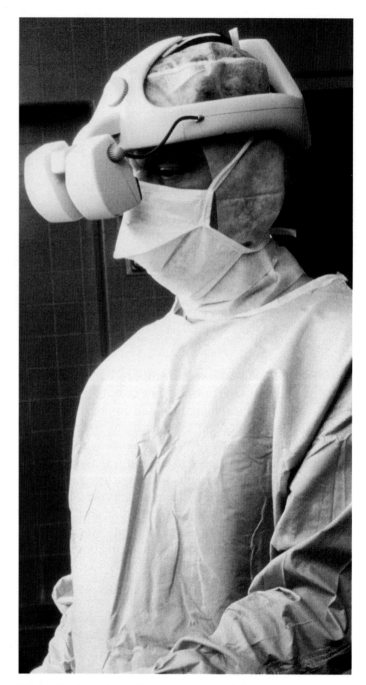

Figure 23–1. Interactive, voice-controlled, three-dimensional (3-D) viewing headset (Vista Technologies, Carlsbad, CA). The headset provides 3-D endoscopic microsurgical viewing of the operative anatomy. The radiographic, computed tomographic, and magnetic resonance images and stereotactic guidance views can all be simultaneously projected onto a portion of the visual field, permitting the surgeon to examine the surgical trajectory and pathology without turning away from the patient during the surgery.

gical dissection from one location while the patient is on the opposite side of the planet. In addition to other endoscopic microscopic procedures, Zeus is currently being investigated to enable a fully endoscopic approach for coronary artery bypass graft (ECABG) procedures. For a surgeon's hands, Zeus accomplishes what a microscope does for a surgeon's eyes.

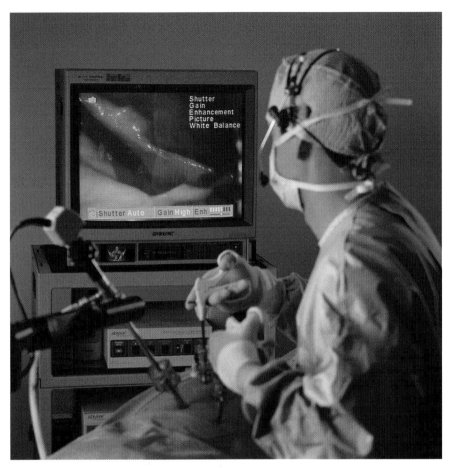

Figure 23–2. A voice-activated robotic arm functions efficiently to hold and reposition the endoscope intraoperatively. This system is called the Automated Endoscopic System for Optimal Positioning (AESOP). [With permission from Computer Motion.]

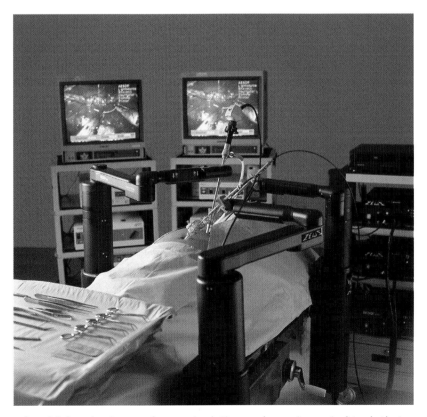

Figure 23–3. Zeus consists of multiple robotic arms for manipulating endoscopic surgical tools that can be used to suture tissue, dissect tissue, and suction. The precision robotic arms can eliminate tremor and scale movements to perform microsurgical anastomoses and microdissection. [With permission from Computer Motion.]

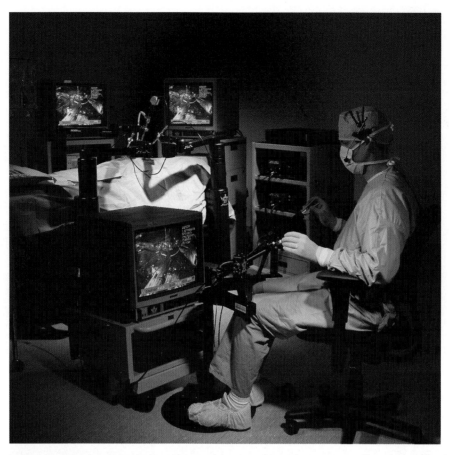

Figure 23–4. While seated at a control unit and observing a video monitor, the surgeon directly manipulates the robotic arms of Zeus. [With permission from Computer Motion.]

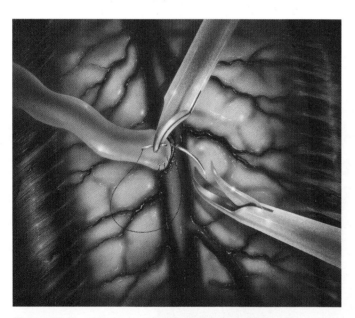

Figure 23–5. A microsurgical vascular anastomosis is performed using Zeus. [With permission from Computer Motion.]

Another recent robotic development (HERMES, Computer Motion, Golita, CA) uses speech-recognition technology to give the surgeon direct voice control over all aspects of the operating room. The surgeon can then perform the procedure more effectively with a smaller surgical team. Through the microphone headset, the surgeon can control most of the equipment in the operating room: light sources, camera, insufflators, pumps, drills, energy sources, videocassette recorders, slide and photographic equipment, suctions, electrocauterization tools, and so on. The status of the devices can also be displayed on video monitors to obtain visual feedback regarding the devices' functioning during a procedure.

Robotic surgical systems and computerized interfacing have tremendous potential for improving a surgeon's performance and efficiency by increasing the ability to perform a wide array of endoscopic microsurgical procedures (Fig. 23–6). Surgical tools and biomaterials (i.e., multiarticulated tools and multiple purpose tools), spinal instrumentation to correct spinal deformities endoscopically, bone reconstruction methods (i.e., bone cement, bone morphogenic protein), retractors, and other devices are also being developed for endoscopic use.

NEW SURGICAL TECHNIQUES

The indications and range of procedures performed using thoracoscopic approaches to the spine will continue to evolve and expand. Dural closure techniques

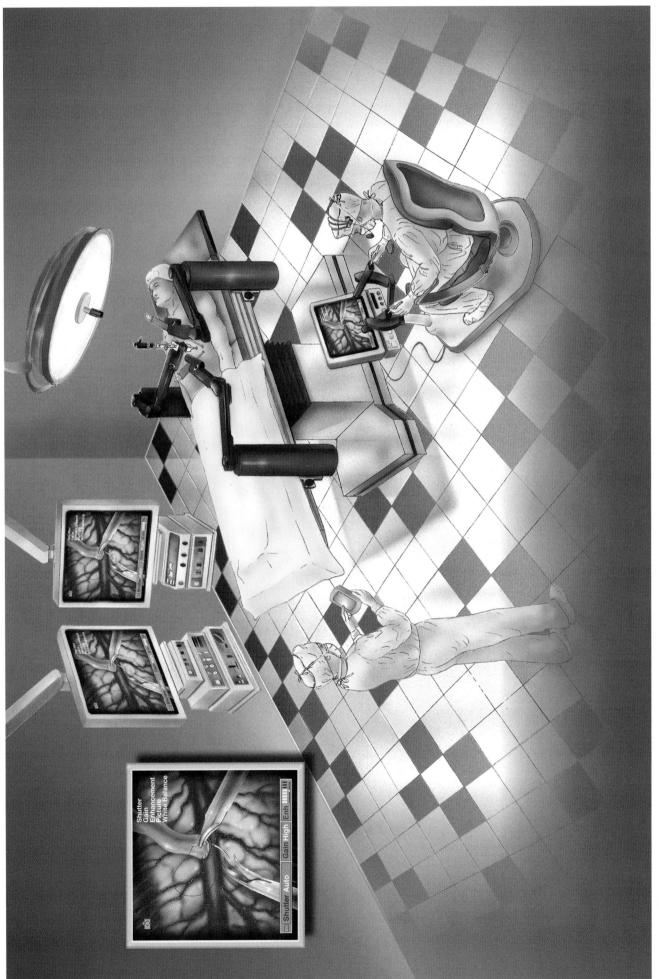

Figure 23–6. Artist's concept of the operating room of the twenty-first century, where the major components of endoscopic surgery will be controlled using robotics and computer-assisted surgical adjuncts. [With permission from Computer Motion.]

(suturing and sealant methods) will allow intradural procedures to be performed solely by endoscope. Developments in methods for repairing the diaphragm (e.g., suturing, stapling) will increase the application of endoscopy to pathology affecting the thoracolumbar junction. New anterior spinal instrumentation will allow more reliable corrections and fixations of thoracic spinal deformities to be performed solely by an endoscopic approach without the need for posterior spinal instrumentation.

CONCLUSIONS

The feasibility and safety of thoracoscopy for the treatment of spinal disorders have been established. Retraining and the dedicated acquisition of new surgical skills are required to perform these techniques safely. The growth of thoracoscopic spinal surgery is tremendously exciting. It is an honor to be participating in the evolution of techniques that can profoundly benefit our patients, preserve the effectiveness of surgery, and reduce the incidence of patients' complications.

Index

Page numbers followed by "t" indicate tables. Page numbers followed by "f" indicate figures.

Access, dissection tools, 36–47
  hemostatic tools, 41–43, 43–44f
  portals, 36, 37–38f
  soft-tissue dissection tools, 36–41, 38–43f
  spinal dissection tools, 44–45, 45–48
  ultrasonic scalpel, 43–44, 44f
AESOP, voice-controlled robotic arm, 356
Anatomy
  thoracic, thoracoscopic perspectives, 49–56
  thoracic spine, 57–67, 125–127
Anesthesia, 79–82
  biopsy, vertebral lesions, 214
  intraoperative management, 83–84, 84f
  intraoperative monitoring, 83–86, 84–85
    cardiopulmonary parameters, 84
    motor evoked potentials, 85
    somatosensory evoked potentials, 84–85
  intubation, 80–81
  lung deflation, 80–81
  monitoring, intraoperative, 79–80
  postoperative care, 82, 85
  preoperative evaluation, 79, 83
  preparation, 79
  thoracoscopic spine surgery, 79–82
  ventilation, 81–82
    volume therapy, during operation, 82
Anterior correction, endoscopic, idiopathic scoliosis, 183–211
  complication, 204–207
  postoperative management, 202
  preoperative management, 184–185
  results, 202–207
  surgical technique, 185–202
    discectomy, 185–186
    instrumentation, placement of, 186–202
Anterior release, spinal deformities, 161–181
  advantages, 172–175
  complications, 169–172
    bleeding, 169–171
    dural tear, 171
    lung tissue trauma, 171
    lymphatic injury, 171

    spinal cord injury, 171
    sympathectomy, 172
  disadvantages, 172–175
  operating room setup, 162
  procedure, 162–169
  team coordination, 162
Arteries, thoracic spine, anatomy, 60f, 62f, 65–66
Arthrodesis, disc space, 293
Articulations, thoracic spine, anatomy, 63–65
Automated Endoscopic System for Optimal Positioning, 356
  AESOP, voice-controlled robotic arm, 356
Autonomic ganglia origin tumor, thoracoscopic resection, 267

Biopsy, vertebral lesions, 213–220
  contraindications, 213
  indications, 213
  preoperative planning, 214
    anesthetic considerations, 214
    diagnostic imaging, 214
  surgical technique, 214–220
    lower thoracic spine, approach to, 217
    midthoracic spine, approach to, 217
    patient positioning, 214–217
    portal placement, 214–217
    thoracoscopic paraspinal tumor biopsy, 218–220
    upper thoracic spine, approach to, 217
    vertebral body, disc space biopsy, 217–218
  thoracoscopic anatomy, 213–214
Bleeding, as complication of anterior release, spinal deformities, 169–171
Bone grafts, vertebral body reconstruction, 294–295
Bony architecture, thoracic spine, 57–63, 58f–64f
Broad-based disc herniation, calcified, thoracoscopic microsurgical discectomy, 233

Canal exposure, 134–142
Cardiopulmonary parameters, anesthesia, intraoperative monitoring, 84
Central thoracic disc
  calcified, thoracoscopic microsurgical discectomy, 225–233

Central thoracic disc *(cont.)*
  soft
    herniation, thoracoscopic microsurgical discectomy, 23
    thoracoscopic microsurgical discectomy, 233
Chylothorax, with thoracoscopic microsurgical discectomy, 241
Classification, of thoracoscopic spine procedures, based on difficulty of procedure, 22
Cleaning lens, 32t, 32–33, 33–34f
Closure, portal sites, 121
Color image generation, 29–32
Contraindications, thoracoscopic spine surgery, 88
Corpectomy, thoracoscopic, 271–291
  clinical results, 274–277
  illustrative case, 273–274
  indications, 271
  preoperative planning, 271
  technique, 271–273
  thoracoscopy, thoracotomy, for corpectomy, compared, 277–279
Costotransversectomy, 237
Credentialing, for thoracoscopic spine surgery, 19–26

Defogging lens, 32t, 32–33, 33–34f
Diagnostic imaging, biopsy, vertebral lesions, 214
Digital color image generation, 29–32
Disc fragment, retained, with thoracoscopic microsurgical discectomy, 241
Disc space arthrodesis, 293
Disc space biopsy, 217–218
Discectomy, thoracoscopic, microsurgical, 221–244
  broad-based disc herniation, calcified, 233
  central thoracic disc
    calcified, 225–233
    soft, 233
      herniation, 23
  chylothorax, 241
  clinical outcomes, 236–243
  diagnostic imaging, 222–223
  hemothorax, 241
  illustrative cases, 225–235
  indications, 221
  infection, 241
  intercostal neuralgia, 241
  misidentified level, 241
  neurological deterioration, 241
  retained disc fragment, 241
  subcutaneous emphysema, 241
  surgical approaches, 222
  surgical technique, 223–225
  thoracoscopy, 237
Dissection, access, tools, 36–47
  hemostatic tools, 41–43, 43–44f
  portals, 36, 37–38f
  soft-tissue dissection tools, 36–41, 38–43f
  spinal dissection tools, 44–45, 45–48
  ultrasonic scalpel, 43–44, 44f
Dissection tools, access, 36–47
Dural closure techniques, 358–360
Dural tear, as complication of anterior release, spinal deformities, 171

Education
  techniques, endoscopic skills, 20
  for thoracoscopic spine surgery, 19–26
Emphysema, subcutaneous, with thoracoscopic microsurgical discectomy, 241
Endoscope holders, 33, 34f
Endoscopic anterior correction, idiopathic scoliosis, 183–211
  complication, 204–207
  postoperative management, 202
  preoperative management, 184–185
  results, 202–207
  surgical technique, 185–202
    discectomy, 185–186
    instrumentation, placement of, 186–202
Endoscopic imaging tools, 28–31f, 28–36
  3-D endoscopy, 33–36, 35–36f
  cleaning lens, 32t, 32–33, 33–34f
  defogging lens, 32t, 32–33, 33–34f
  digital color image generation, 29–32
  endoscope holders, 33, 34f
  illumination, 32, 32f
Endoscopic skills, educational techniques, 20
Endoscopy
  contemporary, 4
  development of, 7
  history of, 1, 2t
Equipment, for thoracoscopic spine surgery, 27f, 27–48
Extradural tumor, thoracoscopic resection, 245–266

Foramina, thoracic spine, microanatomy, 69–78
Fragment, of disc, retained, with thoracoscopic microsurgical discectomy, 241

Ganglioneuroblastoma, thoracoscopic resection, 268
Ganglioneuroma, thoracoscopic resection, 268

Hemostatic tools, 41–43, 43–44f
Hemothorax, with thoracoscopic microsurgical discectomy, 241
History, thoracoscopic spine surgery, 1–5
  endoscopy, 1, 2t
    contemporary, 4
    time line, 2
    twentieth-century, 1–3, 3f
    video-assisted thoracoscopy, 3–4
Holder, endoscope, 33, 34f

Illumination tools, 32, 32f
Image generation, digital color, 29–32
Imaging tools
  cleaning lens, 32t, 32–33, 33–34f
  endoscopic, 28–31f, 28–36
    3-D endoscopy, 33–36, 35–36f
    defogging lens, 32t, 32–33, 33–34f
    digital color image generation, 29–32
    endoscope holders, 33, 34f
    illumination, 32, 32f
Infection, with thoracoscopic microsurgical discectomy, 241
Insertion, portal, 109–113
Instrumentation, for thoracoscopic spine surgery, 27f, 27–48
Interbody fusion, after thoracic discectomy, 293–294

Intercostal neuralgia, with thoracoscopic microsurgical discectomy, 241
Internal fixation techniques, thoracoscopic, 323–354
  illustrative case, 324–325
  screw plates, 323–325
  screw rods, 325–354
Intradural tumor, thoracoscopic resection, 247
Intraoperative management, anesthesia, 83–84, 84f
Intraoperative monitoring, anesthesia, 83–86, 84–85
Intrathoracic neurogenic tumors, thoracoscopic resection, 245–269
Intubation, anesthesia, 80–81

Laboratory models, thoracoscopy, 22t, 22–26, 23–25t
Laparoscopy, thoracoscopy, compared, 10–12
Left middle thorax, anatomy, 54–55, 56f
Left upper thorax, anatomy, 54, 56f
Lens
  cleaning, 32t, 32–33, 33–34f
  defogging, 32t, 32–33, 33–34f
Ligaments, thoracic spine, microanatomy, 69–78
Lower thoracic access, portal configuration, 117–121
Lower thorax, right, anatomy, 52f, 54–56f
Lung
  deflation, anesthesia, 80–81
  mobilization, spinal exposure and, 127–129
  tissue trauma, as complication of anterior release, spinal deformities, 171
Lymphatic injury, as complication of anterior release, spinal deformities, 171

Mediastinal anatomy, thoracoscopic perspectives, 49–56
Methylmethacrylate, vertebral body reconstruction, 295–321
Microanatomy, thoracic spine, foramina, ligaments, 69–78
Microsurgical discectomy, thoracoscopic, 221–244
  broad-based disc herniation, calcified, 233
  central thoracic disc
    calcified, 225–233
    soft, 233
      herniation, 23
  chylothorax, 241
  clinical outcomes, 236–243
  costotransversectomy, 237
  diagnostic imaging, 222–223
  hemothorax, 241
  illustrative cases, 225–235
  indications, 221
  infection, 241
  intercostal neuralgia, 241
  misidentified level, 241
  neurological deterioration, 241
  retained disc fragment, 241
  subcutaneous emphysema, 241
  surgical approaches, 222
  surgical technique, 223–225
  thoracoscopy, 237
  thoracotomy, 237
Middle thorax
  access, portal configuration, 113–117
  left, anatomy, 54–55, 56f
  right, anatomy, 51–54, 52–53f

Misidentified level, with thoracoscopic microsurgical discectomy, 241
Monitoring
  anesthesia, 79–80
  intraoperative, anesthesia, 83–86, 84–85
Motor evoked potentials, anesthesia, 85

Nerve
  sheath tumors, thoracoscopic resection, 268
  thoracic spine, anatomy, 60f, 62f, 66, 67f
Neuralgia, intercostal, with thoracoscopic microsurgical discectomy, 241
Neuroblastoma, thoracoscopic resection, 268
Neuroectoderm origin tumor, thoracoscopic resection, 267
Neurofibroma, thoracoscopic resection, 268
Neurogenic sarcoma, thoracoscopic resection, 268
Neurogenic tumors, intrathoracic, thoracoscopic resection, 245–269
Neurological deterioration, with thoracoscopic microsurgical discectomy, 241
Neurovascular elements, thoracic spine, anatomy, 65–66

Open surgery, thoracoscopic surgical skills, compared, 12, 13–16f
Operating room setup, 95–102
  anterior release, spinal deformities, 162
Operative approaches, to thoracic spine, compared, 9

Palmar hyperhidrosis, thoracoscopic sympathectomy, 148
Paraganglioma, thoracoscopic resection, 268
Paraganglionic system origin tumor, thoracoscopic resection, 267
Patient positioning, 102–106
  biopsy, vertebral lesions, 214–217
Perioperative management, thoracoscopic spine surgery, 87–93
Peripheral neuroectodermal tumor, thoracoscopic resection, 268
Plates, for thoracoscopic internal fixation, 323–325
Pleural dissection, 125–142
Pleural mobilization, 131–133
PNET. *See* Peripheral neuroectodermal tumor
Portal configurations, 113–121
  for lower thoracic access, 117–121
  for middle thoracic access, 113–117
  for upper thoracic access, 113
Portal insertion, 109–113
Portal placement techniques, and portal selection, 107–124
Portal positioning, 107–109
Portal selection, 107–124, 109
Portal sites, closure, 121
Portals, 36, 37–38f
Postoperative care, 82
  anesthesia, 82, 85
Postoperative management, thoracoscopic spine surgery, 87–88
Preoperative assessment, thoracoscopic spine surgery, 87
Preoperative evaluation, anesthesia, 79, 83
Pulmonary complications, thoracoscopic spine surgery, 89

Radicular canal, thoracic, microanatomy, 70–76, 76f
Reconstruction techniques, thoracoscopic spinal, 293–321
  disc space arthrodesis, 293
  interbody fusion, after thoracic discectomy, 293–294

Reconstruction techniques, thoracoscopic spinal *(cont.)*
  thoracoscopic anterior release, spinal deformity, 293
  vertebral body reconstruction, 294–321
    reconstruction
      with bone grafts, 294–295
      with methylmethacrylate, 295–321
Release, anterior, spinal deformities, 161–181
  advantages, 172–175
  complications, 169–172
    bleeding, 169–171
    dural tear, 171
    lung tissue trauma, 171
    lymphatic injury, 171
    spinal cord injury, 171
    sympathectomy, 172
  disadvantages, 172–175
  operating room setup, 162
  procedure, 162–169
  team coordination, 162
Retained disc fragment, with thoracoscopic microsurgical
    discectomy, 241
Ribs, vertebrae, thoracic spine, articulations between, anatomy,
    58f, 64–65, 64–65f
Right lower thorax, anatomy, 52f, 54–56f
Right middle thorax, anatomy, 51–54, 52–53f
Right thoracic outlet, anatomy, 49f, 49–50
Right upper thorax, anatomy, 50–51, 50–51f
Robotic arm, voice-controlled, 356
Robotic devices, 356
Rods, for thoracoscopic internal fixation, 325–354

Scalpel, ultrasonic, 43–44, 44f
Schwannoma, thoracoscopic resection, 268
Scoliosis, idiopathic, endoscopic anterior correction, 183–211
  complication, 204–207
  postoperative management, 202
  preoperative management, 184–185
  results, 202–207
  surgical technique, 185–202
    discectomy, 185–186
    instrumentation, placement of, 186–202
Screw plates, for thoracoscopic internal fixation, 323–325
Screw rods, for thoracoscopic internal fixation, 325–354
Skill development, education in, 20t, 20–22, 21f, 22t
Soft-tissue dissection tools, 36–41, 38–43f
Somatosensory evoked potentials, anesthesia, 84–85
Spinal canal exposure, 134–142
Spinal complications, thoracoscopic spine surgery, 89
Spinal cord injury, as complication of anterior release, spinal
    deformities, 171
Spinal deformities, anterior release, 161–181
  advantages, 172–175
  complications, 169–172
    bleeding, 169–171
    dural tear, 171
    lung tissue trauma, 171
    lymphatic injury, 171
    spinal cord injury, 171
    sympathectomy, 172
  disadvantages, 172–175

  operating room setup, 162
  procedure, 162–169
  team coordination, 162
Spinal dissection tools, 44–45, 45–48
Spinal exposure, 125–142
Spinal localization, 130
Spinal surgical approaches, thoracoscopy, compared, 8–17, 9t,
    9–11f
Spinal thoracoscopy
  future developments, 355–360
    education, 355
    scientific assessment, 355–356
    technology developments, 356–358
  instrumentation, 360
  new surgical techniques, 358–360
    new dural closure techniques, 358–360
    new methods for repairing diaphragm, 360
  robotic devices, 356
  robotic surgical system, 352–358
  voice-controlled robotic arm, 356
Subcutaneous emphysema, with thoracoscopic microsurgical
    discectomy, 241
Sympathectomy
  anterior release, spinal deformities, 172
  thoracoscopic, 143–160
    surgical technique, 144–147

Team coordination, anterior release, spinal deformities, 162
Thoracic anatomy, thoracoscopic perspectives, 49–56
Thoracic discectomy, interbody fusion after, 293–294
Thoracic outlet, right, anatomy, 49f, 49–50
Thoracic radicular canal, 70–76, 76f
Thoracic spine
  anatomy, 57–67
  arteries, anatomy, 60f, 62f, 65–66
  articulations, anatomy, 63–65
  bony architecture, 57–63, 58f–64f
  foramina, ligaments, microanatomy, 69–78
  ligaments, anatomy, 63–65
  nerves, anatomy, 60f, 62f, 66, 67f
  neurovascular elements, anatomy, 65–66
  operative approaches, compared, 9
  surgical anatomy of, 125–127
  veins, anatomy, 60f, 66
  vertebrae, ribs, articulations between, anatomy, 58f, 64–65,
    64–65f
  vertebral arches, articulations between, anatomy, 61f, 64
  vertebral bodies, articulations between, anatomy, 61–62f,
    63–64
Thoracoscopic access strategies, 107–124
Thoracoscopic anterior release, spinal deformity, 293
Thoracoscopic corpectomy, 271–291
  clinical results, 274–277
  illustrative case, 273–274
  indications, 271
  preoperative planning, 271
  technique, 271–273
  thoracoscopy, thoracotomy, for corpectomy, compared,
    277–279
Thoracoscopic internal fixation techniques, 323–354

illustrative case, 324–325
screw plates, 323–325
screw rods, 325–354
Thoracoscopic microsurgical discectomy, 221–244
broad-based disc herniation, calcified, 233
central thoracic disc
calcified, 225–233
soft, 233
herniation, 23
chylothorax, 241
clinical outcomes, 236–243
costotransversectomy, 237
diagnostic imaging, 222–223
hemothorax, 241
illustrative cases, 225–235
indications, 221
infection, 241
intercostal neuralgia, 241
misidentified level, 241
neurological deterioration, 241
retained disc fragment, 241
subcutaneous emphysema, 241
surgical approaches, 222
surgical technique, 223–225
thoracoscopy, 237
thoracotomy, 237
Thoracoscopic paraspinal tumor biopsy, biopsy, vertebral
lesions, 218–220
Thoracoscopic resection, intrathoracic neurogenic tumors,
245–269
Thoracoscopic spinal reconstruction techniques, 293–321
disc space arthrodesis, 293
interbody fusion, after thoracic discectomy, 293–294
thoracoscopic anterior release, spinal deformity, 293
vertebral body reconstruction, 294–321
reconstruction
with bone grafts, 294–295
with methylmethacrylate, 295–321
Thoracoscopic spinal surgery, guidelines for, 19–20
Thoracoscopic spine procedures, classification, based on
difficulty of procedure, 22
Thoracoscopic spine surgery
complications, 89–93
contraindications, 88
credentialing, 19–26
education, 19–26
equipment, 27f, 27–48
instrumentation, 27f, 27–48
intrathoracic complications, 89
neurological complications, 89
perioperative management for, 87–93
pleural, and intrathoracic complications, 89
postoperative management, 87–88
preoperative assessment, 87
pulmonary complications, 89
spinal complications, 89
Thoracoscopic surgical skills, open surgery, compared, 12,
13–16f

Thoracoscopic sympathectomy, 143–160
surgical indications, 143–144
surgical outcomes, 147–159
surgical technique, 144–147
Thoracoscopy
advantages of, 17
clinical indications for, 8t
development of, 7–8
disadvantages of, 17
general principles, 7–18
laboratory models for, 22t, 22–26, 23–25t
laparoscopy, compared, 10–12
other spinal surgical approaches, compared, 8–17, 9t, 9–11f
in spinal surgery, 8, 8t
thoracoscopic microsurgical discectomy, 237
thoracotomy, for corpectomy, compared, 277–279
video-assisted, 3–4
Thoracotomy, 237
thoracoscopy, for corpectomy, compared, 277–279
Thorax
lower, right, anatomy, 52f, 54–56f
middle
left, anatomy, 54–55, 56f
right, anatomy, 51–54, 52–53f
upper
left, anatomy, 54, 56f
right, anatomy, 50–51, 50–51f
3–D endoscopy, 33–36, 35–36f
Time line, thoracoscopic spine surgery, 2
Tools, dissection, access, 36–47

Ultrasonic scalpel, 43–44, 44f
Upper thorax
access, portal configuration, 113
left, anatomy, 54, 56f
right, anatomy, 50–51, 50–51f

Vascular mobilization, ligation, 133–134
Veins, thoracic spine, anatomy, 60f, 66
Ventilation
anesthesia, 81–82
volume therapy, 82
Vertebrae, ribs, thoracic spine, articulations between, anatomy,
58f, 64–65, 64–65f
Vertebral arches, thoracic spine, articulations between,
anatomy, 61f, 64
Vertebral body
reconstruction, 294–321
reconstruction
with bone grafts, 294–295
with methylmethacrylate, 295–321
thoracic spine, articulations between, anatomy, 61–62f,
63–64
Video-assisted thoracoscopy, 3–4
Voice-controlled robotic arm, 356

Zeus, 352–358